Pain

Pain

A Political History

KEITH WAILOO

Johns Hopkins University Press

Baltimore

Johns Hopkins University Press
2715 North Charles Street
Baltimore, Maryland 21218-4363
www.press.jhu.edu

Library of Congress Cataloging-in-Publication Data

Wailoo, Keith, author.
  Pain : a political history / Keith Wailoo.
      p. ; cm.
    Includes bibliographical references and index.
      ISBN 978-1-4214-1365-5 (hardcover : alk. paper) — ISBN 1-4214-1365-5 (hardcover : alk.
paper) — ISBN 978-1-4214-1366-2 (electronic) — ISBN 1-4214-1366-3 (electronic)
    I. Title.
  [DNLM: 1. Health Policy—history—United States.   2. Pain Management—history—United
States.   3. Analgesics—United States.   4. History, 20th Century—United States.   5. History,
21st Century—United States.   6. Pain—psychology—United States.   7. Politics—United
States. WL 11 AA1]
  RB127
  616'.0472—dc23   2013034071

A catalog record for this book is available from the British Library.

*Special discounts are available for bulk purchases of this book. For more information, please
contact Special Sales at 410-516-6936 or specialsales@press.jhu.edu.*

Johns Hopkins University Press uses environmentally friendly book materials, including recycled
text paper that is composed of at least 30 percent post-consumer waste, whenever possible.

To my exemplary parents, Bert and Lynette Wailoo

Contents

....

Pain

Between Liberal Relief and Conservative Care

In the 1990s, talk-radio stars like Rush Limbaugh and Laura Schlessinger—the brash and arrogant voices of American conservatism—rose to fame by rejecting presidential candidate and later president Bill Clinton's liberalism. Like many tough-talking conservatives, Schlessinger singled out for special abuse four words Clinton had uttered during the 1992 campaign: "I feel your pain." The phrase became a frequent object of scorn for those who doubted the liberal's ability to feel another's pain and who (in the name of conservatism) held an opposing political worldview. Schlessinger responded caustically to Clinton: "I'm not here to deal in feelings. 'I feel your pain' is bullshit." Limbaugh, who routinely praised the virtues of the individual and of the free market and decried the malfeasance of government, championed himself as a moral force against Clinton's liberalism. In 1996, Limbaugh's television program showed footage of Clinton leaving a memorial for his commerce secretary, Ron Brown, to illustrate liberal deception. The footage showed the president first laughing until, when he saw the camera, he became somber and even wiped away a tear. To the derisive laughter of his followers, Limbaugh warned, "This is the best illustration of the fake and phony characteristics of this man, the disingenuousness of him, and this says it better than most." Behind such claims of compassion, Limbaugh asserted, lay a vast agenda of deceit with implications for policy and society: "Just keep this in mind, today it's the pharmaceutical manufacturers, the cable TV industry, insurance companies, physicians, and chief executive officers of major corporations [Clinton is] targeting. Tomorrow it could be you."[1] For such conservative commentators, the fraudulence of pain—that is, the fraud of people claiming to be in pain, the fraud of politicians claiming to

1

feel others' pain, and the charade of government programs claiming to help people when they only promoted dependence—was galling.

As political pundit E. J. Dionne wrote in 1996, it had become "easy to parody Clinton's willingness to translate 'I feel your pain' into an eclectic and philosophically promiscuous mix of policies that play well in the polls." In other words, these arguments (both Clinton's pain-speak and conservative portrayals) were not all rhetoric and political stagecraft—they informed policy. Indeed, from the mid-twentieth century, liberal government expansion had been informed by the goal of relieving pain in society, with compassion for disabled individuals driving the development of disability policy and concern for the elderly in pain driving Medicare politics. Pain and policy comingled. Meanwhile, the conservative movement ascended, using as political fodder the argument that liberal politicians' supposed concern for the pain of others was an elaborate fraud. Mocking Clinton and defending Limbaugh, one letter writer took issue with what he saw as the Left's code words and the harm done in the name of liberal compassion: "The left is so fond of accusing conservatives of using code words. 'Civil rights' have become the biggest code words of all, standing for reverse discrimination, quotas, affirmative action, race-based set-asides . . . In this 'I feel your pain' society, white males are the only group it is legal to discriminate against." An editorial writer, Paul Taylor, similarly caricatured liberals as two-faced whiners: "In 1992, the whiners achieved the latest in a string of dubious political victories by electing a president who is forever reassuring them: 'I feel your pain.' Naturally, this makes them whine even louder."[2] Pain defined a fundamental political divide.

This angry caricature of compassionate liberalism as deceitful and destructive predated the 1990s. Indeed (as the pages following will show), the claims made about pain and about people in pain were central to the ongoing battle between liberals and conservatives stretching back to World War II. Long before Clinton, conservatives had alleged that excessive "bleeding heart" compassion and the government programs that supported it had led American society down the road to dependence, welfare, fraud, and fiscal wreckage. If pain afflicted America, they alleged, the liberals had indulged it or caused it. The political Left had built a robust system, for example, of taxpayer-financed government disability benefits catering to people who claimed pain as their primary ailment, they had encouraged a culture of complaint and easy relief, and (so the argument against Clinton went) they had done this under the dubious guise of feeling the pain of others. That many in America believed in Clinton's compassion, voted for him, and elected him president, made the claim all the more infuriating.

Conservatives in the Clinton years were mostly refining old arguments on liberalism, pain, and fraud that had been honed in earlier eras. When Ronald Reagan became president in 1981, he too took a stand on pain. He assured Americans that "in this present crisis, government is not the solution to our problems, government IS the problem."[3] By March 1981, people literally *claiming* to be in pain and seeking Social Security disability benefits for alleged chronic conditions found themselves in the crosshairs of the Reagan revolution. The president turned to Richard Schweiker, his secretary of Health and Human Services, to oversee a purge of half a million people from the disability rolls, "weeding out ineligibles." Officially, the concern was not pain but pain fraud—benefits extended to people on the basis of their subjective complaints. Of course, the Reagan war on pain fraud was a war on liberalism itself; it was a policy response to the rise of disability benefits, the advent of Medicare, and the growth of a welfare state organized around misguided compassion. Reagan had spent decades insisting that government programs like Medicare and Aid to Families with Dependent Children (welfare) bred paralyzing dependence and that excessive regulation and taxation penalized hardworking people. The system, as built by liberals, undermined freedom and free enterprise. Nothing attracted more derision from Reagan than the claim that bloated government and the welfare state knew people's pain. Limbaugh's accusation, then, merely added another chapter in a long narrative, continuing a line of conservative skepticism about the excesses of liberal society.

Was this critique correct? Was it an accurate portrayal to say that liberalism originated in and expanded on the deceitful claim to compassionately feel the pain of others? Or was this critique merely a caricature? The pages ahead tell the story of liberalism, conservatism, and the politics of pain—not merely at the level of rhetoric but as ailing bodies, broken lives, illness, and disability that vexed government and politicians from the post–World War II era to the present.[4] Ironically, another Republican president, Dwight Eisenhower, had launched such debates by signing in

1956 a new Social Security disability law that created the groundwork for subjective suffering to be alleviated at state expense. Eisenhower's other challenge had been veterans' health care and disability benefits—with the American Medical Association (AMA) howling that the expanding Veterans Administration (VA) system was merely socialized medicine and the veterans' lobby countering that relief was the soldier's right. Even as early as the 1950s, the politics of pain was fractious.

This volume stands alongside other scholarship that convincingly argues that the mobilization of strong emotions underpinned historical shifts away from welfare-oriented policies and that in the liberal-conservative debate "it is not dependency that is the problem, but fear and hatred of dependency." Building on this politics of emotion, this book traces how, over time, the powerful question of other people's pain became a recurring site for political battle. In those battles, as we shall see, theories of pain—medical, psychological, economic, and other views on aches and anguish—became weapons; often the courts would be the site of conflict and resolution. In looking at U.S. political history through the topic of pain, the book offers an approach informed by the history of law, medicine, and government, yet it is grounded in the history of the experiences of people. In looking at political history through pain, one can see how those experiences became ideological and political fodder. The book also advances a strong claim: that the complex interaction between liberalism and conservatism can be better understood by considering where politicians, lawyers, scientists, sociologists, and sufferers stand on this question of pain, compassion, government, and relief.[5] Over time, I argue, pain—and whether subjective pain is real pain—came to represent not just a clinical or scientific problem, but a legal puzzle, a heated cultural concern, and an enduring partisan issue.

In the end, the conservative critique of liberals' views on pain made artful, effective political theater—a damning accusation in the broader 1980s vilification of liberalism. Yet Reagan was correct in one sense: there was in fact such a thing as a *liberal pain standard* that had been developed within disability policy, in medicine and science, and in government during the decades before Reagan became president, and there was, in his own time, a severe backlash aiming to impose a *conservative standard* for judging pain. Looking beyond rhetoric and caricature, this book narrates the drama of pain in America—a political history in which Reagan's presidency was a dramatic fulcrum.[6]

This history of liberalism, conservatism, and pain contains many rich ironies. In 2003, police in Florida accused Rush Limbaugh of "doctor shopping"—that is, using his Latina housekeeper to obtain from multiple doctors hundreds of prescriptions for the painkiller OxyContin to feed a secret drug habit. For political commentators, it was a crime that seemed to undercut conservative beliefs at their core. Just as Clinton's "I feel your pain" had been Limbaugh's gain, now the tables were turned. Limbaugh had railed against bleeding-heart liberals as too soft on criminals and too concerned about the pain of others. In court, however, Limbaugh's attorneys embellished their client's own pain. Playing the victim card, they noted that "Limbaugh did not go to these doctors to seek pleasure. He went there to relieve pain. He had a serious hearing loss and went deaf. He had major surgery, and you'll see in these records the details of that surgery and the pain that he went through . . . He went to this other set of doctors because of his spine. In 1998 his coccyx bone was removed and it was found that he had cysts in his spine. He was being treated for the pain regarding these conditions." Moreover, his attorneys shifted the blame away from Limbaugh himself—pointing to the drug to which he was addicted and the medical advice he had received as the problem:

> The doctors counseled him that there could be psychological and
> physiological dependence on pain medication. This was hardly a
> surprise. But they had to make the decision about using the medication
> or suffering the pain. They used a drug called OxyContin which
> everybody has talked about, which came into effect, I think, in 1996
> was issued by the drug company. Today it is listed as the most
> potentially addictive medication that is legally available. It is being
> investigated in Congress, in the FDA and there's a huge number of
> lawsuits that have been filed against the pharmaceutical company for
> the issuance of OxyContin.[7]

The fact that this fierce advocate for conservatism, rugged individualism, and law and order was hooked on painkillers and that his attorneys looked to government and lawsuits for answers even as he railed against governmental dependence and social engineering posed a contradiction on many levels.

Was Limbaugh merely being duplicitous, and did his duplicity expose the contradictions of the conservative position? This book argues, in part, that his addiction to painkillers was more than lies and contradictions; it was a natural by-product of the deregulated, market-oriented world that Reaganism created. As an OxyContin addict, Limbaugh was the beneficiary of a drug market revolution that had been unleashed by the conservative deregulation of the industry that started in the 1980s. He was, in a sense, both the beneficiary and the victim of those forces. He was also the face of a new pain and abuse problem that blossomed in the wake of conservative government. By 2000, the Drug Enforcement Administration (DEA) had named the diversion of prescription drugs into the illicit drug market as the leading abuse threat in the nation—with OxyContin pushing aside heroin, crack cocaine, and ecstasy as the drug problem for this era. The rise of OxyContin abuse showed how the pain market and American consumerism had changed since the Reagan revolution, with direct-to-consumer advertising and the rise of Internet pharmacies putting painkillers more easily within the consumer's reach. In an age where advertising flourished and regulation lagged, Limbaugh's mode of relief was an obvious and troubling consequence. Conservatism's conceit was that liberalism indulged complaints; wherever true pain existed in society, private enterprise was envisioned as the best remedy. Limbaugh's OxyContin addiction suggested otherwise, marking another turning point in the politics of pain.

In the chapters ahead, Eisenhower's conflicted disability politics (chapter 1), the expansion of liberal government in the name of remedying pain (chapter 2), Reagan's attempt to purge the disability rolls in the 1980s and the curious rise of "fetal pain" (chapter 3), the politics of pain, disability, and Physician Assisted Suicide in the Clinton era (chapter 4), and the 2003 Limbaugh OxyContin case (chapter 5) are re-examined not as medical stories but as important markers in American political history. Whether and to what extent was it possible for Bill Clinton, Ronald Reagan, a physician, or a judge (or any person) to know another's pain? The question went to the emotional core of a public policy dispute that lasted decades. Should social policies be driven by compassion toward such pain?

Did the market provide better relief than government? These questions became hot-button political problems for Americans debating the "welfare state" and questions of citizenship and government. Pain's reality—which pains were real, which were false, and who was the best judge—was a recurring question. Pain's variety—which were severe, which were mild—bedeviled observers from the age of Dwight Eisenhower's disability law to the era of Barack Obama's Affordable Care Act, which contained its own pain-related provisions. Pain perception inflamed politics and vexed policy makers and social scientists. And, as we shall see, given these recurring and intractable disputes, it has been the courts (far more than physicians) that have decided, time and time again, how to measure distress and how to define the right to relief.

In American politics, pain comes in such variety—the pain of the disabled person seeking benefits, pain associated with fibromyalgia, the pain of the dying patient, the pain of the child, and so on—that the question of pain's legitimacy is open to a stunning array of manipulations.[8] All pains are not the same or equally deserving of relief. When, for example, Larry Kudlow, President Reagan's former economic advisor, admitted in 1994 to a drug and alcohol addiction, news reports rendered him sympathetically—not as a fraud or a man seeking wanton pleasure. He was portrayed as an ambitious and fiercely competitive man—the quintessential entrepreneur driven by a will to succeed. The very qualities that conservatives prized had, in the conservative pain narrative, led him to painkillers. Kudlow attributed his slide into drug use to the "pressure to produce" on Wall Street. "You think you're a superman," Kudlow explained. "You think you can do anything." This drive and hubris threw him, he admitted, into drugs' embrace. In this telling (as in the Limbaugh coverage years later), the nature of the pain for which the man sought relief was assumed to be excruciatingly legitimate pain.[9] Thus, when we examine the history of pain and relief in America, we must attend to the persistent problem of whose pains are being discussed and how those pains are rendered. The conservative critique of compassion in Reagan's time was not just a critique of pain itself; it was a criticism of particular people (minorities, women, AIDS sufferers, and so on) associated with and benefiting from the nation's liberal turn in the 1960s and 1970s and defending liberalism into the 1980s. As we shall see, the question of who is the modal, or standard, sufferer—whose pain matters and occupies center stage (soldiers,

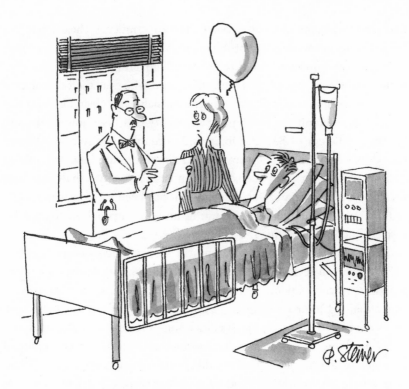

*"We can give you enough medication to alleviate
the pain but not enough to make it fun."*

FIGURE I.1.   Peter Steiner's cartoon captures an enduring tension at the heart of
pain and politics—the line where relief becomes pleasurable.

New Yorker, February 21, 2000.

workers, women, black people, and so on)—also tells a political story of
America's recent decades, as does the question of who is qualified to
judge real and imagined pain.

Whether people in chronic pain have been granted a hearing or some
measure of legitimacy as true sufferers depends on contextual factors—
the political and economic milieu of the time, the social status and context
of the suffering, and the meanings associated with the particular pain experiences. Over the decades, the face of pain keeps changing, shaping the
terms of the political debate along with it. Elderly pain carried a particular valence in the 1960s, as did the pain of sickle-cell disease in African

Americans; the pain of housewives in the 1950s meant something different from the pain of industrial workers. Specific economic and demographic trends have driven pain into the foreground of politics: the persistence of industrial labor as a source of disability, the steady rise of white-collar sedentary work and its own implications for pain, and the growth of the elderly population and its infirmities. Wars, too, have shaped the character of anguish and the demands on government for relief. Since the 1950s, then, aches, hurts, and chronic anguish have come in multiple forms—low-back pain, injury-related pain, and headache predominated at first, but arthritis and cancer-related pain rose, decade by decade, in importance. New maladies and complaints, like fibromyalgia and even "fetal pain," rounded out the American pain profile by the late twentieth century, raising new questions about false and true pain and making pain management all along the life course—from birth to death—into a fraught political exercise.

The problem with pain in America is that there are so many different kinds of hurt—with so many questions swirling around each—and that the political milieu determines the meaning of complaint. For a growing government, one question came to dominate: Did the person in pain deserve disability benefits, and, if so, how long should these benefits be granted? This question became a central worry of conservatives, who were concerned about the perverse incentives of welfare, the citizen's capacity for fraud, and the rise of government dependence in lieu of market labor. For them, the pain of the hardworking businessman or woman warranted far more sympathy than the pain of the industrial laborer. Pain, in the conservative and liberal worldviews, raised different worries about the market, government benefits, rights, and citizenship. From the 1950s through the 1980s and still today, conservatives worried—as the ranks of people with disabilities swelled—about whether subjective pain was real pain and whether chronic pain was a symptom of underlying maladjustment. More recently, religious conservatives have turned the pain of the fetus into potent politics. For liberals, by contrast, the pain of the terminally ill cancer patient seeking "death with dignity" has served similar functions by politicizing pain in ways that mesh neatly with liberal values and commitments.

This history of pain focuses on both the political sphere and the medical realm—and also on how closely they have been conjoined. It examines the micropolitics of doctoring (that is, whether caregivers offer liberal, conservative, alternative, or radical care) and the macropolitics of what pain means in the United States. Writing in 1977 on pain management, sociologists Anselm Strauss and Shizuko Fagerhaugh distinguished between these two kinds of politics, noting that "political processes are involved in the interaction surrounding patients in pain. By political processes we do not mean the activities that spring most readily to mind, namely party politics or the vying for votes by aspirants to public office." The sociologists called attention to politics on a more intimate level—"such political actions as persuading, appealing to authority, negotiating, threatening, and even employing force in order to get things done."[10] This small clinical world with its micropolitics of pain would be their focus. Other scholars defined pain politics more broadly. Philosopher Martha Nussbaum observed that compassion has long been "a central bridge between the individual and community . . . a way of hooking the interests of others to our own personal goods." Political debates about the future of the good society, Nussbaum insisted, revolve around pain and compassion, with many modern moral theories seeing compassion as "an irrational force in human affairs, one that is likely to mislead or distract us when we are trying to think well about social policy." When Nussbaum wrote these words in the 1990s (as we shall see), this claim had reached a crescendo; so much of American political turmoil was framed in these stark terms of compassion, pain, welfare reform, and so on.[11] The pages ahead investigate just how these two worlds of pain and relief (the medical and the political, the micro and the macro) have informed one another, shaping each other's ideologies, intersecting with the law, and constraining the possibilities of relief.

Reagan's conservative pain standard and Schlessinger's diatribe against Clinton's "I feel your pain" rhetoric were not new inventions; they both responded to an ideal going back almost two centuries before World War II that had been central to the formation of the liberal state and its commitments to its citizens. In the writings of eighteenth-century conservative icon Edmund Burke, pain stood at the center of matters of social order. For Burke, pain had a fundamentally transformative and beneficial aspect. Unlike the experience of pleasure, which Burke saw as fleeting and superficial ("when it is over, we relapse into indifference"), the pain experience left a lasting and sublime mark on the person. Tolerable pain that did not threaten life, for him, was a virtue: "If the pain is not carried to violence," Burke wrote, "and the terror is not conversant about the present destruction of the person . . . they [pain and terror] are capable of producing . . . a sort of tranquillity tinged with terror; which, as it belongs to self-preservation, is one of the strongest of all passions."[12] To appreciate the lessons of pain, in other words, one needed to tolerate it and to look past distress to the larger message it carried for the sufferer—opening the doors into the sublime itself. Thus, at the start of the conservative intellectual tradition, pain had its value and redemptive virtue—in much the same way that some ardent Christians might say that pain redeems and brings the Christian sufferer closer to the experience of Jesus Christ. In contrast, for John Stuart Mill (one of the architects of modern liberalism and born early in the nineteenth century, a decade after Burke died), pain had no such redemptive value. For "according to the Greatest Happiness Principle [that he espoused], the ultimate end . . . is an existence exempt as far as possible from pain, and as rich as possible in enjoyments . . . This, being, according to the utilitarian opinion, the end of human action, is necessarily also the standard of morality."[13] (Here too, ardent Christians could point to Jesus as a model—not to his suffering and his redemption but to his compassion toward and relief of those who suffer.) Seen in this light, the political battles over pain in American society continue a moral struggle with deep roots in Western religion, politics, and society. The pain debates of the past sixty years joined this long philosophical and spiritual discussion—a discussion informed by new developments in medicine, drug policy, science, and government, which crosses back and forth into the legal realm.

Pain and its relief defined a high-stakes challenge—a topic not easily controlled by politicians, physicians, judges, or any single group; for that reason, it has incited a steady struggle over who has the right, jurisdiction, and authority to say who is in pain: doctors, sufferers, pharmaceutical companies, politicians, the federal government, the states, lawyers, or judges? Even as pain medicine has emerged and grown as a clinical specialty during the past seven decades, physicians were never in true control and always looked to others—the drug enforcement agencies, police, courts, disability activists—for guidance. Thus, while it is tempting to see the history of pain relief as a medical story in which ascendant doctors and scientists (rather than the courts) should have authority and control over the question of who was in pain, in truth, the politics of pain has always been deeply contested. Doctors, as we shall see, have played critical roles—advocating for sufferers, inventing new theories of pain, endorsing relief practices, and bridling against legal constraints. But these experts have largely conformed to the cultural trends of their time. In the politics of pain, politicians and ideologues have often led the way, creating new rules about whether pain should count as disability. Often, it has been the courts, not scientists or physicians on their own professional terrain, that have settled questions about the validity of chronic pain, the criteria of disability, and the citizen's right to relief. As we shall see in the pages ahead, these ambiguities over who owns the topic (and over whether it was a moral problem, a political challenge, a legal question, a personal dilemma, a pharmaceutical opportunity, or a medical problem) made pain a fraught and contentious field.

ONE

The Trojan Horse of Pain

....

But come now . . . and sing of the building of the horse of wood . . . led up into the citadel as a thing of guile . . . So there it stood, while the people talked long as they sat about it, and could form no resolve.

BOOK 9, *ODYSSEY*

For Lieutenant Colonel Henry Beecher, soldiers' pain was a paradox. Treating men gravely wounded on the Italian war fronts in the mid-1940s and at the Anzio beachhead, Beecher, a medic who later became a renowned pain specialist, marveled at how "strong emotion can block pain." Gravely wounded GIs (in fact, as many as three-quarters of them) did not request morphine, he found, despite being in severe pain and often near death. What allowed these badly injured men, subjected to almost uninterrupted shellfire for weeks, to show surprising optimism and even cheerfulness? With this question fresh in mind, the war doctor came home understanding that pain was far more complicated than most people thought and that the capacity of men to withstand wrenching anguish was a profound mystery. In time, pain would become not merely a bodily paradox but also a profound political one.

A decade later, Louis Orr viewed the GI through a different lens. Orr insisted that, once safely at home, the veteran had become a whiner, a complainer, and "a Trojan horse" opening the way for socialized medicine. As a prominent physician in the American Medical Association hierarchy, his pronouncements carried political force. The medical organization had successfully opposed President Harry Truman's plan for national health insurance in the late 1940s, and it remained alarmed about any proposals to expand insurance and benefits—both to veterans and to the general population. Writing in the late 1950s, Orr saw the veteran's complaint in this political light, as an excuse for government encroachment into private health care. In the years since the war ended, he insisted, the GIs' complaints of disability had grown out of proportion to their actual injuries. Orr alleged that the trend had been encouraged by veterans' groups (such as the American Legion) lobbying Congress to liberalize disability benefits. The result was incessant coddling and crippling dependence on government, particularly within the Veterans Administration health-care system. These developments, Orr feared, were leading America to the brink of socialism.[1]

What had happened to shift the profile of the GI and his pain so dramatically from the hardened fighter on the Anzio beachhead in 1946 to the chronic complainer on the VA ward in 1957? Had the soldier's marvelous endurance on the front lines been converted into a societal weakness by life at home? Was it true, as Orr and the American Medical Association contended, that expanding government benefits; creeping, coddling liberalism; and social indulgence were to blame? It was not just that memories of the soldiers' heroism had faded in the intervening twelve years: the disability and pain debate of the 1950s concealed within it an ideological skirmish about liberalism and the legacy of New Deal policies, about social accommodations and postwar citizenship, about disability provisions for the general population, and about the future of the nation itself. The case of these soldiers (and the civilians they would become) sits at the core of this chapter in American pain and politics. As we shall see, the debate on the soldier's complaint was a battle in the larger social conflict, one that would expand and transform beyond veterans per se and become a raging political war shaping American society for decades to come.

Context mattered in assigning a meaning to pain; Henry Beecher knew this. There was something in war's setting that gave a man a strange ability to tolerate long-bone fractures, penetrated abdomens, head wounds, and other severe injuries. For a civilian similarly injured in a car crash on his way to work, Beecher reasoned, the accident marked the "beginning of a grave disaster." But war wounds were different. At first, fighters barely even notice injuries. Why? The soldier downplayed his torment because "his wound suddenly releases him from an exceedingly dangerous environment, one filled with fatigue, discomfort, anxiety, fear and real danger of death, and gives him a ticket to the safety of the hospital," Beecher speculated. "His troubles are about over, or he thinks they are." Removed from the immediate threat of death, "it is not difficult to understand their relief on being delivered from this area of danger," Beecher observed.[2] However traumatized, soldiers' minds now turned to thoughts of going home, and thus they seldom asked for morphine, Demerol, or other painkillers.

The case of a husky nineteen-year-old soldier with a lacerated spine from a mortar shell gave Beecher his first view of these paradoxes of pain and social setting. The soldier "complained bitterly" about the pain, appearing to be wild from it, convinced that he was still being driven through with his own rifle. In reality, his back was gravely wounded. In the unruly triage procedure, the man was not given morphine—the most commonly used opiate—but whatever was at hand (in this case, a strong barbiturate sedative, sodium amytal). The sedative, which did nothing at all for pain, had a striking effect: "his color improved," the young man relaxed, his blood pressure rose, and he "turned for the better." His manic state had not been due to pain, Beecher concluded. Once sedated, a euphoric state set in; this was its own painkiller. Interviewing many such men, Beecher found that pain ranked low among their worries. In shock or euphoria or perhaps dreading death, they complained of strange things like unquenchable thirst, which usually "rose to first place as a cause of suffering."[3] But what would happen with a change of context? How long would a body's ability to relieve itself in this way last? What would happen to these men at home if the torment returned, if it persisted, or if the scars did not heal?

At home, these soldiers in anguish looked entirely different and would come to occupy an important place in American politics. How the soldier-civilian handled his pain became not just a medical problem but a challenge for government. If such men did not recover fully, they came to the VA—a once small, but now growing, branch of the postwar federal establishment—for help. With the VA's expansion, the notion that the veteran's chronic complaints and his lingering health troubles might be legitimate disabilities that warranted social compassion and long-term compensation quietly crept into American political consciousness. War kept these issues in the foreground. Memories of the world war faded but the Korean War erupted in the early 1950s, and the logic of pain and disability became surely tied to injury abroad and the growth of government care for returning soldiers.

For a nation on constant war footing, veterans' disability and pain were morally and fiscally troubling. What form of public and medical accommodations would the ailing GI receive? When was injury truly disabling? When was pain too much for a normal man to tolerate? While ongoing care for injured veterans might today seem uncontroversial, at the time, it was a continuing source of public debate. "Never before in history had a Nation assumed so inclusive a responsibility for its veterans . . . disabled in battle," noted one commentator. In time, these obligations became a burden, and for some observers it also became a severe threat to the country's well-being. "It was inevitable," this same writer noted, "that this burden would undergo a rapid increase as soldiers were returned to civilian life." In 1945, disability claims totaled $336,000. By 1963, expenditures would near $1.7 billion, with almost two million veterans receiving disability compensation. The numbers would continue to rise; the staff of the VA hospitals doubled and doubled again to meet the demand.[4] In the meantime, Beecher would make a career of such mysteries of pain—writing on the placebo effect, on soldiers reporting "phantom" pains in limbs long lost, and so on.

Pressured by veterans' groups to liberalize benefits, the Truman and Eisenhower administrations waded into these dangerous waters, fully aware that charges of socialism might follow. But could disability benefits be limited to soldiers alone? Shouldn't the benefits accorded them be more widely shared? Over the war years, a series of laws had incrementally expanded disability services for soldiers who had service-connected disabilities. Opponents like Orr on the political Right believed that the veterans' case for relief was overstated. Moreover, they feared that this case stealthily laid the groundwork for another liberal agenda: establishing government disability benefits for the general population. The outlines of an American debate emerged, with the soldier's suffering and slow readjustment sitting at the critical nexus. For soldiers and civilians, the issues of chronic illnesses and pain were particularly charged. Were they or were they not related to wartime service? How, if at all, should they be compensated and cared for? How should pain and disability be measured? The state had long been concerned with disability compensation, measured in relation to normative notions of able-bodied citizenship; the medico-political issue carried legal implications for what Barbara Welke called the "borders of belonging."[5] The cost, complexity, and stakes of pain and disability assessment, which had always been large for government, grew exponentially in the post–World War II years.

When Eisenhower came to office in 1953, he faced pressure to liberalize benefits on two fronts—for veterans and for citizens. The "great and growing body of veterans" sat squarely at the center of disability policy debates. America "has traditionally been generous in caring for the disabled—and the widow and the orphan of the fallen," said the president. These commitments would continue, he promised, but they must remain commensurate with injury. Trying hard to bridge the political divide between liberal Democrats' continuing New Deal principles and his own Republican Party's anxiety about the growth of government, Eisenhower hoped the issue would be resolved with such pronouncements—but it was not. Throughout the early 1950s, he faced constant pressure from the Left to expand disability benefits for the general population; in 1956, he succumbed, signing legislation establishing Social Security disability insurance (SSDI).[6] That concession created a new disability benefit within the social retirement system, sparked outrage among conservatives like Orr, and generated an ideological criticism that would last for decades and inform their views on all disability matters; for many critics, such initiatives were Trojan horses, stealthily ushering in socialism under the guise of compassionate relief.

Men Fighting through Pain

The veteran returning from the theater of war was an unknown quantity—a heroic man but also a tightly wrapped bundle of anxiety, depletion, and dependence. The view of many experts in psychology and social adjustment was summed up by Wilma Donahue and Clark Tibbits, who wrote in a volume on disability in 1945, "Whatever military life may have signified in the way of boredom, discomfort, pain, and suffering, for many men it has also meant security and solidarity of purpose." Released now from the constraints of military discipline, what would the soldier become? Some contributors to the same volume worried that the soldier had become a permanent dependent—that many years of being fed, housed, and cared for in the military had done significant damage to his psyche and sense of independence. Many psychiatrists shared the view of Chicago psychiatrist Roy Grinker, who said that the soldier "comes back not a strong hero, but physically and psychologically depleted." If it is true that "angry, regressed, anxiety-ridden, dependent men" were returning to civilian life in large numbers, the future appeared dark indeed. Would they cripple society?[7]

For Orr and his fellow conservatives, this was not a narrow clinical question. The future of the nation now hung in the balance, hinging to a large extent around the ideal of what able-bodied men should be and the reality of how war and hardship had altered them. As legal scholar Charles Reich later observed, the public sector's expansion was creating a new kind of property in the form of social entitlements—built upon a new relationship between citizens and the state.[8] In time, pain would become a precondition of these entitlements. To understand how chronic pain emerged as a political flashpoint, we will take a closer look at U.S. society in Beecher's and Orr's time (from 1945 to the late 1950s), at evolving theories about people in pain, at how the soldier's and the citizen's cases for relief were constructed, at how pain therefore gravitated slowly to the center of American politics, and finally at how by the late 1950s the broad outlines of a liberal pain standard began to emerge.

For critics, the VA was the institutional "ground zero" for a political struggle, as elected officials in the 1940s and 1950s sought to create rules, guidelines, and laws for the determination of disability and the definition of relief, particularly with regard to vague, subjective ailments like chronic pain. Interest groups like the Veterans of Foreign Wars (VFW) and the American Legion regarded pain as a legitimate problem—and relief as a right earned by those who sacrificed. By contrast, the AMA perceived pain and disability through the lens of professional self-interest and political ideology—raising broad questions of welfare, creeping socialism, and the tension between private and public health care. At the same time, however, medical professionals worried that the growing number of synthetic pain drugs—from Demerol to Percodan—might feed another kind of dependence in the course of treating pain. Both public relief and private sector care brought their worries. The path to true relief was not simple and straight. Into this mix of anguish and ideology hobbled more and more people with a wider range of infirmities, and with them came the suspicion from conservatives that much of this new world of pain could be feigned. Little wonder that some saw these persons in pain as a fiscal and administrative problem, others perceived them as legislative and ideological challenges, and yet others saw them as consumer possibilities.

The disabled vet was a particular worry in a society anxious about a return to normalcy. Sometimes, the veteran's problems were physically obvious, and the case for compensation easy to support: the loss of limbs, eyes, and body parts or general disfigurement. But equally often, the damage was hidden: the intense throbbing of internal tissue damage, the effects of concussions and deep scars, and (perhaps most challenging) the psychological damage done by years amid bombardment, killing, and death. Already in 1943 it was clear that "some disabilities resulting from military service leave a man with more or less permanent or recurrent pain or internal discomfort." The end of conflict inspired concern on a grander scale. In the immediate wake of World War II, disability was everywhere. But how exactly should "internal discomfort" be measured? Whether the infirm veteran needed benefits because he *couldn't* work or because he *wouldn't* work drew much attention.[9] The GI's disability was a perplexing issue, creating the framework for social calculations on disability that would move beyond military compensation to civilian life.

Experts from vocational counseling, sociology, and politics voiced deep concern about the damaged soldier's postwar adjustment. "The anticipated civilian world he once knew is found to be different from what he remembered . . . He has been living in a different world. Little wonder that he feels somewhat bewildered, and that feelings of insecurity and anxiety may develop." Government programs answered some needs (offering expansive subsidized education, housing, and other benefits in the GI Bill), putting "a roof over the head of the home-hungry veterans" and alleviating many of their concerns. But the psychological challenges of readjustment were not so easily fixed and became a crucial backdrop to how experts theorized disability and pain. As the editors of *The Disabled Veteran* wrote, the veteran's "sense of inadequacy may be augmented by a reawakening fear that disablement will permanently disqualify him for the competitive existence of a civilian."[10] These lingering problems of war—the lasting ailments, suffering, and disability—could not be put aside easily.

Though the health problems of veterans would have been politically perilous under any circumstances, three demographic pressures made it particularly so in the years immediately following World War II. First, there was the sheer scale of the infirmity of World War II fighters: in 1950, some 215,000 veterans were rated as 50 percent or more disabled, while thousands of others had lesser ailments. Second, the aging of World War I veterans now in their forties and fifties added another 50,000 people whom the VA judged disabled. Third, the start of a bloody campaign in Korea in 1952 exacerbated the problem. The VA was a system inundated with broken bodies. Over these years, a Democratic Congress and President Truman liberalized access—systematically expanding the types of ailments deemed service related and expanding the category of disability. But for Truman, there was a deeper problem: the line between veterans' and citizens' benefits was eroding, not because soldiers became citizens again, but because universal military service meant that any citizen had to be ready to take arms. Before many years, nearly all the population may be veterans or the dependents of veterans, the president acknowledged the year before he left office, and "this means a profound change in the social and economic import of Government programs which affect veterans. It requires a clear recognition that many of the needs of our veterans and their dependents can be met best through the general programs serving the whole population."[11] A better solution than adding further to veteran's health care entitlements would be expanding health insurance for the population at large.

Moves to expand disability programs riled the medical profession, of course—ever fearful of Democrats' plan to establish "socialized medicine" that would compete or do away with private practice. The AMA (a powerful mouthpiece for general practitioners) had been engaged in battle on this front since the end of the war. What Truman characterized as a "Fair Deal" for compulsory health insurance for all, the doctors' lobby labeled "socialized medicine." For the AMA, the creation of benefits for disabled veterans could only be understood as part of a larger ideological attack on free enterprise and private medicine. But the medical grumbling was not only focused on veterans and socialized medicine. AMA doctors were also skeptical about disability in general and what they often saw as a society too quick to coddle any and every man and woman professing pain. Walking the halls at the AMA's annual meeting in 1949, journalist Ray Cromley got an earful of opinions from doctors. They had "nothing but praise for such modern drugs as penicillin and streptomycin," but they were sure that (powerful drugs notwithstanding) "a lot of people just don't want to get well." Such people used vague complaints of "nerves" to hide their laziness. The AMA doctors bemoaned that "modern over-protective attitudes" were eroding a social ethic of self-support, self-care, and independence. Disability, for Dr. Miland Knapp of Minneapolis (a leading authority in rehabilitative medicine), was a by-product of these troubling times. After an injury, he theorized, "many patients develop an attitude of inertia. They believe the surgeon or the insurance company must make them as good as ever. They are inclined to do little or nothing for themselves and expect others to do everything for them . . . Such patients," Knapp speculated, "are likely to develop disabilities out of proportion to their injuries."[12] They needed not compensation or medicine but a good psychologist.

These anxieties, tinged with fears of manhood in decline, had long predated the veterans' battles. In launching a steady social critique, these physicians pointed to a powerful irony about the soldier's readjustment to citizen status: that military service had made these men obedient, hardy, and strong (enhanced their endurance to pain) but civilian society afterward had coddled and weakened them, infantilizing and mothering them and feeding a dangerous dependence. At the 1949 meeting, Dr. Albert Sullivan of New Orleans told Cromley about one case in point—"an ex-Marine who spent two years in the South Pacific without diarrhea. Then he returned to his small home town. He resented being treated as a boy by his parents and came down with chronic diarrhea. His ailment was overcome when he re-enlisted in the Marines."[13] Such strange, apocryphal stories of how masculine strength and valor abroad became sickness at home illustrated the concerns of physicians who focused on coddling and indulgence in the family, in government, and across society.

Such complaints about "disabilities out of proportion to injuries" and the dangers of coddling were part of the postwar era's recurring McCarthy-infused political debates about creeping communism, socialism, and the fate of freedom and democracy. Under pressure to defend the VA system in the Truman administration, one of its advocates insisted that such institutions were not in fact feeding dependence. Rather, they were America's best chance against totalitarianism: "those who consider the quest for social security incompatible with a free society may well be unwittingly giving aid and comfort to authoritarian regimes," said Truman's commissioner for Social Security Arthur Altmeyer. Far from being social-ist, he argued, the VA system and the principle of social security were the nation's best bulwarks against socialism. Terming the welfare state "the great political invention of the twentieth century," Altmeyer boldly de-fended social security as "the instrument of politics that the Communists fear above all else."[14]

Much of this debate about the New Deal's legacy in the postwar years swirled around the question of when a disability was truly service related and when (if related to military service) it was truly disabling. Public Law 748, passed by Congress on June 24, 1948, had already begun liberalizing relief on these questions—creating a statutory list of chronic and tropical diseases that were presumed to be service connected. A long list of ailments with more tenuous connections to military service (including anemia, arteriosclerosis, arthritis, and various bone conditions like osteomalacia, as well as diabetes, cardiovascular and kidney disease, ulcers, and various tumors) had been added to the list of compensable disorders. The AMA had fought against them all. Even the director of the VA testified of his fear that some benefits for chronic conditions would adversely affect veterans' hard-won disability benefits for more obviously service-related conditions. As the 1952 VA annual report noted, there had been "six public laws enacted by the Eighty-Second Congress . . . [in 1951] which liberalized compensation or pension benefits . . . or increased the monthly rates of compensation." These measures expanded access to veterans of earlier conflicts, opening the gates for some non-service-connected disabilities and recognizing new conditions such as multiple sclerosis (with its muscular, speech, visual, and cognitive degeneration) as legitimate when developed within two years of service.[15] With such liber-alized access, the numbers of covered veterans climbed steadily.

For many observers, the term "liberalization" best described what was happening, as too many injuries were increasingly presumed to be service related. As one report later commented, disability relief was a unique entitlement for those who had earned their injuries in actual con-flicts: "peacetime veterans did not receive the same liberal benefits." Other laws in 1950, 1951, and 1953 extended these presumptions of service-connected disabilities to additional disorders such as tuberculosis (if dis-covered within three years after service) and psychosis (if developed within two years of discharge). Driven then by the wars, politics, and shifts in

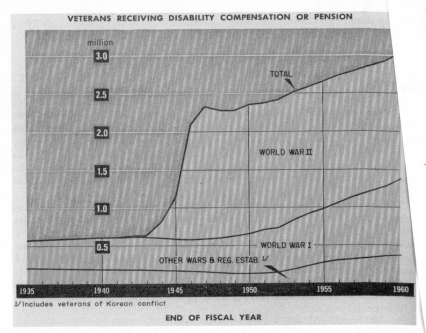

VETERANS RECEIVING DISABILITY COMPENSATION OR PENSION

million

3.0

2.5

2.0

1.5

1.0

0.5

TOTAL

WORLD WAR II

WORLD WAR I

OTHER WARS & REG. ESTAB. 1/

1935   1940   1945   1950   1955   1960

1/ Includes veterans of Korean conflict

END OF FISCAL YEAR

FIGURE 1.1.   The number of veterans receiving disability payments or pensions skyrocketed from just over a half million in 1945 to three million in 1960.

Image from *Annual Report, Administrator of Veterans Affairs 1960* (Washington, D.C.: Government Printing Office, 1961), 54.

such classifications, from 1945 to 1960 the numbers of veterans receiving disability payments and pensions climbed from just over half a million in 1945 to three million in 1960. Expenditures also rose. By 1962, $2.5 billion was being spent on veterans' disability, with "the largest program, both in terms of the rolls and benefit cost, [being] the disability compensation." Instead of dying out or declining, the number of damaged veterans was on the rise. So it was that the veteran's disability (and pain as one feature of his complaint) expanded as a flashpoint in the nation's political discourse.[16]

With Dwight Eisenhower's victory over Adlai Stevenson in 1952, the AMA cheered that the stealthy erosive expansion of the VA would cease. The doctors declared that they had "temporarily won the battle against government control," but they knew that other conflicts would come. AMA leaders would have taken particular comfort in Eisenhower's grim,

ascetic (and old-fashioned) acceptance of discomfort. Speaking in 1954, for example, the sixty-four-year-old president noted that "since the beginning of time men have deluded themselves—or been deluded by other men—with fantasies of life free from labor or pain or sacrifice, of limitless reward that requires no risk, or pleasure untainted by suffering." In the former general's view, the war experience had shattered these beliefs. "From such dreams, the awakening has always been rude and the penalty a nightmare of disillusionment."[17] Ike's view on sacrifice suggested that here was a man who, knowing war, would not allow mere sympathy to drive government expansion.

Rather than championing the disabled and dependent, Eisenhower (like many Americans) chose to valorize those who fought through the worst distress. Marine Private Alford McLaughlin was one of many men the president celebrated. Attacked by hostile forces in Korea and faced with enemy artillery fire in September 1952, McLaughlin received special commendation from Ike during his first year in office. "Although painfully wounded," the president stated, "he bravely fired the machine guns from the hip until his hands became blistered by the extreme heat from the weapons and, placing the guns on the ground to allow them to cool, continued to defend the position with his carbine and grenades." All the while McLaughlin stood up straight and in full view, shouting "words of encouragement to his comrades above the din of battle." This was the image many Americans upheld—of men overcoming agony and distress with "indomitable courage . . . and a valiant fighting spirit in the face of overwhelming odds." And even if people did not know McLaughlin's story, they would recognize the type from comic books and popular films. Many would also know the story of Homer Parrish—the character played by paraplegic veteran Harold Russell—who was one of the lead figures in the 1946 film *The Best Years of Our Lives*. Along with the McLaughlin ideal, Parrish's struggle to return from war and adjust to the stigma of prosthetic limbs loomed large in American views of heroism and disability.[18]

Veterans' disability continued to be a political flashpoint for Eisenhower, putting him in between two fierce constituencies: doctors emboldened by his victory and veterans who saw Ike as one of them. At Eisenhower's inaugural address to Congress in early 1953, the president declared his compassion for veterans and the nation's generosity to fallen men as well as their widows and children.[19] If government had one role

in these times, it was to continue its commitments. Properly caring for those in uniform and appreciating their service, he said, was an honest responsibility of the government. Yet Eisenhower also knew that such commitments could not be without limits and ought not to be extended beyond veterans to the general population. It was a difficult balancing act. On the left, Eisenhower had New Deal Democrats in control of Congress and intent on expanding hard-fought social commitments and pushing for just such an expansion. Complicating matters further, on his right he had two angry groups opposing one another on the disability front—the AMA railing against socialized medicine and veterans' groups, and cold warriors assuring soldiers in Korea that they would receive whatever care they needed at public expense, should they need it, when they came home.

The doctors and the vets—ordinarily united in their support of the Republican Party—were at an angry standoff, one that reflected the broader postwar debate over liberal government. Veterans' groups insisted that disability benefits were not "welfare" payments but justly earned compensation based on a contractual relationship. The Military Order of the Purple Heart laid out the argument: "Holders of the Purple Heart Decoration became disabled because of wounds received in combat with an enemy of the United States. As such we are the recipients of a contractual obligation, between the Wounded Veteran and the Government. This was created, when our Nation, called the boys into the Service and told them that should they become disabled, they would be taken care of, as well as their wives and families." To renege on the contract would be a travesty; the last time it was done, veterans organized a "bonus march" on Washington in the 1930s. Leaders of Disabled American Veterans (DAV) pointed to the nation's involvement in three wars since 1917—two world wars and the Korean War. Maintaining a large military force abroad and providing medical and surgical treatment, insurance, and "compensation for those who were disabled in line of duty" was "part of the cost of war," the DAV insisted.[20]

The AMA did not see disability this way, taking on veterans' groups with increasing vigor. VFW officials were infuriated that the "disgusting . . . ruling hierarchy" of the AMA had attacked veterans' hospitalization programs and accused war veterans (in McCarthy-like fashion) of being creeping socialists and a threat to free enterprise. The AMA spoke for the political Right—a wing of Republicans alienated by Eisenhower's moderation. In 1955, the doctors' organization decried what they saw as socialism by stealth: "continued Federal encroachment into private affairs cannot be advocated logically and consistently by those who, at the same time, voice their opposition to socialism." Veterans' organizations were taken aback by the claim that they were "unwittingly planting the seeds of socialism." The American Legion shot back, blasting the AMA as a "cash-conscious" group who placed "devotion to dollars" over "care for human suffering." VFW leader Wayne Richards had a simple message for the AMA, broadcast in the newspapers: "Lay off." "Instead of exaggerating a few cases of featherbedding" for political advantage, he said, the AMA should leave the VA and the compensatory benefits it provided to veterans out of its war against socialized medicine.[21] But the AMA would not "lay off" and pressed its case against the expansion—focusing its ire on non-service-related veterans' care and compensation. The VA system in all of its dimensions—hospitalization, disability benefits, and treatment for non-service-related ailments—was under extreme demographic, political, and ideological strain.

The moderate Eisenhower faced an impossible political quandary. How would he thread this needle? With one hand, the president warned Americans that citizenship involved a degree of suffering and sacrifice; yet, as an old soldier himself, with the other hand, he insisted that fighters who became disabled in battle had earned the right to relief. Then, to veterans whose injuries had nothing to do with battle, Eisenhower flatly declared that the nation owed them nothing no matter how infirm they became. Vetoing a 1953 bill granting relief to one single Spanish-American War veteran who fell outside the established rules of medical support for a non-war-related disability, Eisenhower voiced compassion but bluntly rejected such "exceptional and preferred treatment." Had the man's case been isolated, the president said, he would not hesitate to approve the bill, but this man was one of "twenty million veterans" whose eligibility for care in federal hospitals was subject to various restrictions. There were "many, many others [who had] been denied similar relief." The toll of infirmity was heavy; if all veterans' ailments were blamed on war, the danger of the system being overrun would be great. To open the doors to all such men would court disaster. "Yielding to compassion or special pleas would eventually destroy the effectiveness of the program," Eisenhower concluded.[22] Thus did Eisenhower portray himself not as the New Deal's nemesis but as its preserving champion.

Pressured hard from both left and right to rethink his disability stand, Eisenhower did what presidents often do amid political turmoil—he found temporary political cover by naming a commission in 1955 to study the problem of veterans' care and compensation. Its goal would be a "constructive reappraisal" of the liberalization of veterans' benefits. He named a trusted military compatriot, General Omar Bradley, to chair the Commission on Veterans' Pensions. Looking back over the past fifteen years of the program, Eisenhower wrote to Bradley, "In 1940 there were only 4 million veterans. There are now nearly 21 million, and the number is increasing rapidly."[23] The prospective burden on government was unsustainable, particularly because of how Democrats in Congress (and Truman) had liberalized services during and after the war to include compensation for non-service-related injuries. Eisenhower tasked General Bradley and his Commission on Veterans' Pensions with finding a new balance.

Eisenhower's appointment of General Bradley to chair the commission acknowledged that the veteran's place in civilian society had become a bellwether political issue. Democrats in Congress, including Senate majority leader Lyndon Baines Johnson and the first-term senator from Massachusetts, John F. Kennedy, were proposing to build on veterans' legislation by extending Social Security disability to all elderly disabled. On the other side, the AMA and their conservative supporters stood firm, charging that non-service-related disabilities were "superfluous care" for veterans and that disability coverage for the elderly was an extravagance.[24] Many observers, then, understood the question of whether the soldier's continuing chronic pain was a true disability to be political and ideological. Every symptom, each ache and worry, every pain-inducing ailment, whether chronic or acute, was now subject to intense scrutiny. Here was the crux of the politics of pain. For liberals looking to the New Deal as a continuing model of governance, the veteran's complaints could become a platform on which broader commitments could be built. But the topic split the Right, with the doctors and veterans squared off for an ideological fight.

At issue was the meaning of "liberalism." Speaking to journalist John Gunther in 1950, Eisenhower claimed to be both liberal and conservative, even as he expressed disdain for both terms. "You know, it's a hard thing these days for a man to believe earnestly and sincerely as I do in what . . . used to be called liberalism, progressivism, political action for the benefit of all, and at the same time not to go whole hog for what are claimed to be panaceas for our ills . . . Then [if he takes that position], he . . . becomes accused of being a darned conservative with no feeling for the people." In contrast to Ike's definition of a conservative as someone who had no feeling for others, Gunther offered another definition—a "liberal is someone who wants to liberate; a conservative is someone who wants to conserve"—and noted that every president had aspects of both in his agenda. Later in the discussion, Eisenhower confessed, "I've gotten so that I hate both terms because those two terms mean all things to all people."[25]

The debate over language illuminated political tensions at the heart of the Eisenhower presidency about the direction of U.S. society. For veterans' groups, government aid aimed to liberate the soldier; disability benefits were akin to the GI Bill and prosthetic devices, allowing men to pursue normal life after the war. Yet even supporters of veterans worried about conserving traditional institutions and values (not only hard work, enterprise, and freedom from government oversight but also the viability of existing government programs). Opponents of liberalizing VA benefits objected that adding more claimants to the VA or Social Security systems would threaten those who already depended upon these programs. Of course, medical opponents had a different, more far-reaching criticism. For them, the term *liberalism* stood in for a range of postwar assaults against their profession and society. As historians like Lisa McGirr have observed about groups coalescing under the banner of conservatism in this era, the term "conservative" came to mean not only defense of "tradition" but also hostility toward welfare, confidence in free enterprise, and deep disdain for expanding government and the coddling dependency they believed followed.[26] As the Bradley Commission began its work, such skeptics (particularly those in medicine) were conditioned to look askance at disability and to judge the pain complainant not as a man in true need but as a liberal Trojan horse.

If public relief for the ailing veterans at the VA provoked controversy, so too did private relief—the kind of relief offered by the booming marketplace in drugs and medical specialization and avidly consumed by a hungry populace. The postwar years were a high point of faith in medical advancement, with specialization and the burgeoning drug market offering new hope to the chronically ailing. A powerful array of sedatives, synthetic opiates, antibiotics, and painkillers had arrived in the war years. Enthusiasm and ambivalence greeted such products, for not everyone, even within the medical profession, thought that those drugs were a godsend. If the 1950s saw rising tensions over public relief, so too did private market relief provoke worries.

The pharmaceutical industry emerged from the war as a major player in American relief, offering a powerful new armamentarium of drugs (Percodan, Demerol, sedatives, tranquilizers, and so on) for the ailing GI, the suffering citizen, and the hard-pressed doctor. Penicillin had been developed in the war and was widely hailed for "performing some unbelievable act of healing on some far battlefront." As one advertisement noted, "Thousands of men will return home who otherwise would not have had a chance . . . When the thunderous battles of this war have subsided to the pages of silent print in a history book, the greatest news of World War II may well be the discovery and development [of] penicillin."[27] Now such products were being put to miraculous civilian uses. Other innovations (Atabrine for malaria, blood plasma preserved and transported to the warfront for transfusion, and painkillers from Percodan to Demerol) were also coming home. The new synthetic painkiller oxycodone, marketed as Percodan by the Endo pharmaceutical company and approved by the Food and Drug Administration (FDA) in 1950, bluntly promised to be less addictive than morphine, thus representing a revolution in pain care. Production of Percodan skyrocketed.[28] But, as in the public sector debates around government relief, skepticism also greeted those who promised private sector relief via aggressive surgery or new drugs. Aggressive marketing and rising consumption filled doctors, politicians, and consumers with hope but also with their own Trojan horse anxieties. Were drugs "miracle workers" in a world in need of relief? Or was this just another guileful promise?

"During the last ten years," announced one journalist in 1960, "the nation has been on an aspirin binge. Consumption of the pain-easing pills has increased four times as fast as the population growth." As he saw it, one reason for the binge was "the general long-term rise in the standard of living. Another is the increased health-mindedness of the American people." Affluence, economist John Kenneth Galbraith observed in 1959, had created new consumption trends—with drug consumerism leading the way out of the Depression and wartime economies into an era of newfound prosperity. This prosperity accounted for aspirin's allure—as if a generation long impoverished, hardened by want, and resigned to wartime rationing and sacrifice had been unleashed to apply salves to its minor hurts. On television and radio, in newspapers and magazines, few Americans could miss the aggressive savvy marketing of relief. Relief was now within easy reach for young and old: "the pill makers have placed their emphasis on speed—fast, fast, FAST, the television commercials insist." Many of the new products overpromised fast relief from anxiety, stress, and grave pain without the fear of drug addiction and dependence often associated with opiates. Many doctors and pharmacists did not quite know what to make of these optimistic promises; others prescribed the new pain remedies, Percodan and so on, enthusiastically. But as Boston psychiatrist Frank Ervin put it later in the decade, "The relief of pain is obviously one of the main functions of physicians . . . Ironically, it's one of the things we do least well—partly because we don't understand it."[29]

Demerol and Percodan quickly engendered new social conflicts over the limits of drug relief—proven effective on the front, promoted aggressively at home as "God's Own Medicine," but increasingly regarded by police and some legislators as a devil in disguise. In 1951, the Senate committee investigating organized crime heard testimony about the drugs' addictive potential and links to a criminal underworld. Testimony from minors, women, and men confirmed the threat. Elsewhere, a former GI described how military service began, for him, an affair with morphine that led him to Demerol. After being bayoneted by a Japanese prisoner, he received a shot of morphine, "my first shot of dope . . . while I was in the hospital . . . After that, I was seeking it on my own." From morphine, he graduated (after the war) to Demerol. The painkiller came to signify an escape. A physician at the hearings also testified how Demerol helped him to cope, at first, with professional stress but soon dragged him into dependence. Promised the gift of relief, he was now plagued by addiction. Playing into many of the fears of the Cold War era, he described the insidious attachment: "He had become addicted to Demerol, a coal-tar derivative, which he took under pressure of too much work and too little sleep. He said he was confident he could use it in moderation, but failed to keep it under control."[30] Already in the early 1950s, then, the unwanted side effects of these relief-oriented products fed into deeper social anxieties about healthy men, women, and children led astray. Americans saw the good and bad in this new economy: they embraced liberal market access to Demerol and Percodan, yet they remained cautious that indulgent consumption carried many hidden costs.

Tranquilizers were the hottest-selling products of the 1950s go-go drug economy, but by middecade they, too, had come under enhanced scrutiny. Between the end of the war and 1960, drug makers produced an expanding array of such tools for fighting minor pain and major anguish and also for regulating anxiety, nervousness, agitation, and related distress. As *Consumer Reports* noted, the popular tranquilizer Miltown "has become the fastest-selling pacifier for the frustrated and frenetic." A backlog of unfilled orders illustrated the high demand. The drug went beyond mere pain management, for it not only relieved "the pain of malignant disease" but also controlled so much more—nausea and general disease. "Most patients who come to see a doctor complain of pain and demand relief from it," insisted Dr. F. M. Berger of the Wallace Laboratories of New Jersey, the producer of Miltown. Speaking before a Congressional hearing, one New York psychiatrist saw the pills as a boon to mankind; it was permitting deinstitutionalization and liberation of the mentally ill and reducing the need for many hospitalizations. A drug associated with the ideals of the 1950s, tranquilizers thus blurred pain relief into a range of more vexing issues from the altering of personality to mood and emotion management and broad social change.[31]

The slippage from pain relief into personality and mood management worried some doctors and drug enforcement authorities and provoked slow political reassessment of the postwar market's drug revolution. Whether the demand for tranquility was stimulated by the industry's aggressive marketing or by unleashed consumerism, drug makers were well positioned to respond to the rising demand for pain relief. In 1956, *Newsweek* reported that 5 percent of all Americans had taken tranquilizers in any given thirty-day period, and drivers, flyers, alcoholics, and heart attack and migraine victims all praised its salutary effects. But by 1957, Minnesota congressional representative John Blatnik (who had also criticized misleading ads for cigarettes and diet pills), opened hearings on the era's popular painkillers, concerned about a trend toward deceptive marketing that played fast and loose with science. For him, it was the private market (and AMA complicity with industry), not government relief, that proved worrisome.[32] Physicians like Louis Lasagna questioned whether the industry made truthful claims about drugs' effects, and, by the end of the decade, Tennessee senator Estes Kefauver opened a wide attack with dramatic investigations of drug industry pricing, side effects, and advertising. For reformers on the left, then, drug-based relief in the 1950s was no less fraught than government disability compensation was for critics on the right. Both forms of relief seemed to have hidden effects; both were caught in a vortex of suspicions about dependence, indulgence, and guile. These questions of relief both touched on the issue of trust—not only whether the complainant could be trusted but who could be trusted to bring true relief, government or the drug companies?

All these issues of soldiers' pain, disability, relief, and recovery became nearly tragic for President Eisenhower when he suffered a severe heart attack in 1955. Recovering from surgery and anticipating a tough re-election campaign in 1956, Eisenhower relied on Demerol, morphine, sedatives, anticoagulants, and other drugs. Reporters pressed the White House for information on the president's mental state (Was he depressed?), his disability (Was it only temporary or enduring?), his recovery, his pain, and his capacity to continue the duties of the office. Meanwhile, his physician, Howard Snyder, worried in a private letter that Eisenhower now saw every pain, no matter how modest, as an ominous sign: "This past week the President has had, toward the latter part of the day, some pains in the right side of his abdomen. These, we feel sure, are due to accumulation of gases in that area in the large intestine. [But] any pain in that area causes the President great apprehension and is so psychologically disturbing that it is quite depressing to him."[33] At this very moment, the Bradley Commission was asking veterans about their experiences recovering from combat-related and non-combat-related illnesses and asking doctors whether "suffering, anguish, and pain" (in contrast to the loss of a limb) were legitimate reasons for disability compensation. If asked, Snyder would have answered yes. For the president, these questions were no longer abstractions; the political had become personal.

Specialists among the Suffering

Standing before the Trojan horse, medical specialists (like the citizens of Troy) were deeply divided about this thing called pain. What was it? How should it be treated, if at all? Almost everything that society offered for relief—disability payments for those who could not work on the public side or drugs and surgery to restore the body's functioning on the private side—had a double-edged quality. A new field devoted to pain theory and management, growing out of the war work of doctors, made sense in this context, and it is no coincidence that 1953 saw the publication of a major work in the field, John Bonica's *Mechanisms of Pain Management*. Working among injured soldiers, Bonica (like Beecher) had seen distress and ravaged bodies up close. His sympathies inclined toward the suffering veterans. Directing the anesthesia and surgery unit at Ft. Madigan Army Hospital in Washington, with its nearly eight thousand beds of injured soldiers from the Pacific theater, the twenty-eight-year-old Bonica noticed "an unusually large number of patients with severe intractable pain." Doing a kind of intellectual triage of pain types, Bonica began to think of pain not as one entity but as many different problems—organic pain being different from psychic pain, and functional pain being distinct from imagined pain. And then there was the vexing mystery of phantom limb pain. For Bonica, this last type was neither feigned suffering nor psychic maladjustment but something more complex, "a fundamentally psychobiological phenomenon." "Though it is a common habit of the mind," he continued, "to think of pain in physical terms and to draw an artificial distinction between what one is pleased to call 'real' or 'organic' and 'imaginary' or 'functional' pain, whatever its source of origin, it is in the final analysis a psychic event."[34]

Such typologies, and Bonica's observations on analgesic effects on each type of pain, formed the basis for a new specialization. To build pain as a specialty, simple theories of perception and personality would not do—such as the view that some soldiers were "can'ts," others were "won'ts," and that some were simply stoic heroes built, like Private Alford McLaughlin, for tolerance and endurance. The pain field's founding theorists and practitioners (Henry Beecher, John Bonica, and others) rejected these simple truisms. After treating and observing soldiers in war, they now sought to make a specialty out of this new and difficult social and psychic problem.

For Bonica, the management of pain through analgesia (drugs used for various kinds of numbing and sensation) opened into the management of mood, hope, emotion, and much more. No one knew better than he that different people reacted differently to hurt and relief, depending on "what the sensation means to the individual in the light of past life experiences and his attitude toward it." Pain sensation, in turn, depended on the person's mood, emotional status, will, cerebral functions, anxiety level, and many other factors. As an anesthesia expert, he knew also that any one drug could have multiple effects in one person and that the same drug had diverse effects across many individuals.[35] Postwar Americans needed relief, but at what cost? Furthermore, finding the right kind of relief for each individual (pain management) was a complex undertaking.

As Bonica left military medicine for work in Tacoma, Washington, these questions of pain and mood management followed him. The 1953 book that followed—years later called the bible of the pain field—outlined the core commitments and practices of the specialist. Pain, after all, was "the leading reason why patients go to doctors," and his publisher hoped that many other physicians would look to Bonica's text for guidance. They were not disappointed; the book was well received, particularly among doctors trying to find their way through the thicket of the new pain-relieving drugs. The expertise Bonica embodied—whether on the benefits of new drugs, on their adverse effects, or on patient complaints—was in much demand. In short order, he also became an expert *for* the pharmaceutical industry—meeting regularly with executives, attending company-sponsored meetings, publishing studies on their new products, and testifying on their behalf at trials about alleged side effects. His was a partnership with industry in the fine art of balancing pain relief and regulating mental states. As he wrote to one executive, "I am anxious to use this drug not in postoperative patients but in patients with inoperable cancer pain. As you no doubt know, many of these pa-

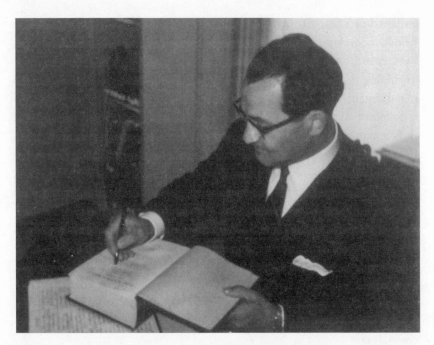

FIGURE 1.2.   John Bonica, later regarded as the "father of pain medicine," pictured in the 1960s signing one of his widely read analgesia textbooks.

Image courtesy of History and Special Collections for the Sciences, UCLA Library Special Collections.

tients are depressed mentally because of their hopeless prognosis. This, in addition to the depressant effect of narcotic therapy which is frequently used for pain relief, takes a very heavy psychological toll."[36] For Bonica, managing pain, mood, side effects, expectations, and disability were as one—making his work on behalf of patients and industry complex.

As he moved deeper into the field of pain management, however, Bonica realized that surgeons had already carved out a place for themselves in the management of pain and mood through aggressive brain surgery, especially the lobotomy. Surgeons had their own well-developed theories about people in pain—who they were, the organic origins of their complaints, and why such neurosurgical therapies as lobotomies worked best. Neurosurgeons' faith in lobotomy as the best medicine for the patient suffering in excruciating, intractable anguish had similarly been shaped by their experiences in World War II. Like Bonica and Beecher, the neurosurgeons had gathered new insights managing the traumas of war wounds. In war, the field had developed a set of radical surgical practices in the name of saving lives, emerging confident that "the neurosurgeon plays an important part in ridding these patients of pain." One noted prewar pioneer in the pain management/lobotomy field, surgeon Walter Freeman, agreed that "there is no fine dividing line" between organic pain and imagined pain. Following in Freeman's bold footsteps, 1950s surgeons answered the double-edged problem of how pain sensations could be both anatomical in origin and personality based with their own double-edged therapy. In some people, said physiology professor George Wakerlin, the lobotomy resolved the mystery. Once patients were lobotomized, he argued, "pain ceases to be bothersome, altho [sic] it is still felt, when the front part of the brain is severed in an operation called a lobotomy. This disconnects the anatomical switchboard thru [sic] which the pain signals are dispatched."[37] Across these fields, there was much disagreement about what pain was and what were its underlying mechanisms. But few could dispute that lobotomy worked against pain, particularly if the goal was to subdue the complainant.

Although lobotomy had become deeply controversial as a mode of pain relief and would soon embody much about the era's surgical hubris and excess, in early 1950 such surgeries still dominated medicine's approach to pain, particularly in terminal cases. The decision to conduct the lobotomy operation in an advanced cancer patient was fraught. But its advocates insisted that the procedure was humane, compassionate, and nothing less than a therapeutic triumph over a tortured existence. Freeman described one woman given a new life, free from worry, who had once suffered from disabling, intractable pain owing to an abdominal disorder. Many earlier operations had failed. But after Freeman's excision ("boring two holes in the skull above and to the front of the temples and severing the fiber between the thalamus and the prefrontal lobe"), the woman recovered dramatically. Before the operation she had screamed in pain when touched, said Freeman, but now the woman was able to "leave the bed of pain to which she had been confined for two years" and was "free of any feelings of intense pain" and even gainfully employed as a bookbinder. Moreover, this kind of relief—a profound surgical modification of feeling—lasted. He told of other sufferers relieved by the operation, such as the jeep driver who had lost his arm in an accident and "complained of extreme pain in the stump (a not infrequent complaint in such cases)."[38] He too had been helped dramatically by the lobotomy.

Neurosurgeons were sensitive to the accusation that the operation left people as "vegetables," but this was untrue, Freeman argued.[39] For men like Freeman and for many Americans, lobotomy stood not at the forefront of medical barbarity but as a symbol of humane, compassionate care—a practice that restored people in tortured disability to full functionality, freedom from anxiety, and a fuller health than they had ever had before.

In the micropolitics of medical procedures, new professional divides and subtle tensions were opening up in the 1950s—with the rifts between surgery and drug remedies defining alternative paths in the quest for relief. In an era of heady postwar specialization, each specialty sought to remake the body in its own way. Better living through chemistry or through lobotomy—these were only two of the ways that, as David Serlin has noted, postwar medicine made new inroads in rehabilitating bodies and identities. For surgeons, technical precision was the key to restoration. Harvard neurosurgeon James C. White argued for cutting pain transmission pathways selectively and deliberately. Severing neurological pathways saved sufferers from multiple threats to mood and personality—"from prolonged suffering, the deterioration of drug addiction, or ultimate suicide." Cutting such conduits for pain also radically altered the personality of the sufferer—"so that pain to him became a sensation rather than a constant threat." The technical challenge, White explained, was "to cut the pain tracts so completely that pain is permanently relieved" but also selectively so that bladder control and muscular strength was not adversely affected. In the view of such practitioners, lobotomy even constituted a humane, "legal alternative to euthanasia"—easing the cancer sufferer out of life not with sedation and drugs but by removing the worry centers of the brain, diminishing anguish, and allowing the disease to take its course with suffering removed. As White saw it, "lobotomy [was] justified when there is no other solution."[40]

Some surgeons also argued that the costs of lobotomy were low when weighed against its alternative: the high social and moral cost of using drugs for pain and feeding addiction. Here was yet another calculus of relief, surgical radicalism to make anguish bearable, to rescue people from torture as well as from addiction. Harvard's White, who had spent the war years with the U.S. Navy treating spinal cord and neurological injuries, insisted that neurosurgery was the preferred solution to precisely those kinds of pain, "unbearably severe and resistant to all known methods of medical treatment and to operation on the underlying causative factor," that lent themselves to opiate addition. This type of trouble was increasingly common "in the aged or in young people after certain injuries and diseases [including] the intense burning pain which may follow an eruption of herpes zoster (shingles); cancer . . . gunshot wounds and other injuries of the spine; and the pains experienced by amputees." In these conditions, morphine was an obvious choice, but its downside of dependence was well known. Surgeons claimed (and many experts agreed) that the operations they endorsed, if performed smoothly, could return people who once had been disabled, pained, and addled by morphine to productive work and happy, satisfying lives. Indeed, one new study on lobotomy ("cutting the channels to the front of the brain") showed how a person with intractable pain was simultaneously relieved of his hurt and cured his addiction to forty-two grains of morphine daily.[41]

Lobotomy as pain relief worked in a perverse way; lobotomized people often reported calmly that they were still in pain, but they simply did not complain about it. This observation only added to the fascination with pain and perception as things of mystery. If the culture of complaint was a problem, surely here was a solution. People suffering in chronic distress emerged from the operation tougher than before, more able to endure hardships, and more tolerant of anguish. In some ways, the practice fit neatly into the era's belief in toughening up chronic complainers and hardening them to life's cruelties. Among the procedure's "interesting effects on personality" was its effect on worrying. As one journalist noted, pain became "a sensation rather than a horror. It gives people a little 'thicker shell' but doesn't make vegetables out of them, contrary to popular opinion." Surgeons knew that this thickened shell could be seen as dehumanizing but insisted that observations of lobotomized patients showed only that "certain aspects of personality and perceptual style, which are changed by a prefrontal lobotomy carried out for the relief of pain, are precisely those that differentiate within the normal population those who can tolerate pain well from those who suffer greatly from it." In this view of lobotomy, the line between the naturally pain-tolerant individual and the lobotomized person was blurred. Essentially, "a person who is exceptionally tolerant of pain has the personality and perceptual style of the individual after a prefrontal lobotomy, whereas one who cannot tolerate pain resembles in personality a patient before prefrontal lobotomy."[42] But, to nonsurgeons the practice was clearly troubling and double edged, and Freeman constantly defended against charges of radicalism.

This was the medical field that John Bonica entered. In favoring drugs, he became a modest reformer—believing that neurosurgery's "destructive procedures" should be employed only as the last resort when pain proved intractable to all other measures. In medicine as in society, then, pain was a Trojan horse containing many hidden dangers. If one were in chronic pain, finding true relief—whether by surgical mood manipulation, drugs, or disability compensation—would be treacherous and contentious whichever way one turned. For many observers delving into the mysteries of pain, the greatest mystery of all was the complainant; and by the mid-1950s, much of the new pain field's theories, speculations, and worries surrounded the complainer him- or herself.

One prominent physician, Ian Stevenson, warned that the blockbuster drugs of the era, rather than relieving worry and distress, only masked underlying problems in people's lives. Tranquilizers and pain-relief drugs allowed people to enter a drug-induced haze, to escape caring and responsibility: "Tranquilizers, like alcohol, numb not only psychic pain, but also love. Thus the widespread use of these drugs expresses—and may also dangerously promote—both the loneliness and the callousness of our crowds." He warned, "A chemical suppression of psychological difficulties remains a concealment whether with just a little vermouth or with a shiny tablet." If not handled carefully, drugs—like surgery—had a stealthy power to destroy.[43]

The Bradley Commission and the Cash Value of Pain

When General Omar Bradley's Commission on Veterans' Pensions began its work in 1955, among the many questions it tackled was how to rate the soldier's pain as a disability. Was the pain complaint a true disability or an excuse for shirking responsibility? If it was truly disabling, what was pain worth in dollars? The GI's complaint balanced on a tightrope. Here was the commission's dilemma: "If too high, the payment might encourage malingering; if too low, it would simply be a relief grant . . .

This problem has vexed our legislators and public administrators from the earliest times."[44]

Compensation for ailments, including pain, involved a difficult political and moral accounting—translating suffering into cash. "Our central purpose has been . . . developing a monetary payment sufficient to enable the veteran to readjust financially in his home community," one 1956 commission report stated. With sixty-six regional offices and many smaller units around the country doing disability determination, creating uniformity was one challenge.[45] Also vexing were the ailments that did not fit neatly into the VA's mind-body disability categorization. The system recognized impairments of the body (loss of arm, eye, etc.), and of the mind (categorized as psychoneuroses); the challenge was how to tailor the payout not only to the type but also to the degree of disability while paying heed to the broader social good. Across its thousands of pages, the Bradley report made clear that these were not medical questions but political ones.

Who knew for certain whether the veteran's chronic affliction with, say, tuberculosis or arthritis really originated in the trenches, in exposures to pathogens abroad in cramped bunkers, or back at home? What kind of expert could judge the origins of these complaints? To tackle this quandary, the commission asked 153 eminent physicians for help. Most of the responding doctors were skeptical that the current disability determination system was based on sound medical evidence. Too often, they believed, the veteran had been given the "benefit of the doubt," especially in diseases of unknown etiology like arthritis. This needed to be revisited. Chronic disease was a particularly perplexing problem; "one-half of the 153 respondents believed that the presumption of service connection" was not based on "accepted medical principles." Slightly more than a quarter believed otherwise. The others hedged. One doctor expressed the skepticism of the majority: "I would change the whole system to one where there is no presumption in any case."[46]

"In your judgment, should factors other than loss of earning capacity such as pain, suffering, social handicap, and mental anguish be compensated?" Bluntly, the commission put this question to the doctors. The question unleashed a torrent of deeper anxieties—starting with their distrust in subjective complaints, moving on to their belief that rewarding pain complaints encouraged deceit, and then ending with what many saw as the true problem: the skewed social incentives and overliberalization of the postwar years. "The day has long passed when earning capacity is the sole yardstick," noted one supportive respondent. "These and other factors are of equal or greater importance." This respondent spoke for a solid majority (55 percent), who believed that if pain from injury continued long after the war, then, yes, it should be compensated—that is, "unless objective findings by a competent physician negate them beyond reasonable doubt."[47]

But in the commission's poll of doctors, 41 percent insisted that accepting pain as a disability pushed them (as reluctant gatekeepers to the public purse) and society into the dangerous terrain of rewarding malingerers. For the skeptics, accepting pain as a disability grated against their views on fairness, feasibility, and human duplicity as well as the male soldier's adaptability to hardship. Pain was easily feigned, and its features were "vague, subjective, readily simulated [by deceitful claimants], and difficult to evaluate." The category of pain, they insisted, was "imponderable," "impossible to calibrate objectively," "too difficult to evaluate fairly," "practically unfeasible," and "an insurmountable task," even if "from a humanitarian standpoint" it was proper to treat it as a disability. Rather than accept immeasurable pain as a reality that might throw their commitment to medical objectivity in doubt, many chose instead to doubt there could be such a thing as disabling pain—primarily because of the impossibility of measuring it fairly. Faced with unfeasibility of measurement, one doctor concluded flatly, "Give medals, ribbons, etc.; but not pension." Furthermore, another specialist noted, compensating for pain only favored men who were quick complainers and penalized "the adaptable sturdy characters."[48] These anxieties reflected, of course, underlying social codes about masculinity and deeper worries about whether idealized sturdy men should express pain, deny it, or cope with it.

Furthermore, many physicians argued that providing monetary awards for pain and anguish opened the door of relief to hordes of complainers. These doctors harped not only on the difficulty in measurement but also on the capacity for manipulation when a dollar value was put on such vague ailments.[49] "These subjective complaints are extremely difficult to evaluate fairly; they are prone to lead to gross exaggeration," noted one physician.[50] Dr. Norton Canfield spoke for many others when he insisted, "These conditions are too hard to measure and to place a dollar value on them is not reasonably possible."[51] This monetization of pain gnawed at many of the respondents. The irony, they insisted, was that only the complainers would be paid for their pain while hardier souls would tolerate their hardships without payment. As Walter Burrage put it, this was an unconscionable payoff: "in practice the complainer commonly is 'payed off' [sic] while others 'carry on.'"[52] This was the doctors' deep enduring conceit about the Trojan horse of the soldier's pain. The entire system was not lifting men up but rewarding the wrong kind of men while dragging them down into a pit of government dependency.[53]

How much discomfort or distress should the nation ask a citizen, called to serve, to bear in service of country? In the end, the commission's ambivalence on the question captured society's quandary. One on hand, the Bradley report appeared to take a hard line on this question—insisting that "the performance of citizenship duties cannot be expected to be painless or free from sacrifice . . . Our national survival requires that all citizens do their part and make whatever contribution they are required to make." Therefore, not all veteran pains and bodily sacrifices should result in financial compensation. On the other hand, the report also acknowledged the need for a supportive system for the truly disabled man. As it noted, the expectation of sacrifice "does not mean that military service must be rendered without compensation or that maintenance should not be provided to those who are invalided . . . as a result of military service." With extraordinary sacrifice came the rightful expectation of long-term support. But then, pivoting once again, the report commented, "It is fallacious to . . . claim that just because the uniform was worn for awhile [sic] the Government owes the former wearer a living. Much of the pain and suffering of military service . . . cannot be compensated."[54] Here was an articulate ambivalence befitting the time. The report covered all sides of the question, illustrating why the pitched battles being waged by doctors and veterans would not be settled quietly or easily.

By asking doctors to itemize and "rate" particular ailments for their levels of disability, the commission learned that their ideologically sharp views softened when it came to the specifics. Everyone agreed that at one end of the spectrum were major disfigurement, immobility, and loss of multiple limbs. In such cases it was easy to declare the vet disabled without criticism or continuing judgment. But what about cases where those disabilities were less graphic, where recovery was possible even if very difficult, or where clear evidence of anatomical damage was lacking? Scars, for example, came in many forms—from the minor kind to major disfigurement. Not all scars warranted compensation. But for some doctors, the pain associated with the scar needed to be taken into account in the calculus of disability. As one wrote, "The compensation of wound scars at 10 percent cannot be related to impairment of earning capacity and indicates that an allowance for pain and suffering has been included." One VA rehabilitation specialist observed, "Scars about the face, severe neuralgias, and upper extremity amputees should be entitled to extra compensation." As questions of pain became more specific in relation to the body, then, the report produced much evidence supporting the VA, the veterans' groups, and liberal New Deal politicians committed to expanding disability benefits by considering "loss of physical integrity, shortening of life, social inconvenience, disfigurement, pain, suffering, anguish, and possibly others."[55]

At the more abstract level, however, many doctors insisted that compensating pain as a disability pointed to an underlying disease: "excessive liberalism." Some survey respondents even dismissed the very concept of disability as a liberal concoction. As the commission report noted, "Some critics of pension legislation . . . viewed this legislation as a move to 'the left,' i.e., a device to weaken the moral fiber of the American people, etc." One respondent, Oscar P. Hampton, saw only the deceitful hand of liberalism at work: "The yardsticks by which total disability is awarded seem rather liberal since the percentage awards throughout the schedule are excessively liberal. I do not believe there is medical validity for the liberalizing provisions." For Hugh Morgan, the problem was that liberalism threatened to bankrupt the system altogether: "in order to conserve this for deserving veterans it is all the more important to exclude the now [i.e., newly] eligible who could bankrupt and destroy the undertaking." Going even further in castigating dependency, Hedwig Kuhn dismissed the idea of disability outright: "I doubt if there are very many people in the world who are truly disabled," he barked. Technology and medical innovation, he thought, was lightening the burden of afflicted people: "Even a polio victim in an iron lung is not truly disabled if he has imagination. He can even support himself by writing music, writing books, talking into dictaphones and what not." The belief that effective treatments were at hand informed such skepticism. If a "crippled" man had prostheses and an "imagination" in Hedwig Kuhn's view, why would he ever need benefits?[56]

As to the question of what ailments could be considered service connected, the doctors' views were at once politically attuned and clinically informed. Yet their theories of disease and disability were shifting—particularly as once recalcitrant conditions seemed, in the context of postwar medical innovation, to be more treatable. Tuberculosis is a case in point of what some physicians saw as disabilities yielding to cures. As Dr. John Minor argued, "Modern developments have had a marked effect on the problem of disability, the best example of which is furnished by tuberculosis with the shortening of hospital and institutional or home care time, early return to activity, etc." The miracle drug penicillin and other antibiotics were laying siege to TB-related disability. But Walter Bauer knew that there were new, chronic diseases gaining prominence in the wake of TB's decline: ailments like arthritis, multiple sclerosis, and cardiovascular disease. The question before the commission was whether these maladies, new and old, were service related. "It is not possible to be definite in many of these instances . . . when the illness manifests itself after separation from service," wrote Bauer. The evidence could not speak for itself, so like many of his colleagues he relied on his views about the soldier. "Since all questionable problems of this type are settled by giving the veterans the benefit of the doubt, it is the latter policy which really underlies the presumption—not a group of medical facts." In judging the soldier's pain, then, doctors confronted several political assessments: first, whether a "grateful and efficient country" should give the veteran the benefit of the doubt; second, how to connect the new, late-manifesting chronic diseases, ailments with uncertain etiology, directly to the war; and, third, the social impact of converting disability ratings into monetary benefits.[57]

In the end, the Bradley report captured the ambivalence of the moment—even as the politics of disability was taking a dramatically liberal turn in a Congress consumed by health-care intrigue. The commission called for caution in further expanding veterans' benefits. Eisenhower (himself ill, recovering from the heart attack, and running for re-election in the summer of 1956) was not inclined to take any major steps on questions of civilian or veteran disability. But, heading into the elections, he found himself boxed in by an energized and Democratically controlled Congress pushing to expand disability benefits. Two formidable demographic pressures kept health politics before the Congress: ailing veterans and the growing number of older Americans lacking the resources to purchase health care in a booming market. As historian Philip Fungiello has noted, the crafty Senate majority leader saw the political opening. Johnson understood that disability among the elderly was a wedge issue for Democrats heading into the elections and pushed hard for a bill establishing a new Social Security disability entitlement. Johnson's maneuver forced Republicans into choosing between compassion for all disabled citizens (not only veterans) on one hand or allegiance to the AMA on the other. Eisenhower opposed the legislation, hoping to bottle it up in committee and to keep it from the floor of the Senate. Johnson, however, skillfully maneuvered a successful committee and Senate vote, and the bill's narrow passage forced the president to sign or veto a sweeping new law establishing benefits for disabled Americans. Political expediency prevailed. Ever ambivalent and caught between true conservatives and ardent liberals, Eisenhower signed the law, much to the AMA's dismay, even as he agreed with them that its effects could be dire. He promised steady monitoring of the program, he pledged efficient and effective management of the disability plan, and he said that future policies must place greater emphasis on helping "rehabilitate the disabled so that they return to useful employment." Signing the law, Eisenhower fell back on the language of security, hoping that the legislation would "advance the economic security of the American people."[58] *Security*, Eisenhower hoped, was a potent political watchword (social security, national security, economic security) that all Americans could rally around—whether they were New Deal liberals or right-wingers.

There is no question that the law ushered in a new era in disability relief and altered the landscape of the nation's pain politics—for citizens, for veterans, for the VA, for physicians, and for the practice of disability administration that would grow in its wake. The law also pushed doctors, reluctantly and often angrily, into new roles as "raters" of disability and adjudicators of pain. It was a role for which by their own testimony many were unsuited, both because theories of disability and illness were in such flux and because of their sharp professional animosity to the law. There was no consensus on the criteria for disability and little agreement on relief. Yet, who else but physicians would rate disability? From here on, adjudication about the nature, severity, and effects of impairment would unfold with all parties—patients, doctors, bureaucrats, and often judges in the courts—cognizant of the economic and political stakes. But even after the law was passed, skeptics did not cease warning about the dangers of subjective evidence in disability determination; the problem would never go away. Nor would their complaints subside about the cost of this new social commitment, whether through the VA or through Social Security. At the VA, the burden expanded; by 1958, disability compensation cost $1.4 billion for two million veterans. "Requests for reconsideration [of rejections] jumped from 13,500 in 1955, to 44,610 in 1956, to 64,678 in 1957, to 92,664 in 1958."[59] By 1960, the new disability provision was also stressing the system with sharp increases in requests for benefits, increased numbers of rejections, and an expanding bureaucracy to manage requests, rejections, and appeals.

On the Management of Spoiled Identity

The pain complaint became, then, a complex cultural symbol in the 1950s. In the wake of the new disability benefit, an angry critique of people claiming to be disabled (and those claiming pain as their disability) sharpened. It proved impossible for AMA leaders not to see the soldier as part of an elaborate charade, but the hostility to disability claimants went deeper. For many physicians, a web of postwar developments—the booming drug market, the rise of government disability benefits, the actions of disability lawyers, and the commodification of pain relief (that is, its translation into monetary benefits)—made them profoundly uneasy about the pain topic. Out of their critique would emerge a distinctive and stigmatized pain persona—a stock figure standing in for government corruption and personal deceit, and focusing their tirade.

Writing for the AMA in the wake of the disability law's passage, Louis Orr launched a blistering counterattack against the president. Having fought fiercely against Truman's national health-care plans, the doctors' lobby had not expected this from a Republican administration. Betrayed by Eisenhower, Orr exclaimed, "We look about us and realize that right here in our own back yard, without any prodding from planners and socializers, we have allowed politicians to create a Trojan horse of ominous dimensions." As the AMA chair of the Committee on Medical Service, he saw Ike's concession as conjoined with the expansion of veterans' health, which led "to Socialized Medicine and Socialism by way of the Veterans Administration." Orr's essay was later published simply as "The Trojan Horse." As he saw matters, the VA's slow expansion was a sneak attack on free enterprise itself. Accusations of socialist infiltration, of course, had been the stock in trade of Senator Joseph McCarthy's "witch trials." But in 1956, with McCarthy only recently disgraced, the AMA took up the flag, insisting in its own inflammatory fashion that these silent threats to democracy were real. Truman's 1949 proposal for national compulsory health insurance had failed, but now these many "so-called fringe measures" (as Orr put it) intruded the federal government into medical education, insurance, and medical care.[60]

To Orr, wars and the subsequent elevation of the needy GI in postwar American civilian life were a subterfuge for the slow creep of social dependency. In the previous two decades, wars had produced a fourfold increase in the number of veterans; at home, their numbers constituted a profound threat. Orr found society's increasing commitment to non-service-related injuries particularly outrageous. Of the half a million veterans the VA treated in 1951, "85 percent of them had non-service-connected disabilities"; the numbers were increasing. The future looked bleak, for "if we have any more 'small' wars like Korea . . . then our veteran population will again increase rapidly, and the entire problem will be compounded many times over."[61]

For decades, the AMA and the VFW (a powerful veterans' lobby) had been at odds over the question of who was disabled. Since World War I, the AMA had consistently battled to block expansion of the VA's care for veterans with non-service-connected disabilities. By law, the VA was permitted to care for such cases only when beds were available. In the aftermath of World War II, however, the power of the veterans' lobby grew, as did their support for the VA system. Once small, the VFW had seen a "meteoric upsurge" in membership after the war, with two million new members; and it now rivaled its big-brother organization, the American Legion (although, as one observer noted, the VFW was "neither as influential as the Legion nor as affluential"). After the Second World War, it is revealing that the littlest brother making up the "Big Three" veterans' lobby was the DAV, "which has sprung up after World War I, and now numbered some 130,000—its numbers doubling since Pearl Harbor."[62]

Answering Orr's attack, Robert Bell, physician and medical consultant with the VFW, recalled the heroic memory of the men who had fought, sacrificed, and still carried the scars of their service. For Bell, fair compensation for heroic sacrifice was the key issue, not socialism and stigmatized identities: "the factor that has changed is the large increase in number of war veterans due to three great wars within the span of almost one generation." Government's commitment needed to match its wartime demand on citizens, for, despite the three great wars, "it is difficult to perceive how anyone can read into this program a trend to socialism." Bell characterized Orr's fears as grossly exaggerated. Furthermore, he insisted, the toll of chronic illness in the system was far lower than Orr alleged. In Bell's telling, the nation was deeply in the GI's debt; they "offered their maximum gift at a time when the country was endangered, and under this program they are only being accorded limited health benefits in their hour of individual need." Not only were they worthy of care and compassion but it was "the height of folly to endanger a restricted but humane policy and program which so fully expresses the goodness, the humanity, and the moral leadership of this great country."[63]

Orr responded by taking issue with Bell's liberal vision of the soldier's pain as worthy of the largesse of relief. Wasn't pain and sacrifice a normal duty of citizenship? "The performance of the DUTIES OF CITIZENSHIP cannot be expected to be painless or free from sacrifice," he contended. Here was the crux of the disagreement. Pain and sacrifice were expected of all citizens; to expect otherwise led the nation down a dangerous path. But disability relief now allowed the Trojan horse through gates; and, in its shadow, the ideological scaffolding of an American pain and disability debate came into view. Complicating the debate was the fact that the line between citizen and soldier had eroded. As the Bradley report eloquently noted in 1955, "Changes in the nature of warfare are making the old concept of 'veterans' obsolete. Peacetime conscription, total war, and the threat of atomic warfare tend to blur or erase the line between the man in uniform and the civilian."[64] Now with the passage of SSDI, other groups (the elderly, children, women, African Americans, workers, and so on) who, critics charged, had even less of a claim for relief than veterans were swept into the controversy. The alleged character of *their* pains and disabilities (Were they heroic? How much had they sacrificed?) would become a moral and political battleground. All pain of course was not equal, but now the medical expert was compelled to "rate" differences in disability and pain. The soldier's anguish and the aging citizen's complaints needed to be measured, using monetary yardsticks. New pain complaints would appear as well. Claims of pain specific to black Americans (such as sickle cell anemia, discussed in the following chapter) would carry yet another set of political meanings. Which of these complaints were real? Which deserved relief? How much relief? In the shadow of the disability law, these questions came to define a major political rift—with one side wishing to expand services in the name of compassion, and the other warning of a coddling, creeping loss of social vigor and values in society.

Pain became a signifier with potent political and psychological meanings. For many physicians writing in the late 1950s, the pain complainant became a tainted symbol of much that was wrong with society—a particularly vexing type of what sociologist Erving Goffman called "spoiled identity." To California psychiatrist Henry Albronda, people who complained about chronic pain were maladjusted; they should be studied with caution and listened to with sympathy, but they should never be offered quick relief. Two political developments concerned him: not only had the federal government liberalized disability relief, but so too had his home state of California. Had the war years taught Americans nothing about pain? Studies showed, he said, that even during the war, the "psychosomatic backache" was the most common type of "functional backache among troops"—originating from anxiety and nervous energy. Speaking at a pain symposium in San Francisco in 1957, he grouped migraine headache, cardiospasm, and low back pain with all these vague "problems of psychogenic pain."[65]

Albronda drew a direct line from the war to the postwar pain complaint—as if civilians had learned from the vets' poor example. He had emerged from years caring for soldiers at war with hardened skepticism. Compassion only made people in chronic pain complain more, he insisted. The hidden truth was this: many were simply maladjusted malingerers. He pointed to earlier studies showing that "all patients who complained of phantom limb pain had considerable psychopathic disturbances . . . Men who had dominant psychopathic traits and reacted poorly to their disability tended to be more demanding and complaining than those with sound personality before the injury." In persistent chronic pain sufferers, "masochistic self-punishment underlies [the] chronic painful condition." Their sickness, in other words, went deeper, to a fundamental psychic imbalance.

The conditions were ripe for a psychological theory of pain complainants not as sympathetic heroes but as pathological; their indulgence emerged as a major social threat. For Albronda, Orr, and others, the soldier's professed pain had opened the way for government to become a destructive parent. Patients, doctors, politicians, and others were guilty, in this view, of nurturing the pain complaint, expanding access to free care, and exaggerating the severity of slight ailments. Reflecting also a Freudian turn in postwar psychiatry, Albronda saw excessive mothering in childhood as the real origin of the pain complaint. Parents (like government) needed to be on high alert lest chronic complainers get too much attention, gain easy relief, and grow to take advantage of others with their selfish dependence. "In most families," Albronda stated to his colleagues at the pain symposium, "the young child soon learns that his cries of pain bring solicitude, and later he runs to his parents for comfort whenever he is hurt."[66] Whether in the family or in society, providing impulsive relief for every complaint was deeply misguided.

The expansion of disability benefits catalyzed this critical theorizing about pain, with doctors like Albronda describing the new pain persona as a thick web of repression, self-deceit, and fantasy. They had been conditioned by society to be plaintive, and they were being rewarded for this destructive behavior; this was the beginning of a conservative critique that would simmer and boil over the following decades. The pain complaint may develop, he noted, "in the child who secretly enjoys seeing the punishment of siblings, then punishes himself by fantasy for enjoyment . . . Or," he added, "the child brought up to repress feelings of hatred may as an adult use complaints of pain to cover his hostile feelings toward an associate." In contrast, "a well-integrated, adaptive person can disregard the not overpowering peripheral stimulus," he wrote.[67] Professional self-interest and frustration with the gatekeeper role led many such doctors to the same conclusion—that the pain complainant was a symptom of something deeply wrong with the government and society that produced him or her; pain was not a problem to be taken at face value or remedied impulsively with drugs or medicine. It symbolized what we might call a crybaby society.

Doctors were not alone in seeing the moral and economic stakes of illness and in theorizing pain; observers like economist Barbara Wooten, sociologist Talcott Parsons (writing on the "sick role"), and many others saw that shifts in the burden of responsibility were afoot. "The concept of illness expands continually at the expense of the concept of moral failure," wrote Wooten in *Time* magazine in 1956, "The significance of this question of who is sick and who is sinful cannot be laughed off as 'merely semantic.'" The war experience of soldiers was one arena of debate, but now a new national debate about citizens was replacing it. There are "practical consequences" to "drawing the boundary between health and illness in one place rather than another," Wooten observed. Were complainants sick or sinful? she asked. And who would carry the burden of their care?[68]

A bevy of specialists, new theories, and entire industries (not to mention new government programs) were emerging around the treatment and management of pain in this era; but if pain was being turned into profits and revenues, the process was a complex one. The case of arthritis highlights just how many economic interests and tensions this commodification of pain provoked. As the *New York Times* explained, arthritis "attacks the aged, the young and those in their middle years. It causes not only physical suffering but also economic and social hardships." By some estimates, it affected eleven million adults and children, caused eighty million lost workdays, and (most troublingly) made "300,000 workers totally unemployable each year; it robs them of more than $1,000,000,000 a year in wages." The search for pain relief, as the chair of the Arthritis and Rheumatism Foundation saw it, also drove millions of Americans into the arms of charlatans and quacks, where desperate people spent $250 million a year on fake cures and promises of relief. But even legitimate and proven pain relievers, like the booming tranquilizers, were subject to growing criticism, with *Time* magazine calling them "don't-give-a-damn pills" because of their ill effects on people's consideration of one another.[69]

With quacks selling false relief on one side and government offering disability benefits on another, doctors stood at the center of an often frustrating pain relief economy, but so too did lawyers. Thus, pain forced physicians to contend, for example, with personal injury attorneys like Melvin Belli (a man who earned the nickname the King of Torts for his pioneering work in personal injury law). Writing in 1951, Belli commented that "pain is not a readily measurable commodity. Trial juries and judges may never be able to return verdicts for seemingly identical injuries with the precision that a cigarette machine vends an identical package for an identical coin." Not only did pain thresholds vary from one individual to the next, Belli knew, but the economic consequences of pain varied and received different payouts: "a disabling injury to the wage earner may be more financially catastrophic than the same injury to a non-working housewife." As an advocate for injured people in the private tort system, Belli had known for some time what doctors who had been pulled into the disability system were only just realizing—that "pain . . . may depend upon counsel's imagination and vividness of portrayal by demonstrative evidence." As J. L. Barritt, the San Francisco-based medical director of the state's Industrial Accident Commission, noted, the doctor faced a dilemma when it came to assessing the thresholds, the character, and the evidence of subjective pain.[70]

With all these economic, moral, legal, and medical theories and agendas surrounding them, people in pain stood at a troubling political nexus; many were accused of a perverse and deceitful commodification that put the nation at risk. "No one but the patient himself knows exactly how severe his symptoms are. They are in a way his stock in trade—as yet unpriced," noted Barritt. It was doctors and lawyers—called upon to study ailing people and characterize disability—whose theories, battles in the courts, and final judgments could turn this "unpriced" stock into a compensable disability. In dramatic courtroom settings, pain was becoming *commodified*—a term drawing our attention, as I've written elsewhere, "to the processes by which bodily experiences such as pain are assigned value (monetary and otherwise) by physicians, patients, insurance companies, and others." Men like Barritt, however, voiced unease and resignation with this new task of "distinguish[ing] between the subjective *complaint* and actual subjective *disability*."[71]

Who could blame physicians for being frustrated with policing pain and managing relief in postwar society? The new political economy asked much more of them than they could comfortably deliver, not only about the measurement of pain but also about monetary compensation for subjective illness. Writing in 1957, one Southern California doctor felt pressured by insurance companies for accuracy: "the increasing attention given in recent years to the question of insurance coverage for the expenses of sickness has caused the public and insurance companies to be more conscious of the cost of medical care." For insurers, the stakes were clear: defining where sickness ended and malingering began was a crucial business problem.[72] The rise of both private insurance and public compensation of the VA variety raised worries over so-called perverse incentives—whether payment for sickness encouraged people to prolong their disability. For professionals, other incentive problems appeared. For surgeons now fighting with insurance companies to be paid for their procedures, few compensation issues were as contentious as whether operations for back pain would be reimbursed by insurance plans. This was the new pain relief economy at work, as doctors were drawn, by force of law, into the era's disability debates. In recoiling from these postwar trends, some physicians expressed their frustrations with government, private insurance, and the gatekeeper role through their disdain for the complainant.

"Pain presents us with a series of paradoxes," wrote physician Louis Lasagna in introducing a special 1956 issue of the *Journal of Chronic Disease* devoted to the problem of pain. Pain is widely experienced, "yet pain is almost impossible for anyone to define adequately."[73] Absent consensus, the politics of pain meant that some medics like Lasagna gravitated toward compassionate relief while others like Albronda saw complainers (not pain per se) as the problem. Pain in all its confusing duplicity had arrived—a mysterious, worrisome presence in postwar society. Lawyers, insurers, drug marketers, and scholars, too, gathered around pain, regarding it with puzzlement and wonder, unable to see inside and worried about the dangers or profits lurking within. From this point forward, the question of pain would never stand apart from these economic and social interests—drug companies pushing their brand of relief, and private insurers and government administrators weighing their commitment to care against their fiscal concerns and the needs of veterans, the aged and other groups. But it was the physicians who worried loudly about the spoiled and suspect identity of the person in pain. In the shadow of two wars, contending with an aging society and fearing a postwar expansion of government many deemed to be a socialist threat, many of them saw the pain complainant as a tainted symbol of the indulgence, permissive social conditioning, easy access to welfare, and excessive liberalism that was destroying the nation. In time, this argument became the cornerstone of a conservative critique.

Pain, the Trojan Horse

The kind of care provided to the person in pain was not merely a medical concern: it was cultural and political issue through and through.[74] By the early 1960s, many Americans (lawyers, physicians, bureaucrats, patients) understood disability and pain in broad moral terms. The grassroots conservative movement that was stirring, ultimately bringing Ronald Reagan to the California governorship, tapped into this belief that people were turning professed pain into profit and that the liberalization of government benefits (in the name of better health care) did nothing except feed social dependence. "In our society the virtues of self-reliance and independence are so highly valued that many people feel a great deal of shame and humiliation at the idea of having to be taken care of," wrote one physician in his state medical journal in 1963. His topic was not welfare or taxes, but pain management, cancer care, and the peculiar psychology of the cancer patient. People used pain selfishly to get what they wanted from others, he noted, since "conflict over dependency may lead to a demand that the physician get him well. This demand may be expressed through an increase in the intensity of pain as a way of saying, 'Do something to get me well.'" Dependence bred its own selfish focus on pain: "it is also possible that the patient feels such a sense of guilt about the need to depend on others that his pain becomes a method of self-punishment and also a way of saying to himself, 'Look—I'm justified in having to depend on others because I'm suffering so much.'"[75]

These psychological theories about the person in pain had taken root in the contentious postwar years of hope and Cold War anxiety. These years saw the construction and reconstruction of the psychological motivations of such people. Pain "may become the sufferer's chief occupation," Albronda warned, a self-sustaining social pathology, with the doctor as unwilling accomplice. Compassionate responses only indulged complainers and fixed their underlying neuroses in place. The "medical relief of such severe pain, unless accompanied by early diagnosis and careful personality assessment and therapy, will only lead to another pain complex," he insisted. Other critics loudly echoed the California psychiatrist, worrying that relieving pain too easily masked underlying problems. But what were such practitioners to do when faced with a person in chronic pain? "Listen without anger to the patient's undue complaints and gain his confidence," Albronda urged. But also "understand that unwise probing, injecting, massaging . . . in trying to relieve pain that is psychically perpetuated serves to fix the neurosis and lessen the chances for cure."[76]

Psychologizing of the pain complaint became common fare as critics linked liberal medicine to an insidious social and political threat. When the doors of the wooden horse swung open, Louis Orr and others saw hordes of people with chronic headaches, backaches, and arthritis. In the case of people with arthritis, the social threat came not from the disease per se but from the so-called arthritic personality—men, and also women, who were allegedly maladjusted, hostile, and prone to complain. Experts would create an elaborate psychological profile of these guileful, infiltrating, warriors: "factors such as repressed hostility, poor marital, social, and vocational adjustment, and obsessive-compulsive character structures are among the reported manifestations of psychological maladjustment in these patients." These people were prime targets for manipulation by a government that coddled them so much that they ceased to take action for their own lives.[77] Physicians in the AMA saw themselves as leading the way by ringing alarm bells; but they were not alone, as other experts also worried about the hidden costs of new disability exemptions.

Who was the pain complainant? Was he or she truly deserving of relief? These questions, which had opened with soldiers and now applied more broadly, gained poignancy because of the political debate over liberal relief. As the influential sociologist Talcott Parsons theorized, "The privileges and exemptions of the sick role may become objects of 'secondary gain' which the patient is positively motivated, usually unconsciously, to secure or to retain." Experts had first worried about soldiers; now women more and more appeared as another vortex of concern. "The patient with painful degenerative knees is usually a female, and she is often obese," observed the Cleveland-based orthopedic surgeon Frederic Rhinelander in a 1960 issue of *Arthritis and Rheumatism*. "She is generally middle aged, and she is apt to be much worried about her condition," he continued. Such people posed an organic as well as a moral problem.

For them, even mentioning the word "arthritis" could foster intense fear of permanent dependence, so "at the outset, she must be assured that she does not have 'arthritis' (in the sense that she fears that she is not on her way to becoming a deformed cripple). She must be assured that her joints are simply wearing out a bit prematurely, and that the process can be alleviated by simple measures." To even use the term, he implied, could create the dependence that so many people feared. A Michigan epidemiologist offered another theory—arguing that angry men who repressed their hostility were particularly prone to arthritis.[78] Whether the typical arthritis patient was a skittish woman or an angry repressed man, the need for a theory of pain that took into account perception, gender, identity, and psychology seemed clear—not just for the good of the patient but also for the good of society.

Asked by the Bradley Commission to assess pain, anguish, and suffering as a compensable disability, many physicians were hostile because they understood the political stakes. Speaking passionately against liberalization, they opposed the idea on practical as well as political grounds.[79] "It would be an insurmountable task to rate pain, suffering, social handicap, and mental anguish," wrote William Altemeier.[80] Like Louis Orr, a chorus of such men saw pain as a ruse. The outlines of a great American pain debate were now evident. The stakes and major players were in view. It had begun with the ailing, wounded, or perhaps arthritic veteran. Were his illnesses connected somehow to mortar shelling on the beaches of Anzio, or was his pain a sign of social weakness? In this dispute, pain was a Trojan horse because indulging such complaints would open the way for all kinds of abuse, dependency, and social pampering. The fragile, coddled pain complainant had emerged as a stock figure in the conservative attack on liberalism and liberalization.

TWO

Opening the Gates of Relief

....

Call no faith false which e'er hath brought relief to any laden life.
SIR MORRIS LEWIS, "TOLERANCE"

When President Dwight D. Eisenhower signed the new disability law (SSDI) in July 1956, he opened a gateway to relief for Texas resident Rosie Page and thousands of others. A middle-aged mother, Page had entered the workforce during the World War like thousands of other American women; she continued working after the war. After four years as a packer in a Texas manufacturing plant, in 1959 she began feeling stiffness and aching in her hands and neck. By the time she quit work soon afterward, Page was in extreme pain and extraordinarily nervous as well.[1] Forced to quit one manufacturing job, Page tried another, but pain and the question of her nervousness stalked her every move.

Often tranquilized, nervous, and out of work, Page turned to the federal government, seeking disability benefits and relief through the Social Security disability program that Eisenhower had reluctantly established. Rejected by the agency, she appealed, setting her sad case on a momentous legal journey. Her case was a vexing puzzle. Did her pain have origins in her "nervousness"? Did it truly prevent her from working? Was she, in fact, disabled and thus owed relief under the new law? As doctors, lawyers, and federal bureaucrats weighed Page's complaint, her pain would be slowly transformed—from a personal struggle into milestone in the era's debates over disability and citizenship. The *Page v. Celebrezze* case, as it came to be known, would be followed by anyone who looked to government to open the gates to true relief. Page's claim opened an opportunity for other plaintiffs, lawyers, and judges to craft new policy at this juncture where questions of health collided with problems of work and citizenship.

Page had lots of company in her quest for federal relief. Pain hobbled the elderly with arthritis and burdened thousands of wounded war veterans. It haunted the lives of athletes, housewives, politicians, and other people in a society that was being transformed by more wage-earning women. Pain bothered men like Philip Kerner, a sixty-five-year-old World War I veteran with diabetes, who had recently won a ruling that put the burden on the government to prove the case against his disability. In an aging society, it ate away at the savings of retirees like seventy-year-old Edwin Brinkley, who pressed the visiting Senate Special Committee on Aging to visit the prescription counters of Fort Lauderdale, Florida, "and see the oldsters having to pay exorbitant prices for the necessary remedies to relieve their pain." The answer Brinkley hoped for was Medicare— the battle over which would go on for another three years. Americans like Page, Brinkley, and Kerner seemed to be facing a rising tide of crippling arthritis pain, migraines, back pain, cancer-related pain, and unspecified subjective pains. Here was a society apparently in an epidemiological and social transition—making an affluent turn, leaving behind an era of high mortality from infectious disease, and entering a new era when a host of chronic degenerative ailments became society's chief burden. Chronic, degenerative disease was "a price we pay for living longer," noted one health institute's report, and chronic pain was one of the tragic perils of progress especially for a society being altered by aging and work.[2]

The battle over Page's pain introduced into the legal record the many questions swirling around the government's promise of relief. First, was the pain real? Second, could the federal government be trusted to deliver relief, and could it do so without condoning dependency, fraud, and socialism? Third, might the booming market in pain drugs be a better pathway to true, lasting relief? These questions linked Page's pain to the most turbulent political questions of the 1960s—government's role in ensuring equal opportunity, in safeguarding the most vulnerable, and in regulating industry so that it would be a promoter of good and not a means of exploitation. As the decade of the sixties opened, a familiar partisan debate continued: some saw government relief as a false promise; others saw market claims to provide "fast relief" with new drugs—Demerol, Miltown, Percodan, and so on—as a sham exploiting the vulnerable. Could claims of relief from these products be validated, trusted, or embraced? Here too government in the 1950s and 1960s was asked to speak to the pain problem. The decision before Americans was whether pain complaints of people like Rosie Page should be borne silently and stoically or whether such citizens in distress should be supported by law and relieved by a sympathetic government. The problem of pain was in a sense a question of trust. Who could be trusted to know and relieve another's pain and to handle this growing problem of relief?

Five years after Eisenhower signed the disability bill establishing SSDI, the task of judging Page's pain fell on President Kennedy's Department of Health, Education, and Welfare (HEW). As the federal bureaucracy turned its attention to plaintive people, it became deeply engaged with a task that would haunt the expansion of liberal government—the challenge of distinguishing people with true pain from "chiselers," HEW secretary Anthony Celebrezze's term for people seeking undeserved government handouts through deceit and fraud. It was Celebrezze's job to police the boundary between deserving pain and undeserving fraud—and after HEW administrators turned down Page's disability claim, he followed suit, rejecting her appeal. The issues embedded in pain management were profound in their moral, fiscal, and civic implications. Underpinning the question of what a compassionate, liberal government owed to such citizens was the problem of evidence. What sufficed as evidence to validate a person's need? Another question shadowing the rise of liberal governance was dependency and how the government would safeguard against the twin dangers of pain relief—on the one hand that its policies would produce dependency, on the other that hucksters and scam artists would inevitably arise, preying upon the vulnerable with their false promises of other forms or relief. As a "nervous" housewife, Page's case was one among a flood of new challenges for government as the decades opened.[3]

How far would liberal government expand? How much should the gates of relief be opened, and for whom? The key to the health of liberal reform was distinguishing honest need from fraud. During the 1960 election, Kennedy had criticized his opponent Richard Nixon's apparent disregard for disability, reminding voters that "in 1949, 79 percent of the House Republicans voted against any inclusion of disability benefits under social security, and [then-senator] Richard Milhous Nixon was among them. Why he would ever discuss social security and try to defend his party's record on this matter—I don't understand." SSDI has since become an established entitlement. But once in office Kennedy took up the challenge of governance, seeking to both expand and to manage those commitments—for example, finding money for mental health reform and further liberalizing disability benefits, while practicing fiscal restraint and managing the requests of thousands who had filed SSDI requests and appeals.[4] Page's story of woe, nervousness, and hardship was many things wound tightly into one person—her pain was at once a sensitive administrative and political concern, a contentious clinical dispute, a fiscal worry, and (in a sign of the growing role of the courts and law in this momentous decade) a vexing legal problem.

"If Pain Is Real to the Patient"

Medical experts sharply disagreed about the legitimacy of Page's complaint. Their differences illuminated just how difficult it was for authorities to reach consensus or to judge pain by standards untouched by cultural biases and social considerations. Her own osteopathic physician had diagnosed her condition as osteoarthritis "with significant rheumatoid arthritis in the fingers of both hands." She had complained of back pain so bad that it stopped her from doing housework or climbing stairs, but HEW examiners found "the spine showed only minimal arthritic changes." Examiners for HEW did find X-ray evidence confirming arthritis in her hand, but they found no "objective evidence to support complaints of pain in areas other than the hands." But one sympathetic physician watching Page very closely concluded that she was no fraud, simply because of how she moved—her movements were a portrait in honest fragility. She rotated her neck slowly and carefully, with limited range; she raised her shoulders only slightly when asked to do so; and she walked unsteadily with assistance from her husband and daughter. Another expert contended that Page showed signs of "severe anxiety state with conversion hysteria." It was a damning analysis, as "hysteria" was widely recognized as a dismissive label for the emotional, complaining woman. Taking all of this into consideration, the agency was never convinced about the severity of these pains.

When HEW called upon an orthopedic surgeon, he also offered a psychiatric diagnosis akin with the hysteria diagnosis—finding no objective X-ray results at all and concluding that Page's problems were entirely psychological. Setting the tone for HEW's rejection, he observed that "claimant 'had a marked psychogenic overlay of her symptoms.'" The pain complaint, he insisted, had a genesis in the woman's hostile, defensive reaction to being challenged: "there was not 'full cooperation' between the doctor and Claimant . . . rather 'there was a great deal of hostility' based on her belief that she was being deprived of disability compensation."[5] Concerned about the absence of clear objective evidence and bothered by the woman's attitude, HEW rejected Page's request. When the HEW Appeals Council followed suit, Page's next delicate step (accompanied by her lawyer and family) was into the federal courts.

In court, her case came before Judge John R. Brown, a Republican who had been appointed to the federal circuit by Eisenhower eight years earlier. Given his political background, Brown might seem an unlikely person to originate a sweeping liberal interpretation of Page's condition as true pain. But Republican commitments were different in Eisenhower's time than today, with moderation verging on liberalism a powerful force in the party; in any case, the politics of pain did not align so neatly with party ideology. Like Eisenhower, Brown took a moderate view informed less by right-wing ideology than by a broad philosophy on government, morality, and social policy regarding the nation's most vulnerable citizens. A former clerk later recalled, "The one statement I remember most was his repeated insistence that we are our brothers' keepers, a stereotypically Democratic notion." But as a lifelong Republican, the judge "would always add that our brothers and sisters had no right to demand to be kept."[6]

Brown had carried this outlook on moderate intervention into his rulings on African American voting rights in the South, siding with blacks' complaints against state-imposed voting restrictions. The parallels between the *Page* case and voting rights lawsuits were clear—both hinged on whether the courts would condone or condemn government barriers to full citizenship. In a time when, as Attorney General Robert Kennedy insisted in 1963, "those of us who are white can only dimly guess at what the pain of racial discrimination must be," one question before the courts was how government should legally remedy such professed pains. Brown's *Page* ruling called for an interpretive leap. No one could truly know how much pain Mrs. Page was in. Her case called on those who would judge to weigh objective evidence, to consider the science, to assess the cost, but also to "climb in [her] skin and walk around it in," as novelist Harper Lee had written a year earlier.[7] Across the political spectrum, this was the political and judicial challenge—building a liberal, compassionate society based on intersubjective understanding.

The question was not only whether Judge Brown would see the world from Page's viewpoint but whether he would command HEW to sympathize with her pain. Ruling on Philip Kerner's behalf in 1960, New York circuit judges earlier had insisted that HEW could not dismiss the pleas of the aging diabetic veteran lightly and without amassing evidence of his nondisability. Whether Brown was swayed by these earlier arguments, by his "brother's keepers" convictions, or by the display of evidence in the case record, he pushed the Kerner decision further. He took Page's side; he acknowledged that there was a yawning gap between the lives of judges like him and those living with hardship, infirmity, and want. His ruling affirmed dramatically that the lack of "objective clinical and laboratory findings" was no grounds for dismissal: "if pain is real to the patient . . . , the disability entitles the person to the statutory benefits even though the cause of such pain cannot be demonstrated by 'objective clinical and laboratory findings.'"[8] Charges of excessive liberalism and judicial activism would follow, but Brown remained content that he had done the right thing for Page and for society.

Brown's 1963 *Page v. Celebrezze* ruling that Page's subjective complaints were real and deserving of compensation upended revered legal opinion on such matters dating to the 1930s. Decades earlier, the eloquent and influential Judge Learned Hand had made a hard distinction between pain and *disabling* pain. The two were not the same, he insisted, nor should all cries of pain be nursed and given solace. In his 1937 opinion in *Theberge v. United States* (written in the midst of a long, deep economic depression), Hand insisted that "a man may have to endure discomfort or pain and not be totally disabled; much of the best work of life goes on under such disabilities."[9] Notably, the ruling read like a tough-minded formula for coping in hard economic times. Hand's opinion had become much quoted, with even the HEW Appeals Council citing this long-standing view in its rejection of Page. Not only did pain have a positive value, but HEW also raised the objectivity question—insisting that Page's complaints were "inconsistent with or out of proportion to the objective clinical and laboratory findings." HEW's argument drew heavily on Hand's austere sense of pain as omnipresent, necessary, and even conducive to one's best labor. More than twenty years after Hand's ruling, grim endurance remained a cardinal virtue.

Judge Brown rejected this old view of hardship as the kind of theory that befit a harsher more rigid bygone era. Page's pain was born of another moment, and it was "true pain" even if it did not have the requisite objective features that Hand wished to see. Furthermore, Brown rejected outright the notion that "the best work of life" could, and should, be done amid distress, discomfort, or necessary hardship. Over the next years, just as other judges had once followed Hand's lead, jurists of this new era would follow Brown.

With his momentous statement, "if pain is real to the patient," the Brown ruling established a liberal pain standard in American litigation and jurisprudence.[10] This was a far-reaching, idealistic claim: that felt pain could become an entitlement and that the experience itself triggered compassion and financial support. A generous theory of felt pain as true pain emerged—in law, in medicine, in government, and in society. This theory grew more capacious through the decade, resonating with the era's fitful ideals of expanding equality and citizenship. Brown insisted, "This notion that pain must be endured, that pain, no matter how severe or overpowering, is not disabling unless it will 'substantially aggravate' a condition is 'contrary to the standard announced in' cases from this and other Circuits"[11] As his brother's keeper, the Republican judge pushed the logic of liberal relief toward a new precedent.

Over the next decades, legal scholars later observed, "a significant number of federal [disability] cases were decided in which the alleged disability was wholly or substantially related to pain." Rather than dismissing such pains out of hand, the court now threw these complex conditions back to HEW—with the command that subjective pain must be taken seriously. As the U.S. solicitor general assessed matters in 1965, "HEW tries literally hundreds of these disability cases. It would seem that more and more of them are being taken to court and that in a goodly percentage of the litigated cases (particularly in depressed areas of the country) the

Secretary's decisions are being reversed." In the wake of such rulings came a sweeping liberal expansion; claims grew and the disability program swelled to thousands, tens of thousands, and then hundreds of thousands. In time, these cases occupied the attention of judges throughout the federal circuit. As well, a growing cadre of medical experts, lawyers, government officials, and other experts in the sciences would be drawn into the judging of pain and disability in the legal arena. One might think of this development as the slow expansion of a bureaucracy of relief spanning the 1960s and 1970s.[12]

Private Ailments into Public Anguish

Was pain "real" if it was not detectable by X-ray analysis? Was psychosomatic or psychoneurotic pain eligible for compensation? If so, what levels of relief should be granted to those infirmities and for how long? Evaluating pain in the wake of the *Page* decision demanded a new breed of pain experts, or perhaps even a team of them. Coming out of medicine, law, sociology, and other fields, they were thrust onto a large stage, where their judgments on pain causation, their demonstrative evidence, and their theories of pain psychology and personality would be used to navigate between the era's liberalizing tendencies and simmering conservative discontent. As the U.S. solicitor general saw it in one 1965 HEW dispute, all cases of disability posed challenges: "In all but the extreme cases it is very difficult to determine whether a man is truly disabled. Many subjective and intangible factors, as well as so-called objective medical evidence, play a role in the appraisal of a man's condition. Almost invariably there is considerable conflict in the expert testimony."[13] Determining true pain from false pain became a recurring flash point of political controversy—every case raised questions of perception and personality, and beneath the accumulating claims for relief lay troubling issues of welfare, citizenship, the size and scope of government, and the very future of the society.

In the early years of the 1960s, many patients and their attorneys were gaining the upper hand in disability compensation cases, even as pain remained a contentious issue in medical-legal debate. The famous trial lawyer Melvin Belli effectively used what he called "demonstrative evidence" to win over juries in cases involving pain and suffering; other lawyers spoke of "projecting trauma." The new trend in court was using charts, graphs, X-rays, and other images to win over juries in disability and liability cases. Doctors despised the tactics; Belli understood why. Physicians found their authority challenged in these courtroom battles; they regarded men like Belli as wolves "circling the wounded deer ready to leap for the jugular." But Belli had discovered a winning strategy— producing victories in suits for injury and securing disability claims for plaintiffs in an era when the law had opened the door to public relief. As governments in the United States and the United Kingdom extended disability benefits to their citizens, Belli wrote, expertise in debating disability was needed from personal and industrial liability cases to government compensation cases: "the doctor and lawyer can for himself see which way the socialistic wind is blowing, can read the cases, and can place his own bet whether, in the next ten years, his fees will be coming from private but rich Mrs. Throckmorton or even richer but public Uncle Sam."[14]

Journalists, social scientists, and others were also busy spinning theories of pain that intersected with the legal debate and that shaped shifting sensitivities about a diversifying cultural and ethnic landscape. The media seemed fascinated by pain's many mysteries beyond the soldiers who had occupied center stage in earlier years—questions like whether women felt pain the same way that men did, whether different ethnic groups (Italians, Irish) tolerated pain differently from one another, and why some people complained more than others. One 1962 *Popular Science* article sped readers through new findings on the hardy, stoic Eskimo (citizens in the newest, fiftieth state), noting grandiosely that "decidedly, Eskimos . . . have been known to hack off a gangrenous foot to save a leg—and do it without wincing—but it's not uncommon for a gray-flannelled Madison Avenue executive to shudder at the first sound of a dentist's drill digging into a heavily novocained tooth." Such overstated gaps in pain tolerance confirmed a worry of the era—that civilization had bred in men a kind of weakness unknown to the primitives. In India, paradoxically, the fact that "Indian fakirs snuggle down on beds of nails—seemingly in comfort [could be] explained on the basis of hysteria—a kind of emotional frenzy that may act as an anesthetic." Here was yet another moral about pain: that hysteria did not only feed a culture of complaint but could also in the Near East build a wall against pain. Many such anecdotes found their way from research into popular reporting, underscoring that the American fascination with pain was not only narrowly judicial. Not only judges and lawyers but also social scientists and the broader media worried about the toughness of some citizens and the oversensitivity of others—and the implications of pain endurance for the nation.[15]

If anyone could judge pain and analyze pain complaints, it was the young, disabled sociologist Irving Kenneth Zola. Echoing an emerging point of view, he insisted that "real" pain was as much a cultural construct as a scientific one. "Today's chronic disorders do not lend themselves to such easy conceptualization and measurement as did the contagious disorders of yesteryear," Zola wrote. Stricken with polio at age sixteen, he walked with braces and was already on his way to developing disability studies as an academic field. His interviews with two groups of ethnic Americans (Irish and Italian) led him to appreciate the diversity of the pain complaint. Zola found that Irish subjects carried their burden stoically, tending to "deny that pain was a feature of their illness" far more than the Italian Americans. The study of illness and complaints thus merged into the study of cultural norms, for, as Zola put it, whether a symptom found acceptance in a particular society depended on "the 'fit' of certain signs with a society's major values which accounts for the degree of attention they receive."[16] Pain behavior, in short, was cultural.

Across several expert communities, the pain debate was now fully engaged—and turning into a distinctive cultural debate. By focusing on the culture, psychology, and consciousness of the complainant, a tragic variety of human suffering came into view. "To most people, pain is a simple idea, offered readily but often difficult to define," observed one neurosurgeon later in the 1960s. But "the physician must remember that pain is a concept, one with wide connotations" in which the anatomical transmission of the pain stimulus was "separate and distinct from its interpretation by the conscious mind." As a surgeon put it, "The former represents pain, and the latter, suffering." The legal world—with its battles over awards for pain and suffering and its systems for assessing damages in injury cases—was far ahead of the medical sciences. "In these respects," the neurosurgeon observed, "courts of law, which clearly recognize these terms, appear to be more cognizant of the problem than the medical profession at large."[17]

Theories of pain and disability were varied and unsettled, and they embraced fascinating questions of psychology, the human mind, and perception. As early as 1960, Henry Beecher had observed that placebos could actually be effective painkillers, under certain circumstances. The notion that pain could be controlled with a sugar pill took researchers deeper into the complexities of perception, individual personality, and how previously existing stress could accentuate someone's cry of pain. Forced to broaden its perspective, pain scholarship expanded to incorporate psychology, sociology, and other fields concerned with perception. Drug biology could never explain it all, since even when someone took a pharmacologically active drug like morphine, Beecher contended, "the power attributed to morphine is . . . presumably a placebo effect plus its drug effect." This kind of scholarship suggested that faith, culture and belief, and positive personality traits could explain drug action; for, as Beecher noted, "Placebos work best when administered with an air of hope and confidence to an extroverted sort of patient who feels a real need for relief of his symptoms." Beecher's view of pain as linked to personality and experience became a new standard reference in press accounts and medical writing and also in court arguments and rulings. Pain theory in the 1960s would move deliberately, relentlessly, toward appreciating the power of the subjective, the mind, psychology, and perception in pain and its control.[18]

Fascination with how people coped with pain and hardship ran the gamut from mundane interest in how a child learned when to complain to concern with spectacular feats of pain tolerance—issues equally of interest to parents, lawyers, scientists, and social commentators. On the mundane end, scientists speculated that average people acquired their pain tolerance from parental conditioning. Critics of the loosening of social mores wondered whether "permissive" parenting (for example like that apparently promoted by the popular pediatrician Benjamin Spock) laid the groundwork for indulgence and adolescent complaint. Or was it true, *Science Digest* wondered, that "a person's reaction to pain may often depend on how he saw his parents behave under similar circumstances when he was a child"? Through spanking, for example, a child was thought to acquire the "'conditioned anxiety' that keeps his behavior as an adult within socially acceptable bounds."[19] The debate over spanking and pain (and Spock) was another dimension of a postwar debate that fragmented along cultural, and often generational, lines. Wasn't imposed pain, in some ways, beneficial? Americans raised amid Depression-era hardship, war, and want might have recognized and even endorsed Judge Hand's view—that some degree of pain was essential to becoming a "normal" well-adjusted citizen—but in the postwar years, many Americans surely found the promise of a new pain-free life for children and adults to be appealing.

In an era of prosperity and growing middle-class comfort, cultural feats of pain tolerance could be graphic and shocking. As historian Karen Halttunen has argued, Anglo-American middle-class sensibilities have long been shaped by "spectatorial sympathy" for the pain of others. Watching Buddhist monks and nuns stoically burn themselves in Vietnam protests, American scientists marveled that mental training could so thoroughly sever the link between body and mind and between stimulus and perception. A science writer remarked on the "serenity" in their faces, asking, "Do they not feel the pain, or is their control so extraordinary that they can freeze their facial muscles into a mask of nonexpression?" In a context of war and social turmoil, the question ("How much pain can you stand?") had no objective answers.[20] How people handled their own pain, whether they faced discomfort with grim determination or with cries of anguish, protestation, and demands for relief—these matters wove hardship and tolerance seamlessly into pressing discussions of the era about protest, groups' rights, and social recognition.

Somewhere between the spectacular and the mundane, "new" pain syndromes migrated into popular discussion shaping and reflecting the sensibilities of the 1960s. Readers of the *Chicago Defender* in 1962, for example, were asked to consider the case of a boy named Calvin who suffered from sickle cell disease, an African American ailment defined by "recurring joint pains" that carried its own powerful political meanings. For fourteen years, Calvin carried his burden of recurring pain, then his ailment deepened, and he finally succumbed to it. By the mid-1960s, news of the condition had spread beyond medical journals or the black press. Sufferers with this "common Negro disease" had become symbols of a change in perception—their plight was covered in the mainstream media and turned into a broader plea for racial recognition, intersubjective understanding, and pain relief. "Nor is 'suffer' too strong a term for what victims of sickle cell anemia go through during a crisis of the disease," noted the *New York Times* in 1965. With widening reports, the pain of this chronic disease became a metaphor tied to social recognition and political appeals for urgent relief. Sickle cell was only one example of "new" syndromes and disorders that became political in a cultural sense, linking clinical pain to the civic ideals and demands of African Americans. It was a public anguish calling not only for sympathy but also for the creation of new institutions (in health care and in government) where relief and compassionate care might take center stage.[21]

As a symbol of pain honestly felt, seeking true relief, Rosie Page was supported by and supported in turn what seemed like a legion of sufferers. A truly open society should be compassionate to their needs. Their subjective pains were real pains; their private ailing was now understood as social suffering. Public anguish appeared in a bewildering variety of forms—housewives, working men and women, athletes, African Americans with apparently "race-specific" complaints like sickle cell disease, and disabled warriors (from the Korean conflict and, after 1965, from Vietnam). Most notable of all was arthritis, which commanded a great deal of attention and provoked contradictory theories about another group, the elderly, and about the gates of relief and the capacity of a prosperous, liberal society to care for its people.[22]

Arthritis and the Expanding Government of Relief

The most prominent of the newly visible pain syndromes was arthritis, an ailment that cut a wide and worrisome swath through society. By mid-decade, it starkly illuminated the government's pain relief challenge. Not just a disease of aging, arthritis affected children, athletes, and poor people as well. The Los Angeles Dodgers star pitcher Sandy Koufax had "the most famous arthritic elbow in sports history," receiving almost daily cortisone injections. When the illness forced his retirement in 1966, arthritis solidified its role as disability threat to the ablest of men. Former president Eisenhower (still an avid golfer) had it in his wrist. It was also diagnosed among children; the poor were said to suffer disproportionately. As the *New York Times* informed its readers in 1965 and as health officials warned, arthritis was a multifaceted crippler. As the *Times* put it, "Arthritis cripples more persons in low-income families than in other groups . . .

of the 13 million Americans with Arthritis, 50,000 were school-age or preschool children."[23]

Despite arthritis's ability to cut across the life course, its impact on the elderly commanded special public concern in the early 1960s. The ailment illuminated a growing demographic challenge (the care of the elderly), and it framed the middecade debate about society's commitment to the aged. As this kind of pain rose to prominence among all the others, it called on government to act, even as the private sector (particularly the booming pharmaceutical economy) also promised relief. Both versions promised compassionate fast relief. At the same time, both stood accused of a deceitful fraud.

Advocates of social insurance for the elderly (emboldened by the election of President Kennedy in 1960) saw the elderly arthritic sufferer— alone and vulnerable to exploitation—as the strongest case for continued health-care reform. In their name, liberal Democrats pushed Eisenhower's disability relief to new levels. The political maneuvering that ultimately produced Medicare and Medicaid legislation in 1965, with its health coverage for people over age sixty-five and for people living in poverty, preserved this image of arthritis. As Democrats pressed for reform in the early 1960s, frequent congressional hearings highlighted how the elderly with arthritis were viciously victimized by both pain and by health quackery. As the chair of the Senate Special Committee on Aging stated in January 1963 hearings, in the "era of the hard sell . . . the senior citizen is particularly vulnerable to the spiel of the pitchman. When he is ailing and in pain . . . he will listen to a glib promoter who has 'the sure cure' for arthritis . . . The young have time to recoup from financial folly . . . The results of fraud upon the elderly are particularly tragic."[24] Lacking health insurance (and often uninsurable), older Americans tended also to be poorer and were thus the primary face of health vulnerability.

While new programs like Medicare and Medicaid absolutely expanded the scale of government's concern about elderly pain, other initiatives of the era focused on preventing pain-relief fraud. Liberal concern about pain fraud in this era extended to the predatory danger of marketed relief and thus focused on the private sector and the need to protect vulnerable citizens. The challenge of pain relief was multilayered. Midway through the decade, the U.S. surgeon general labeled arthritis "a billion dollar crippler"—doing damage on two fronts, first because of lost work hours and second by turning these productive citizens into disabled dependents of the state. Furthermore, such problems of disability and poverty were intimately intertwined, as two legal analysts observed: "Not all who are poor are physically handicapped, and not all who are handicapped are poor. But the two conditions—poverty and disability—are historically so intermeshed as to be often indistinguishable," explained Floyd Matson and Jacobus tenBroek. For some other experts, echoing the conservative critique, it was the specter of fraud perpetrated *by* the complainant, not *upon* him, that warranted attention. For such critics, the person with arthritis had underlying psychological problems—repressed hostility, poor social adjustment, and obsessive-compulsive character. But for Democratic legislators pushing for Medicare legislation in 1964 and 1965, the fraud of deepest political concern was the more heinous problem of hucksters and drug marketers promising fast relief and preying on poor, gullible older Americans. For those involved in the government of pain relief, arthritis sufferers constituted both a multimillion dollar drug market—and also a problem keeping regulators on their toes alerting "the public to what was termed 'the $250,000,000 racket in misrepresented drugs and products for arthritis.' "[25]

The worry over pain-relief fraud originated in the era's relentless and wide-ranging drug innovation—with the pharmaceutical industry boom in drugs provoking a good deal of regulatory worry. Americans' reprieve from the 1962 thalidomide scandal highlighted the wisdom of robust regulation; in that case, a drug promising nausea relief for pregnant women instead caused thousands of birth defects in Europe but not in the United States, where the drug had not been approved by the Food and Drug Administration (FDA). Still, the existing FDA regulations required only that drug manufacturers demonstrate safety, not that drugs—for pain or anything else—be effective. With the government now in the business of acknowledging pain and regulating on the basis of drug effects, distinguishing between legitimate pain relievers and fraudulent remedies was a new problem for regulators, not just for consumers. A wide range of products from large and small drug houses (such as Liefcort, chloroquine, dipyrone, dimethyl sulfoxide (DMSO), and indo-methacin) sat on the fringes of the legitimate market.[26] The market itself was unsteady. As the *New York Times* reported in 1966, of the thirteen drug companies that had sold "dipyrone under various trade names as a pain killer and antirheumatic drug," most had left the market by late 1964 when the FDA reported on the drug's side effects. Complicating the situation and turning the tables on government as protector, a subset of users desperate for relief were leaving the U.S. to find the drug elsewhere; their supporters now warned that government regulation (in the name of protecting the public's health) was actually keeping wonder drugs out of the hands of those who needed relief the most.[27] This burgeoning market, with its capacity for both relief and exploitation, kept federal agencies busy, kept lawyers active, and pulled consumers in multiple directions. As Daniel Carpenter has noted, these controversies slowly strengthened the hand of government regulation. A year could not pass in the 1960s without either FDA warnings or Federal Trade Commission (FTC) threats to pain relief hucksters for misleading advertisements.

How should the expanding government police a society and a marketplace increasingly drawn to drug therapy? Rosie Page, herself an arthritis sufferer, had depended on tranquilizers—one of the blockbuster relievers of the 1950s, but one increasingly deemed "habit forming." By the time she approached the government for disability support, skepticism had grown—driven by new studies on their habit-forming potential. Tranquilizer sales were declining under withering scrutiny by Congress and regulators. A 1963 presidential advisory commission characterized them as a "psychotoxic" and fostering dependence, and agencies like the FDA sought to balance oversight with ensuring that innovative drugs produced true relief. As the age of tranquilizers waned, new products (arguably less prone to producing dependence) would emerge to fill the market void. As arthritis sufferers like Page looked to a liberal government for relief and protection, then, pain relief stood as a complex management dilemma in what Philip Rieff would characterize as a "therapeutic society."[28]

DMSO became a textbook example of the promise and peril of the drug economy and of the double-edge challenge of liberal government—to provide aggressive, vigilant regulatory oversight while not standing in the way of valued relief. Was DMSO an exploiter of people in pain, or was this new drug the answer to their prayers? In the mid-1960s, the answer hinged on one's interests and what one thought about the therapeutic state. In February 1965, the media had first hailed DMSO as a miracle drug in reports that often blurred the line between advertising and journalism. Reports proclaimed, "It kills pain, speeds wound healing, reduces inflammation, clears up bruises, serves as a tranquilizer, relieves certain . . . allergies, relaxes muscles . . . and relieves certain types of arthritis." Under the drug's influence, people with bursitis, arthritis, burn pains, and intractable aches reported feeling better; their problems completely disappeared. If pain disability was a growing threat, here was a promising antidote.[29]

Within two months, even as drug maker Crown Zellerbach was expanding DMSO production to meet the growing demand, the popular press changed its tune—now expressing the need for caution and reassessment. It may be "the nearest thing to a wonder drug the nineteen sixties have produced," noted one author, but "more and more people are obtaining some and using it on themselves without medical supervision," and they could be "inviting disastrous consequences worse than their present ailments." What had been a story of a drug's triumph over pain in the market of relief now became, in some eyes, a story of government's failure in policing people and products. In Congress, congressional representative L. H. Fountain voiced his suspicion that the drug houses and their marketers had gained undue influence not only over prescribers and patients but also over regulators. The FDA had approved the drug, even as Fountain and his subcommittee questioned the drug's effectiveness and claimed that many researchers had tested the drug in a willfully illegal and dangerous fashion, endangering the lives of patients.[30]

What society and government seemed to need—at the FDA, at the FTC, in Congress, in medicine, and in the legal world—was more pain managers who could tell the difference between miracle relief and malicious exploitation, who could sort true relief from fraud. Also needed were more pain experts, better theories, stronger evidence on drug effects, and more robust methods for assessing subjective pain and relief. What made the DMSO case especially vexing were the fierce and competing subjective claims—many arthritis sufferers swore that the drug had brought lasting relief to their pain. Meanwhile, the fickle media continued to report on new studies showing serious side effects in laboratory animals and human deaths linked to DMSO. Perhaps, one author now speculated, the popular feel-good wonder drug was "not as wonderful as advertised."[31]

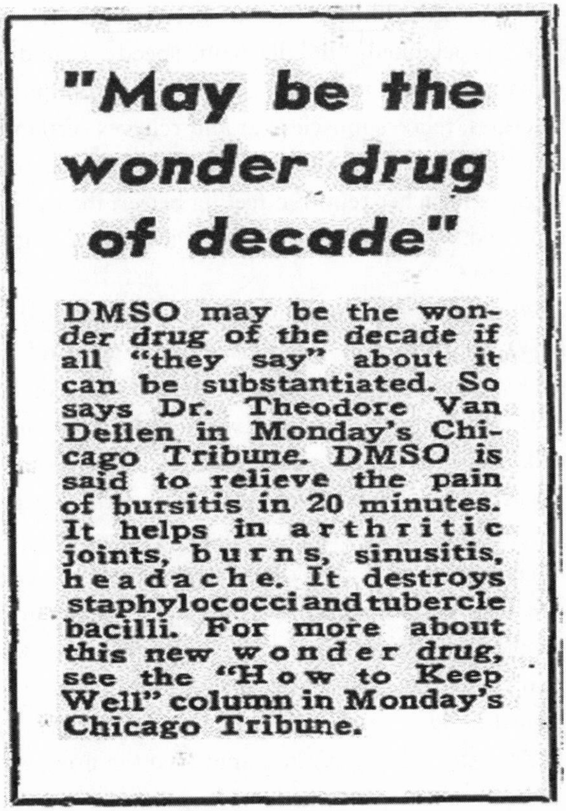

> ## "May be the wonder drug of decade"
>
> DMSO may be the wonder drug of the decade if all "they say" about it can be substantiated. So says Dr. Theodore Van Dellen in Monday's Chicago Tribune. DMSO is said to relieve the pain of bursitis in 20 minutes. It helps in arthritic joints, burns, sinusitis, headache. It destroys staphylococci and tubercle bacilli. For more about this new wonder drug, see the "How to Keep Well" column in Monday's Chicago Tribune.

FIGURE 2.1.   An advertisement touting the "miracle" of DMSO, appearing at the high point of the controversial drug's popular and medical allure.

Chicago Tribune, May 3, 1964, B3.

Relief from the pain of arthritis careened between these political polarities in President Johnson's administration—between calls for growing FDA surveillance of the shady business of relief and defensiveness from a growing government that regulation would not stand in the way of true remedies. FDA official Frances Kelsey, the heroine whose refusal to endorse thalidomide had prevented the drug from entering the American marketplace, took charge of the FDA effort to police suspicious drug claims. By mid-1966 the DMSO drug maker fell under heavy scrutiny, with Congress launching hearings investigating the drug's claims as well as the approval process. After a thorough investigation of DMSO, the

FDA decided in 1966 on a cautious "sensible resumption of controlled experimentation"—allowing researchers who understood the perils to resume testing the drug under strict controls.[32]

DMSO remained in therapeutic limbo—it was not on the market nor available to prescribers nor was it entirely banned. Pushback from industry and researchers was inevitable; from 1966 onward regulators took a defensive posture. Some clinicians praised the drug's power as an alternative to surgery and narcotics. As one researcher noted in 1967, "I practically discarded physical therapy as treatment for acute musculo-skeletal problems, because the rehabilitation of my patients was so prompt." DMSO was every bit the miracle that marketers promised, he said. "There was little or no necessity to prescribe narcotics and tranquilizers, since pain was promptly mitigated following topical application."[33] As an alternative to stigmatized habit-forming painkillers, DMSO had a clear if controversial appeal.

The field known as "pain management" was also in limbo, maturing in this contentious political environment; it is important, therefore, that we see the field not as a medical invention but as a social and political one. Pain management, broadly defined, would henceforth involve negotiating between these competing ideologies of relief and working with the interest groups—physicians, patients, soldiers, police, legislators, and so on—with their own stakes in relief. With DMSO now out of reach and manufacturers and some lawmakers now complaining that it was a "persecuted drug," the FDA was under pressure from patients and some legislators to reapprove the drug in full. Kelsey and others resisted. The stand-off continued through the late 1960s and into the early 1970s. Advocates heralded its power to relieve. Skeptics pointed to its well-established toxicity. The DMSO controversy strengthened the hand of government, but it also encouraged opponents of regulation to portray government as the impediment to relief, not a true solution to people's pain. In their view, the drug was a victim of misunderstanding and persecution—a casualty of an era of expanding, overcautious government.[34]

Government was also in therapeutic limbo, for increased regulation of such substances as DMSO, LSD, and even the birth control pill exposed the gnawing question at the heart of liberal society in the mid-1960s—in a truly "free" society, could government simultaneously protect people afflicted by pain while also being an agent of their self-determination? Was such a balance politically possible? Even more vexing, new social movements pressured regulators as young people's embrace of LSD and marijuana as recreational rebellion and free expression posed new regulatory challenges. Alongside the political Right's distrust of government came another current: a potent libertarian strain from the political Left that also saw regulation as the enemy of freedom. Decisions like the Supreme Court's 1965 *Griswold v. Connecticut*, with the court striking down the state's right to restrict married women's access to birth control, cast the government as an impediment to personal freedom. This argument gathered force not only in industry, among doctors, and youthful protesters but also among people who simply wanted their DMSO.[35]

Radicalizing Relief

That pain management should become a subspecialty in medicine owes much to the contentious questions of suffering, disability, entitlement, and relief swirling around people like Rosie Page. Tort law had long hinged on pain and suffering, but now when people claimed disabling pain or when they sued drug makers claiming to have been harmed by a painkiller's side effects, it was men like John Bonica, the Seattle pain doctor, who were called to give expert testimony about the risks, benefits, and harms. No pain specialist in this era could be merely a clinician, for their insights were crucial in legal and policy disputes over disability, personal injury, and product liability. Bonica's task expanded to include judging true and feigned pain, evaluating a drug's efficacy and its habit-forming potential, judging manufacturers' claims and their products, and helping governments to navigate these expanding problems of relief.[36] Pain experts were gatekeepers to relief in a broad sense.

By the early 1960s, having put out a new edition of his authoritative textbook on pain management, Bonica was leading the anesthesiology program at the University of Washington in Seattle. By 1963, his clinic was becoming recognized nationally as a place where people in pain received a fair hearing. He was said to tackle tough problems that baffled most others specialists. Like the sociologist Kenneth Zola and many others who studied pain, he carried his own burden of pain—in his case because of musculoskeletal injuries earned in his earlier days as a professional wrestler. Bonica carried this burden with grim toughness—as one colleague noted, "We watched him grapple with his pain every day, wrestling it to the mat whenever he had a lecture commitment or a deadline."[37]

A 1963 *Time* magazine profile recounted the route one tortured woman traveled to Bonica's Seattle unit. Like Rosie Page, she had been labeled "hysterical," but in Seattle she found a measure of validation. Her problem had started after a traumatic surgery: "The operation for breast cancer appeared to have been successful, but the patient developed unbearable pain in her right arm. Some of the many doctors she consulted were convinced that her cancer must have recurred—but they could not find it. Others blamed her pain on an emotional ("hysterical") reaction— but they could not help her either." *Time* used her story to suggest that more experts should follow Bonica's model of careful deliberation. His clinic balanced an interest in anatomy with a concern for pain perception and psychology. Neither drugs nor surgery nor psychiatry alone could be the answer. Such cases stood as a "reminder that finding an effective treatment for pain can become one of the most difficult problems of medicine." His multidisciplinary center just getting off the ground, Bonica was said to be asking questions "that many more medical men should be asking themselves."[38] Most important, it seemed that Bonica did not blame and stigmatize, and, as such, his multidisciplinary clinic became a welcome port in the storm.

In this context, the political salience of pain theory grew and tilted toward liberalization. Such a controversial field needed stabilizing theories—not the harshly judgmental concepts of malingering so dominant in the 1950s but new theories that were flexible enough to suit the pain challenges of the times. From the mid-1960s to the early 1970s, a new concept, gate control theory, arose to support the liberalization of the new field. Gate control reinforced many of the tendencies of the era— suggesting, for example, that Rosie Page, Judge John Brown, Henry Beecher, and John Bonica were right to see felt, subjective pain as true pain. The gate control theory was "riding in on the Zeitgeist," one of its inventors, Ronald Melzack, later observed.[39] But in reality the uptake of gate control owed less to a "cultural spirit" whisking ideas along and much more to the fact that the theory resonated on multiple levels with the era's legal battles, cultural critiques, pain relief practices, and liberalizing political commitments.

The revolution in theory began quietly when, in the early 1960s, Canadian-born psychologist Ronald Melzack and English physiologist Patrick Wall invented the gate control concept. Neither man had ever been involved in patient care—they were outsiders to the medical establishment. Both were critics not only of pain medicine's dependence on surgery and drugs but also of pain science and its narrow anatomical bias. At the time, the most preferred medical explanation held to a Cartesian model of pain as something that traveled via nerve impulses to the brain. Melzack and Wall brusquely dismissed this understanding in 1961: "Pain is not a fixed response to a hurtful stimulus. Its perception is modified by our past experiences, our expectations and, more subtly by our culture . . . Pain, we now believe, refers to a category of complex experiences, not to a single sensation produced by a specific stimulus." They dismissed "the concept of a 'pain center' in the brain" as "pure fiction." Not only were multiple parts of the brain associated with pain perception, they argued, but other qualities of the person (mood, psychological state, history, and context) could modify those perceptions.[40]

Borrowing the motif of feedback, information processing, and cybernetics from their colleagues in computer science at MIT, Melzack and Wall's theory offered a new approach informed by a view of the person in pain as a complex processor of information.[41] A great deal of evidence questioned the notion that there was a specific pain pathway or a "pain cell" in the brain—they called this model "specificity theory." If this model was correct, how could researchers explain phantom limb pain, for example? Another theory (so-called pattern theory) suggested that there were no specific pain transmitting fibers, because "all fiber endings . . . are alike, so that the pattern for pain is produced by intense stimulation of nonspecific receptors." As Melzack and Wall saw it, both theories failed to account for such mysteries as phantom pain, placebo relief, and variations in pain perception.[42] The idea in gate control theory that electrical-style gates could close to complete circuits and transmit pain impulse but that those gates could be controlled by multiple means was scientifically vague yet culturally appealing. The theory offered no specificity about actual mechanisms operating these gates in any one person. But that was never the point; everyone's gates operated according to a different logic.

Melzack became the theory's chief entrepreneur as well as an effective critic of the dominance of surgery, psychiatry, and drugs in pain relief. Lobotomy, psychiatry, and drugs were, of course, under attack from other liberal elements that cast medical authority as a form of social control. Melzack believed that these fields dominated as pain relief methods by historical accident, merely because they happened to be well-positioned specialties after the Second World War, just at the moment when pain assumed greater importance in society. Surgeons and drug specialists had seized pain as their own, but the care of pain patients did not belong to them inherently. These accidents of history need not be permanent; "if we can recover from historical accident, these [alternative] methods deserve more attention than they have received." Doctors, pain practitioners, scientists, and others needed to open their minds to unconventional approaches to therapy. This was the cultural work that gate control theory would do.[43] This was no mere theory in the narrow sense but a sociological critique of entrenched power and practice. Pain management was being controlled by economic interests, critics contended. Surgeons, drug companies, and psychiatrists circled around the pain complainant, ready with costly drugs and harmful neurosurgery when other methods would do. If this was the pain economy, Melzack and Wall were not part of it; they had no ties to the pharmaceutical industry, they had no professional interest in being pain managers themselves. In the context of the 1960s, one could see how their arguments might be received as fresh, disinterested, objective, and revolutionary.

Where was the line, then, between true and false complaints? Who could judge the suffering of another? When was extraordinary relief necessary? These questions gathered political force in the 1960s. Asked aggressively, insistently, and skeptically, they amounted to a critique of established medical and of social norms. So while doctors like Robert Shaw of Harvard would decry "pathological malingering" as an evil of the times, the disease "a product of social welfare," other doctors embraced the spirit of liberalism. In Shaw's formulation, even obviously feigned pain (motivated by a person's effort to obtain secondary gains such as disability benefits), could be designated as a legitimate, albeit psychological, disease—"pathologic malingering." But as Shaw himself noted, the doctor's very skepticism of the "sufferer" and his confrontational attitude could

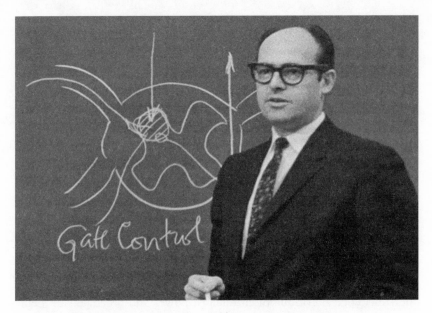

FIGURE 2.2.   Psychologist and pain theorist Ronald Melzack, speaking on gate control theory in a 1965 film, "The Puzzle of Pain."

Image courtesy of National Film Board of Canada.

sometimes make matters worse.[44] This thinking adapted for new times ideas about the personality and psyche of the pain complainant from a decade earlier. But now other physicians, pointing to the work of Melzack and others, contended that pain, all pain, was not a product of indulgence but a response to social oppression and ought to be taken more seriously and relieved.

Already, by the mid-1960s, this new thinking was having a modest impact, which expanded as more and more people cited gate control theory as justification for unconventional thinking and experimentation in relief. Gate control theory offered a new cadre of pain managers a framework for managing the growing diversity of pain complaints, as sufferers navigated the fine line between social sympathy and scorn. Because gate control theory was inclusive, it pushed the managers of relief like Bonica to liberalize their methods. It moved pain managers to consider radical and so-called "alternative" remedies—opening their minds to hypnosis, mind cures, and placebos. In an atmosphere of innovation and social experimentation, the drive toward therapeutic diversity was unavoidable. As one observer later noted, this "more complex view of the pain phenomenon logically opens the way for a much more diversified attack on pain than was formerly customary."[45] This radical idea pushed liberal medicine and liberal law to expand their horizons; even the most far-reaching avenues of relief needed to be explored.

By 1968 (a year wracked by war, protest, race riots, political assassinations, and social turmoil), pain managers across government, law, and medicine grappled openly with pain's many and intersecting complexities. On the heated questions of disability and government, as one scholar noted in 1967, "The three problems which have recently given the courts the great difficulty . . . are 1) the shift of the burden of proof to the Secretary . . . [pressed to prove why any given plaintiff should be ruled ineligible]; 2) the role of pain in disability [following the *Page* precedent]; and 3) the place of so-called personality disorders in the disability scheme." Seeking to call public and professional attention to pain, in 1968 the National Institute of General Medical Sciences threw its resources behind a new film, *Threshold*. Over the next few years, sixteen million viewers saw the award-winning production on television. The film also introduced thousands of dentists, doctors, nurses, and civic groups to the issues now swirling around this controversial field.[46] The profile of pain managers and theorists (Bonica, Melzack, and others) continued to rise, along with the argument for continued liberalization.

By the end of the decade, liberal pain theory opened the way to new forms of cultural understanding bordering on cultural relativism in relief; nothing better captures this trend than Mark Zborowski's 1969 book, *People in Pain*. Zborowski studied Italian, Jewish, Irish, and so-called Old American (Anglo-American) men in a Bronx, New York, veterans hospital and concluded that "cultural relativity, which allows for the acceptance of a pattern of behavior in one group and its rejection in another, is also expressed in attitudes toward pain." What was important to Zborowski, an anthropology student working with luminaries like Ruth Benedict and Margaret Mead, was that these men's cultural identities shaped their perceptions and experiences of pain. He anchored his claims about his subjects by leaning on the insights of Bonica and Beecher and critics of medical authority like Thomas Szasz, who portrayed psychiatric diagnosis as a form of social control. His subjects were men,

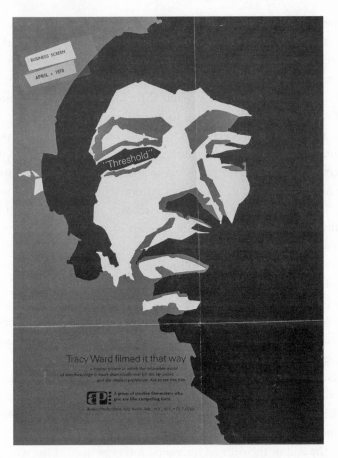

FIGURE 2.3.   Advertisement in *Business Screen* for the widely seen 1968 film *Threshold*, produced by Tracy Ward for the National Institute for General Medical Sciences.

Image courtesy of History and Special Collections for the Sciences, UCLA Library Special Collections.

and he understood that gender norms shaped how and whether they behaved. "Behavior that is appropriate for women or children may be unbecoming for men. According to contemporary norms, soldiers should not cry, but the Greek heroes of the Trojan War shed tears without shame or guilt."[47] For ethnic men, pain meant different things; their pain behavior, Zborowski contended, reflected deeply internalized cultural values and ethnic affects.

Culture, not science, defined what pain meant, who was considered the ideal pain patient, and how he or she would be treated; this was the bold political contention. Zborowski's core proposition was that Jews, Irish, Italians, and Anglo-Americans responded to pain differently, drawing on cultural norms and experiences—the Anglo-American's rational asceticism and trust in expertise, the Jewish veteran's "preoccupation with the symptomatic meaning of pain" and his lack of "anxiety-relieving devices," and so on. Like the sociologist Irving Zola years earlier, Zborowski examined these responses to pain in light of the "transmission of cultural values and norms within society" and "the diversity and relativity of cultural patterns." The danger of Zborowski's analysis was that cultural relativism could blur into outright ethnic typecasting, sometimes becoming one and the same. The Jewish veterans were complainers, made frequent demands on others about their pain; they were also suspicious of doctors. For Zborowski (himself Jewish, having published previously on the Russian shtetl), this understanding should lead not to stereotyping but to sensitivity; ethnicity was a fixed category of identity and a useful framework for understanding and responding to society's diverse pain-relief needs:

> Like the Jewish patient, the Italian patient is often described as a person who makes no effort to control his emotional reactions to pain, who demands attention, and who freely expresses his pain by sound and gesture. On the whole, the behavior of the Italian patients is seen as nonconforming to the standards of the hospital, which emphasizes restraint and self-control. However, in speaking about the Italian patients, members of the hospital staff frequently mention a number of their positive character traits, such as personal warmth, congeniality, and good humor.

Italians were therefore trusting but vocal but also present-oriented—so that when pain diminished they ceased complaining. The Irish veterans, by contrast, tended to ignore pain to such an extent that it did not seem to exist. Like Jews, they were also highly suspicious. The "Old American" was the most stoic and rationalizing of the lot, insisting "that he does not want sympathy or attention, but merely the opportunity to show his working potentialities . . . [He] is the ideal patient, a model used as an example not only by the people who are directly involved in relieving his condition, but also by members of other groups who, although they are also Americans, do not have the adjective old included in their national identification."[48]

The very idea that pain, first and foremost, was culturally defined was disconcerting for any pain manager who believed there should be objective professional guidelines for relief, but the cultural move reflected so much about the era's tensions, as political movements along lines of race, gender, and sexual identity confronted medicine and its norms.[49] As Zborowski noted, "Members of the medical profession are reluctant to differentiate patients according to religion, race, or nationality . . . Therefore, it is not surprising that a number of doctors at first expressed strong disapproval when asked about ethnic differences in response to pain. Some even implied a racist character of the research." The very idea of ethnic pain put doctors ill at ease. Only after Zborowski convinced them that the research did not "threaten their professional and moral integrity" did some cooperate. Then, "many offered information that reflected . . . actual impressions formed during medical practice among the multinational and multicultural population of New York City."[50]

In time, Zborowski's book (standing alongside gate control theory) would become an important support in the pain field's and society's grappling with cultural difference. Attention to culture in health behavior exposed a deep contradiction. On one hand, the book called for cultural sensitivity in medicine and for physicians to pay attention to cultural differences when assessing pain and bringing relief. On the other hand, the book was also a crude work of cultural stereotyping— casting patients as familiar ethnic stereotypes (complaining Jews, stoic Anglo-Americans). In this sense, the book reflects much about the conundrum of how to read pain into culture and culture into pain. *People in Pain* also revealed the forces of cultural relativism pushing American society in new directions and informing these questions of ethnicity, identity, compassion, and relief as the 1960s came to a close. Judging pain was never more complex, for the question of who was in pain now took pain managers deep into the psyche and into the complexities of cultural difference.

If pain was cultural, then what could this mean for relief? By the end of the decade, sufferers and pain managers both saw the radical subjectivity of pain as an open invitation to explore ever more unconventional relief methods—from saline injections into the spinal column to dorsal column stimulation to LSD and acupuncture. The gateways to relief were now swung wide open. Looking back from 1970, John Bonica reflected that the gate control concept was "appealing because it helps explain certain peculiar phenomena of pain." Gate control theory had energized his field. The theory endorsed diversity—welcoming alternative medicines, legitimizing emotions and feelings, and pushing the patient's consciousness into the foreground of legitimate medical and legal discussion.[51]

By the early 1970s, gate control had become a metaphor for an era rich with new therapeutic and political possibilities. It encouraged speculation and individualized relief, from drugs to surgery to hypnosis to many other ways of manipulating the mind and soothing the body. Even those concerned about the hippie-related menace of LSD noted that, among that drug's "bona fide medical uses and benefits . . . , it has been used as a 'death therapy' to help dying people face the end more serenely and with less pain." In its vagueness about what or who controlled the pain gateways, the theory endorsed a laissez-faire, even libertarian, approach to relief. Conventional science seemed unsuited to the task of truly understanding and judging pain. As a Boston psychiatrist concluded in 1971, "In evaluating chronic pain, a search for evidence that pain exists is fruitless and irrelevant." With multiple pathways now posited—neurosurgery, drugs, hypnosis, psychotherapy, and even the use of electrical stimulus—to "switch off" pain—an era of social and therapeutic diversity was at hand.[52]

Like many who had been in the pain field for decades, the British neurology researcher P. W. Nathan was deeply ambivalent about the theory that awakened his sleeping field. An elder statesman in pain research, he scoffed at the theory's unconventional path to popularity, swept into fashion it seemed by the cultural currents of the time. Resting on almost no experimental foundations, the gate control model had an appeal that ran far ahead of the flimsiness of any scientific, clinical, and laboratory findings. Yet Nathan gave gate control theory his begrudging support because, despite its many failings, it had encouraged new pain interventions. The theory *worked*, in a manner of speaking, because it had opened up the field to experimentation that had been wildly productive for pain medicine. "Although the theory has led to the successful treatment of chronic pain, this does not mean that it is correct," he noted wisely. "Ideas need to be fruitful, they do not have to be right. And curiously enough, the two do not necessarily go together."[53] Fruitful it was. Buoyed by the theory, new practices in pain management flourished—the multidisciplinary pain clinic, the idea of patients controlling their own analgesia dosage, and even the rise of alternative relief like hypnosis, acupuncture, and electrical stimulation.

Pain theory had become political, even revolutionary, in several new ways—by challenging professional norms and authority, by encompassing social and cultural suffering more broadly, and by welcoming alternatives and experimentation. Methadone for relief of heroin addiction was one contentious incarnation of this liberal broadening of relief. In 1967, the pain of withdrawal from methadone was seen as far less severe than withdrawal from heroin or morphine—adding to the drug's valorization as an answer the urban heroin crisis. By the early 1970s, critics on the left and right contended that methadone was not a true salve. Commenters on the left argued that the problem of pain ran deeper in society, for addiction itself was a "reaction to the excessive pain of social and economic deprivation . . . anesthetiz[ing] the individual against pain," which methadone could not erase. On the right, methadone as pain relief seemed a charade—substituting one form of addiction for another. So where methadone's advocates continued to argue that the drug provided needed relief from the craving for heroin (without the euphoric high of heroin), detractors saw methadone abuse as a new and growing problem; for them, this liberal therapeutic solution to pain had now become a problem in itself.[54]

By the early 1970s, established pain managers like John Bonica admitted that true expertise on this disputatious topic, pain, did not exist. Speaking in a 1970 CBS television broadcast, "The Mystery of Pain," he admitted that "the response of the individual [to pain] depends on a great variety of factors." Pain response was "influenced by age, by sex, by culture, by ethnic background. It is also greatly influenced by what the pain means to the individual—is it a bad omen, or is it something not so bad." Pain, he noted, was so intimately tied to culture and personality that no scientist could speak on pain better than those who experienced it.[55] Yet, as they watched this radical cultural turn in theory and relief unfold, pain managers grew worried that they might be losing the professional control they had worked so hard to build. Had society become too expansive in its endorsement of liberal relief? Had the gates swung open too wide?

Acupuncture and the Lure of the East

For the pain judges and managers standing watch at the gates of relief, the frustrations of the early 1970s were many. It was one thing to open one's mind to subjective pain as real pain, but it was quite another matter to open the way for all forms of pain (even cultural pain) and all forms of relief stretching beyond the bounds of their professional control. John Bonica's own openness would be pushed to the brink by global events in 1972 when, in the wake of President Nixon's surprise visit to China, acupuncture became a new American fascination. As one news report put it, "Nothing in the American rediscovery of China has excited the popular imagination more than acupuncture anesthesia."[56] For pain professionals, it raised many questions—most importantly about how Western medical expertise and the now established field of pain medicine would respond to this wisdom from the East. Eight years after Robert Kennedy's observations on the unknowable nature of black pain for white Americans, Nixon's trip framed another cross-cultural question: Could Americans understand Chinese pain and incorporate its system of relief?

The détente between President Richard Nixon—who had built his career on anti-Communism since the 1950s—and Chairman Mao Tse-Tung sent ripples across American medicine. The curious case of journalist James Reston, who was part of an advance team before Nixon's visit, put Chinese medical practices in an unexpected spotlight. The journalist developed appendicitis and needed immediate care. Reston's appendectomy was unremarkable, done using conventional Western sedation. Afterwards, however, his postsurgical pain was successfully treated with acupuncture therapy. The case personalized the encounter between American and Chinese cultures. Asked to comment on this new development in pain care, American specialists enjoyed the attention. For many, acupuncture's apparent effectiveness confirmed the wisdom of the gate control theory and its liberalizing influence on medicine. Gate control helped "explain (and legitimate) acupuncture, which most Western physicians had dismissed as a clever trick of autosuggestion."[57] Speaking on such issues, Bonica's status rose; he was now discussed as a founding father of the field. Melzack's stature as a visionary rose as well.

Acupuncture was at once politically fascinating, culturally appealing, and professionally challenging—it was, in short, a quintessential "alternative" to American pain management. It quickly became a cultural symbol in the United States, a reference point in the political conversation on China policy. For those on the left or moderate right preaching a new openness to the Communist East, the method suggested the possibility of an intellectual détente. It embodied a hope. By bridging the East-West divide on the level of pain care, perhaps this ancient, long-hidden knowledge concealed within a secretive Maoist regime might emerge to enlighten the West and the world. This was certainly Mao's agenda. In the United States, acupuncture satisfied another need—a continuing hope for unorthodox, "alternative" breakthroughs in relief that meshed neatly with countercultural, New Age, and "hippie" ideals. As with other forms of disputed relief (methadone, DMSO, and so on), here too the hope for relief married both clinical and political ideals.

Acupuncture—suddenly in great demand by relief-oriented Americans—nevertheless posed a professional challenge for the cadre of pain managers who had defined the field in Bonica's time. Few of these experts had any familiarity with the needle technique, but their patients pressured them to have an opinion on it in a hurry. The letter that Bonica received from a woman named Eileen Mullan, writing from Florida in 1973, was typical. She had tried everything available in the United States to relieve the "terrible affliction" on one side of her head, to no avail: "After years of injections, nerve resections, morphine, electric shock treatments, etc., etc., I finally received some relief. Now I am starting [to experience] the symptoms on the other side of my face and acupuncture has been suggested, the question is, where do I find a qualified acupuncture practitioner? ... I am appealing to you, if it is possible, to recommend someone ... My thoracic surgeon ... does not know anyone." A few months after Nixon's trip, a colleague in Florida wrote to Bonica for help with the rising demand from frustrated patients: "Dear John: I am literally being flooded with requests for referrals of patients to acupuncture centers ... Regrettably, I know of very few physicians who are currently involved in acupuncture. Do you have any information that I can use . . . qualified physicians to whom I can refer patients?" The need for information on the practice was clear to Bonica and the entire medical profession. New regulatory issues had suddenly appeared. What standards should be used to determine whether acupuncture worked or whether clinics would be licensed? Who would control the practice, and what would be its relationship to traditional drug-based anesthesiology? As a recognized leader in the pain field, Bonica was thrown into the public spotlight—peppered with questions of local, political, and global significance. Did the Chinese technique work? Was its popularity driven by ideology or by efficacy? Could it succeed in the United States? How could it be integrated into the American system of relief?[58] The pain expert had no ready answers.

Now a formidable leader of the field, Bonica urgently needed to understand acupuncture in practice—either to validate its effects and to incorporate it into multidisciplinary pain care or to prove that it was another type of quackery. In June 1973, he packed his bags and left for China. His mission, with several other American physicians and officials, took him to Chinese hospitals where he tape-recorded interviews with practitioners, attended operations, spoke with patients, and investigated the benefits and limits of this stereotypically Eastern mode of pain relief seeking a passport to the West.

In China, Bonica learned that pain relief was deeply intertwined with Maoist politics all the way down to the bedside. As an American on foreign soil, he saw acupuncture and pain in China in a political light and in a clinical light.[59] For him, the two were inextricably conjoined. One could not separate claims about efficacy from the political questions surrounding Eastern wisdom and truth contending for Western recognition. Attending one operation, he observed, "We were given a simple gown, mask, cap and sandals and entered and saw first the application of acupuncture on a patient who was to undergo a partial gastrectomy and subsequently a patient . . . 33 years old, who had a diagnosis of tuberculoma and was to undergo a thoracotomy and a possible lobectomy." He carefully documented the procedures: "They placed 2 needles in the paravertebral region, one about the 5th or 6th thoracic level and the other the 9th, with the incision in between. And they had another needle in the right hand focal point and another in the forearm . . . They applied electrical stimulation . . .

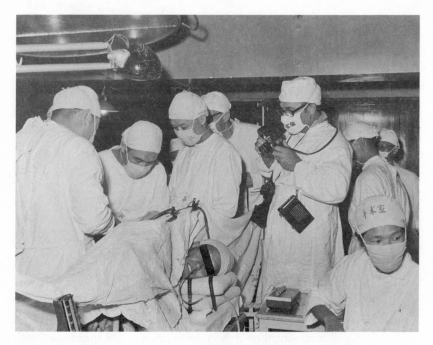

FIGURE 2.4.   John Bonica (standing with camera) documenting acupuncture procedures during his 1973 trip to China, and assessing implications for pain relief in Western medicine.

Image courtesy of History and Special Collections for the Sciences, UCLA Library Special Collections.

and after 20 minutes of this an incision was made." Bonica observed how people treated with acupuncture fared, taking pictures during the operation when allowed to do so.

Watching one alert patient closely, he noted, "Blood pressure rises . . . he showed tenseness in his face." The preparation for the procedure was elaborate. Attendants "had taught the patient how to breathe," and during the operation the "patient continued to talk with the anesthetist who frequently rubbed the center of his nose and spoke in a quiet voice." Yet what was also clear to Bonica was the oppressive weight of ideology in the operating room. When he asked the patient his opinion of acupuncture, he was surprised that "the patient undergoing the lobectomy commented that he was pleased to have the opportunity to participate in this kind of anesthesia which was only due to the progress promoted by Chairman Mao."[60]

Who could ignore this politics of pain? Obviously, pain and relief were deeply embedded in the politics of reform in Mao's China.

Of course, in the United States pain and relief were political as well—but in a way that reflected America's political tensions. Here, sympathetic commentators in the early 1970s read the success of acupuncture as an affirmation of gate control theory and alternative medical trends. As one writer in the *Los Angeles Times* put it, "The gate [control] theory says that nerve signals from the body can be 'gated' or blocked while on their way to the brain where the signals will be interpreted as pain. It is believed that the stimulation produced by acupuncture needles cause the gates to be closed, thus preventing the pain impulses from getting to the brain." Unconventional theory and alternative practice reinforced one another. Gate control theory (still untested) legitimated the practice, and the practice suggested the logic of the theory—it was a neat logic born of these times. While Western researchers agreed that acupuncture worked, there was no consensus on why or how. There were also skeptics. As one observer noted, one theory that could not be ruled out was that "acupuncture analgesia is nothing more than old-fashioned hypnotism." For adherents to gate control theory, the concept continued to show its value by mediating these clinical and political uncertainties surrounding orthodox and unorthodox relief.[61]

For Bonica (having built the pain field through the 1960s), acupuncture was also a threat, for it challenged the American pain managers' expertise and tested the field's openness to further liberalization. It also challenged Americans' openness to alternative medicine and further cultural diversity. When Bonica returned from his own China fact-finding tour, he faced an anxious public and a curious press. Fellow doctors wanted his views as well; the National Institutes of Health formed an ad hoc committee to study acupuncture's benefits, appointing Bonica as its chair. At the same time, state legislators and regulators wanted to know how they should regulate the acupuncture clinics that were popping up. In July 1973, the secretary of Health of South Dakota wrote to Bonica about the pressure he was facing to validate acupuncture in his state:

> I am certain that there will be legislation introduced into our next
> Legislative Session which will deal with acupuncture . . . If you have
> any personal thoughts on what States should do regarding the control

of Acupuncture I would appreciate them . . . I know that Nevada has taken a step which is acclaimed by some and criticized by others [to permit independent practice by acupuncturists] . . . I am not certain that states or governments should take any such action at this time. However, the popularity and the great amount of publicity which the press gives the procedure may dictate action.

Bonica responded cautiously, at first: "The NIH Ad Hoc Committee on Acupuncture which I chair is not involved in legal matters . . . My own opinion . . . is to strongly urge everyone involved in legislation that we do not adopt laws which would permit the widespread use of the technique because it will result in exploitation of the American people." Bonica's home legislature in Washington State took up the issue. The Seattle newspaper headline announced hopefully, "UW Medic Back from China with Prescription for the Future." Was acupuncture that long-awaited pain prescription?[62] If so, how should acupuncturists be licensed and regulated?

Policing now his profession's boundaries, Bonica warned that acupuncture in the wrong hands could lead to fraud and exploitation of people in pain, yet he allowed that the practice had some merits in liberalizing therapy and bringing relief. Interviewed in the Seattle newspapers, Bonica acknowledged that "the Communists have done a remarkable job of improving the health care of the nation" and that "the integration of traditional Chinese medicine, including acupuncture, with Western medicine is working." At the same time, he praised Western medicine's impact in China, adding that about "70 percent of the operations involved Western 'local' anesthesia" and "patients who submit to surgery under acupuncture are talked into it by the surgeon." But, beyond these observations, Americans wanted more from Bonica—they wanted desperately to use his observations on acupuncture to speak to broader issues. For many Americans, the procedure was an opportunity to weigh in on Chinese Communism, on the state of East-West relations, or even on the hope of erasing Cold War divisions between capitalist democracies and Communist totalitarian regimes. For Bonica, however, the politics of acupuncture hinged on its challenge to Western medicine's scientific standards: "the Chinese doctors said they are 'still experimenting'" with the technique, and he pointed to the "great lack of clinical research on the efficacy of acupuncture" in the Western literature.[63] For him, ultimately, this mysterious form of Eastern relief would have to submit to Western methods of scientific scrutiny.

For some observers defending Western standards and values, what seemed like a political infatuation with Eastern theories and practices had gone too far. The *Wall Street Journal*—well aware of the cultural politics of this Chinese invention—extracted only a political message from Bonica's findings. Seizing on his skepticism, they portrayed his lukewarm acupuncture assessment as a warning to liberal China admirers who were too easily infatuated "with China's political and economic wonders." In an article entitled "Needling the China Watchers," its editors opined that "one doctor who recently spent three weeks there reports that twirling those tiny needles isn't all it's made out to be." Eight-five percent of their surgery relied on Western medicine, protested the conservative newspaper. Acupuncture "doesn't entirely remove the pain of an operation . . . and furthermore, the Chinese are getting irritated by the way the Americans exaggerate their use of this technique." In much the same way that acupuncture's virtues were exaggerated, the editors determined that China's economic and political wonders were also exaggerated. "Who knows," they concluded, "maybe in undergoing [so-called] Chinese miracles the patients do hurt after all."[64]

The "Low Back Loser" Returns

It had only been a decade or so since Rosie Page won righteous relief. Within that span, what had begun as a story of bringing relief to her pain-laden life had blossomed into a sweeping cultural and political program of reform, professional growth, and social reinvention. When John Bonica came back from China in 1973, he returned to a liberal society prized for its openness and commitment to compassionate relief. Judge Learned Hand's dictum that all pain was not true pain was a thing of the past—a theory of pain and hardship that befit another, less forgiving time. But Hand's skepticism had not been forgotten entirely. Even in the era bringing Page, gate control theory, DMSO, Medicare, and acupuncture to the forefront of American politics, warnings about coddling, increasing dependence, the "pathological malinger," and welfare simmered—particularly among the more conservative members in the medical profession. Resentment about the era's swelling disability rolls festered. Frustration grew about the compassion-oriented therapeutic society charged with managing pain relief. By the early 1970s, the pain specialists themselves were vocalizing their concerns about hypnotism, methadone, LSD, disability, acupuncture, and other forms of "legitimate" pain relief. For critics, this excessiveness had acquired a name—that name was "liberalism." In this context, the old fear articulated by AMA doctors in the 1950s about the undeserving pain complainant as a fraud resurfaced and took center stage.

Ironically, while in China Bonica rightly interpreted the ideologically charged character of pain and relief; it was obviously a product of that nation's political turmoil. In his field notes, he described how in the early 1960s the use of acupuncture was "abandoned in some (many?) hospitals. From the guarded comments made by several prominent anesthesiologists, I conclude that this disuse was the result of failures in a significant percent of patients, probably due to improper technique." The 1960s in China, he noted, was a time of skepticism about the technique. But during the Cultural Revolution this "'negative' trend of disusing of acupuncture was considered the work of revisionists and subsequently greater emphasis was given to the development and widespread use." Acupuncture was part of Mao's program of reinvention, with purges and propaganda intended to instill faith in a particularly Chinese form of Communism and national virtue. Returning from this front, Bonica noted, "I gained the definite impression that many anesthesiologists are not so impressed by acupuncture but still extol its virtues and exaggerate the number of cases done . . . because this is in compliance with Chairman Mao's teachings and admonitions."[65]

In China, Bonica was an outsider and an ethnographer; at home, he was a professional pain manager and a spokesman for the field. The political contours and hidden agendas of relief in his own country were not as obvious to discern as in China. In his time, a strong liberalizing wind had established his professional practice, in part by blowing open the gates of relief—the 1956 disability law (SSDI), the 1963 *Page* ruling recognizing subjective pain as "real" pain, and gate control theory's validation of diversity and relief. Where there had once been no pain clinics, now there were hundreds across the country. These developments were part of the formation of a liberal American pain standard. Gate control theory underwrote the era's therapeutic diversity, paying professional dividends for doctors like Bonica.[66] Yet, there were limits to this diversity, and growing efforts to stem the liberalizing trend. Only a year before the China trip, Nixon had passed the Controlled Substances Act in 1970 declaring heroin, LSD, and marijuana to be Schedule 1 drugs—the highest form of "controlled substance," having no recognized medical utility. Regardless of what advocates and physicians might say, the law commanded that they had no role in pain control. But even as the Nixon administration declared war on heroin, it sought a middle ground on pain—endorsing, and then later noting the problems with, methadone as form of relief.

Liberal relief would win other victories in the early 1970s, further opening the gates for palliation. Most striking was the advent of on-demand analgesia and patient-controlled analgesia—the stunning notion that hospitalized patients should determine their own level of relief, rather than request relief from doctors and nurses. Its rise signaled that professionals were ceding control to patients, albeit in contained institutional settings. Patient-controlled analgesia advocates saw the simple act of putting the morphine drip into the patient's hand as the surest step to relief; it was also a political shift undermining the traditional authority of the doctor. By 1968, an apparatus Philip Sechzer invented was being used in New York, allowing patients in postoperative pain to treat themselves. As he saw it, every patient could become his or her own controlled experiment. In England at the same moment, researchers were developing a similar "self-service" concept for women in labor pain; in Palo Alto, California, other researchers developed the Demand Dropmaster; and in Canada, another apparatus for demand analgesia was being created.[67] Across these contexts, then, doctors were literally handing the power to patients, so that they might decide how to relieve their own pain. Other innovations, such as Ronald Melzack's widely used McGill Pain Questionnaire, prompted patients to speak for themselves and to describe their pain—was it radiating? spreading? cruel? annoying? terrifying?—and so on.

Skepticism about the claims of people like Page had never disappeared; it lingered and slowly spread among those frustrated with liberalized relief. Bonica's younger colleague, Stephen Brena, had become a skeptic after building a pain clinic in Atlanta. Every city, of course, had its own pain politics shaped by local views on dependency, drugs, and so on. Atlanta (home of a Democratic governor, Jimmy Carter, with eyes on the presidency) was a cauldron of urban-suburban anxieties about race and liberalism's excesses. Working in this context, Brena began writing about a new problem he called "the learned pain syndrome" and described many people at his clinic as exhibiting a kind of "learned helplessness." The concept of "learned helplessness" gave a theoretical grounding to the critique of liberal relief. In seeking to relieve the pain of others, Brena suggested, society had created new forms of dependent behavior (learned pain) and fostered welfare. When Brena shared his concerns with Bonica in 1982, the aging founder of the field responded sympathetically: "I share your concern about the proliferation of so-called pain centers throughout the U.S. and other countries."[68] Bonica, like many Americans, was having second thoughts about bringing relief to so many lives burdened with pain.

The topic of pain, in all its complexity, now contained many of the elements that fractured the political Left and the Right. Calling themselves "neoconservatives," skeptics of social liberalism in the 1970s recoiled against cultural relativism, the expansion of disability benefits and welfare, the false infatuation with Chinese society, and the rise of liberal relief everywhere. Critics charged that American liberals condoned every complaint. They had little patience for those on the far left, like pain reformer Helen Neal, who pushed to bring back heroin as an acceptable form of pain relief.[69] The endorsements of subjective pain as real pain had gone too far, skeptics insisted. The disability rolls were exhibit A in the case against pain. To say that pain was politicized anew in this era is to draw attention to the explicit way in which social suffering—ailments that had defined the post–World War II epidemiological landscape— became an index of party ideology in the 1970s.

How should the people's pain be accommodated? How should their plight be managed? And what price would society pay for compassionate relief? These were no longer veiled political questions; they were explicitly articulated positions defining the political Left and Right. In prosperous times, society would tolerate and even champion liberal relief, but, as the American economy faced inflation, rising unemployment, and fiscal uncertainty, the investigative media (like much of the public) swung toward a hard-edged critique of liberal policies. In a 1972 segment on "low back losers," for example, *NBC News* endorsed the legitimacy of subjective pain and the pain clinic's importance yet also voiced angry frustration about the "losers . . . whose learned pain cost the state of California $102 million a year in compensation." Judges too, sought to moderate liberalism's perceived excesses. In a case involving Manuel Miranda's disability claim, two Republican appointed judges (Bailey Aldrich, a 1959 Eisenhower appointee, and Levin Campbell, appointed by Nixon in 1972) along with Frank Coffin (appointed by the Democrat Lyndon Johnson in 1965), teamed up to articulate a new pain standard. Compassion for subjective pain should have limits, they warned, putting aside the *Page* precedent: "pain is not easily diagnosed, but the Secretary is not at the mercy of every claimant's subjective assertions of pain" when determining eligibility for disability.[70] People in chronic pain were now put on legal and political notice—the gates of relief would not stay open.

When Ronald Reagan—who had spoken for the AMA in 1961 characterizing early Medicare proposals as a socialist assault on human freedom—became president in 1981, eighteen years after the *Page* ruling, the political winds shifted. An argument that the profession had crafted for decades about the fraudulence of pain and liberal governance now had an ardent champion in the White House. Reagan's administration cast a harsh and unforgiving light on those who depended on government and claimed pain as a reason for their disabilities. Hundreds of thousands of people on the disability rolls because of pain were now in the crosshairs of another reform movement. A conservative restoration was on the horizon; the gates began to close.

THREE

The Conservative Case against Learned Helplessness

....

O Liberty, white Goddess! Is it well to leave the gates unguarded?

THOMAS BAILEY ALDRICH,
"UNGUARDED GATES"

Barely two months after Ronald Reagan's presidential inauguration in January 1981, his secretary for Health and Human Services, Richard Schweiker, began purging the Social Security disability rolls
of people claiming pain as their disability. Reagan waged his promised
war on welfare and big government on several fronts, marrying heated
rhetoric with social policy. Reagan once quipped dryly that the ten most
dangerous words in the English language are, "Hi, I'm from the government, and I'm here to help." In a previous run for president, Reagan had
turned one woman—Linda Taylor—into a running commentary on welfare, labeling her as a "welfare queen driving a Cadillac" because of her
extravagant fraud.[1] The charge became a recurring motif, part of the
Reagan formula for vilifying liberals and the federal programs they had
built. In his inaugural address, he continued to press the case—insisting
that "in this present crisis, government is not the solution to our problem; government is the problem."

Once in office, Reagan instructed Schweiker to escalate a review of
all disability claimants—a policy that his predecessor Jimmy Carter had
begun. People claiming pain as the source of their chronic disability came
under special scrutiny at Health and Human Services, a department that
had been created when the former Health, Education, and Welfare department was split into two—Education and HHS. For neoconservatives,
the pain complainant was close kin to Taylor. The affront was not only

the fraud itself but also the gullibility of liberal government in seeking to "help" citizens—which, they claimed, only fed dependence. Consistent with this worldview, HHS became the place where (as one commenter noted) the Reagan revolution "most often collides with the modern social welfare state." This was a pivotal moment, a fulcrum in American pain politics—a time when the accusation of pain fraud figured prominently in the critique of liberalism and when conservatives promised that they had better ideas for managing people in pain.[2]

Schweiker and his Social Security commissioner, John Svahn, shared the conservative view of liberalism as ideologically bankrupt. They believed in the promise of a nation restored by the conservative principles of a smaller federal government, lower taxes, more free enterprise, and fewer regulations on business and industry. Svahn embraced the challenge of "weed[ing] out ineligible Social Security beneficiaries." Over in the White House's Office of Policy Development, Peter Ferrara feared that vague complaints of pain had become a subterfuge for the growth of government. "Over the years, the disability benefit provisions were significantly over-liberalized as compared with the original concept of paying such benefits only for truly permanent and total disability," he wrote. In his view, the decades-long expansion of disability benefits told the story of liberal excesses. Now was the time for a change of course.[3]

The Reagan White House portrayed its disability reforms not as a revolution but as a conservative restoration—as Ferrara put it, to "change back the definition of disability so that it would rest solely on medical grounds and would not take into account vague . . . factors, which are so difficult to determine in a consistent manner." Here was one hallmark of Reagan's formula. His adherents imagined that there had once been a time when objectivity was sacred. Their agenda was merely, they said, a return to these former times. For those frustrated with liberal governance, the appeal to objective reason resonated. A conservative reform would mean creating consistency across disability cases, relying on objective medical evidence rather than subjective complaints, and removing undeserving cheats and frauds from the welfare rolls, all while attacking the growth of government and restoring an old order that, they alleged, had been corrupted by liberalism. Ferrara would have liked nothing better than to get rid of Social Security entirely, but scrapping the New Deal contract between state and citizen was a tall order.[4] Instead, the agenda of Reagan's first term became a slower, more methodical assault—to empty the program of illegitimate claimants.

Over the next three years, HHS's review of the program systemically removed nearly half a million people from the disability rolls, using newly conservative pain standards to weed out pain fraud. For conservatives, pain fraud was not the fraud perpetrated on those vulnerable and in pain (as liberals had once defined it) but was deceit carried out by those falsely claiming to be in pain. Denied coverage by the new administration, one Michigan man, Herbert Tuttle, went to the Lansing office of the Social Security Administration in late 1981. Deeply despondent, he killed himself with a 16-gauge shotgun. His suicide note read, "They cut my Social Security. They are playing God." Others died, ironically, because of "the very disabilities the Social Security Administration believes were not sufficiently serious to keep these people from working." The ensuing battle over pain and disability sent waves of suits into the American courts, and the litigation would consume the federal bureaucracy, the states, and the Congress for the next decade. The arrival of Reagan and his conservative pain standard thus opened a heated policy debate that would redraw the line between true pain and feigned suffering—and the battle over the kind of society America wished to be would stretch on for decades.[5]

The idea that many people feigned pain loomed large in conservative critiques and policies, becoming a major theme during Reagan's first term. As one of the president's supporters later noted in the *Los Angeles Times*, "Reagan attempted to impose rigorous new disability tests on the assumption that many of the so-called disabled were malingerers," many of whom were beneficiaries of rules that had broadened to include "mental disabilities, addictions and subjective states like intense back pain."[6] Framing the issues in these stark black-and-white terms worked politically for Reagan and emboldened his followers. Launching a stinging and dismissive critique of the liberal pain standard, Reagan's mantra was simple: he was attempting to correct the course of the nation with a conservative formula for judging people's pain.

In truth, it was President Eisenhower who had helped open this liberal era, and it was President Carter (whom Reagan dismissed as an arch liberal) who had begun to rethink pain and disability policy along lines similar to Reagan, highlighting how liberalism and conservatism coexisted uneasily from the 1950s into the late 1970s.[7] Elements of the nation's turn to the right were already evident in the Carter years. Rhetorically, however, ascendant conservatives insisted that liberal hypersensitivity to other people's pain had warped American society and infected its laws and government. In short, people claiming disabling pain embodied the problems of liberalism: a love of malingering and refusal of hard work, tolerance for welfare dependence, judicial gullibility, and extreme social indulgence. (So the Right alleged.) Bleeding-heart liberals and activist judges who professed excessive concern for these people were nothing but frauds themselves. They were blinded by excessive sympathy and compassion—to the point of condoning criminality and fraud, accepting the constant expansion of government, taxing others, and producing government dependence. Reagan's critique of welfare fraud resonated with voters anxious about high gas prices, inflation, and fiscal uncertainty and bothered by a host of social issues from the power of unions to racial integration, school busing, and affirmative action. All of these ideological and legal battles swirled around people in pain, feeding their own insecurities and circumscribing the possibilities of relief.

But the liberal society Reagan vilified would not be so easily undermined. The battle over people in pain that started in the Reagan White House and HHS drew a backlash from Congress, resistance from some states, and lawsuits from disability advocates and lawyers. Early in the Reagan revolution, the conservative pain standard was hung up in the courts—themselves being transformed slowly by Reagan's conservative judicial appointments. Liberal commentators and legislators decried Reagan's "purging of the rolls" and the conservative pain standard as a draconian, callous, and inhumane turn away from compassion. Responding to HHS's dismissal of her disability request, one Minnesota housewife, Lorraine Polaski, did not give in. Unlike Herbert Tuttle, she hired an attorney and brought suit against the administration. In time, her case would become a major class action suit putting pressure on the White House, HHS, Congress, and the courts to settle these pain disputes. In its journey through the legal system, the pain debate would become a debate about power, authority to judge, and conservative governance, with the new administration finding itself at odds with state governors and judges who sided with plaintiffs. Even when the judges mandated resumption of benefits, the administration adopted a new executive policy of "nonacquiescence"—attempting to hold this conservative ground as long as they could.[8] Ironically, for an administration that had long decried the role of courts in setting social policy, its purge drove the issue of pain and disability even more deeply into the courts, creating a rich body of law on pain and putting judges more than ever in the driver's seat of determining who was and who was not in true pain and what levels of relief they deserved.

Liberals and Pain Fraud

The policy of "weeding out ineligibles" was not new to Reagan; the ground had been laid by President Jimmy Carter, a Southern Democrat from the moderate wing of his party whose administration was also wary of disability fraud. Well aware of Reagan's stinging welfare critiques in the 1976 Republican primaries, Carter had instituted a continuing review of claimants as president. If there was fraud, he aimed to root it out and reduce the rolls. Carter had arrived in Washington with a vision of moderate technocratic reform, but he soon faced continuing inflation, an oil crisis, and stubborn economic challenges. Reagan's characterization of Carter as a "liberal," in other words, belied the fact that Carter had also stood for reform.

When Carter arrived in Washington, it was not pain per se that concerned him but the fivefold rise in disability payments since the late 1960s and rising instances of welfare fraud. From 1970 to 1975 (on the eve of Carter's election), the number of awards for disability benefits had risen from roughly 350,000 to nearly 600,000. Depending on who was leveling the charge, critics claimed that somewhere between a small percentage and most of these claims were fraudulent. By 1977 and 1978, Carter's secretary of HEW, Joseph Califano, was focusing intently on disability fraud in Social Security as one instance of waste and corruption in government. Carter pushed for modest changes; but, as one editorial noted, Congress, controlled by liberals in his own party, was "so wary of offending beneficiaries . . . [that they] refused to touch even these generous benefits."[9]

Carter's sense that the welfare and disability rolls were expanding was correct, but fraud was not the only (nor a major) explanation. Sixteen years after Eisenhower signed SSDI into law, his former vice president Richard Nixon had signed another round of supplemental security income (SSI) legislation. The Nixon reforms further expanded the disability system, while also consolidating programs like Aid to the Blind, Aid to the Permanently and Totally Disabled, and Aid to the Elderly within the classically defined, worker-oriented, Social Security system. As a result of these expansions, between 1957 and 1982 the program's costs increased from $59 million to $18.5 billion, and the number of eligible insurance recipients rose from 149,850 to 4.3 million. But, perhaps most crucial, under Nixon the economic logic of the program changed. Whereas the old SSDI system had served people who had paid into the Social Security system over the course of their working years through Federal Insurance Contributions Act (FICA) taxes, many of the new people in the new system (aged, blind, or disabled indigent) had not contributed to the system.[10] Here the effects of the liberal war on poverty carried over from the Johnson years into the Nixon presidency. By the early 1970s, both liberals and conservatives had revised and re-revised the economic logic of disability, hoping to bring order and precision to a growing and unwieldy operation.

By the late 1970s, commentators on the left and the right sensed that the growth of the disability rolls was unsustainable. Rather than acknowledge the diverse demographic trends and political decisions that had produced this situation, however, an increasingly vocal group on the right charged that welfare beneficiaries were deceitful, yet rational, economic actors out to maximize profit. Their behavior was said to be distorted by "perverse incentives built into the system." One emerging criticism, for example, was that many people on disability were "eligible for larger payments than their wages." Once they were on disability, the critique went, they were loath ever to work again. According to this critique, disability fraud was created by the system itself. "There is no reason," one 1979 editorial concluded, "to invite fraud by making life more attractive on disability than off." These multiple concerns—the perverse economic incentives, the growth of the programs, and problem of waste, fraud, and abuse—made disability a prime target for reform.[11]

A moderate on this disability issue, Carter was classically liberal on other pain concerns. Pushed by drug reformers to rethink Nixon's war on drugs, for example, the moderate Carter was open to reconsidering the government's strict ban on heroin as a painkiller. But in the realm of disability and welfare fraud, Carter staked out a tougher position, introducing a "welfare policing" system in 1979 called the National Recipient System. One report called it "the largest computer system to check on private citizens ever instituted by the federal government." When combined with the continuing review of claimants, this initiative took earnest aim against corruption, waste, spending, and fraud in government.[12] But would these policies fix the "perverse incentives" in the system? Would they be enough, or had they already gone too far?

Led by Senator Edward Kennedy, the defiant political Left in control of Congress criticized Carter's policies as too quick to cut social welfare programs. Moreover, Carter had infuriated congressional liberals when he decided that pressing for a national health insurance was politically and economically unfeasible. Kennedy criticized the president publicly for a "failure of leadership." By his third year in office, the conventional wisdom on Carter was that the moderate Southerner had tried, but failed terribly, at weaning Congress from its liberal ways—that his efforts had been frustrated by a Democratic political establishment intent on protecting the welfare state it had carefully built. On this topic, the dispute between the moderate and liberal wings of the Democratic Party had grown intense. In Kennedy's view, Carter had betrayed core liberal principles. The senator's anger led him to challenge the president for the Democratic nomination in early 1980, crippling Carter's standing with his own party.[13]

Meanwhile, the political Right continued to lambast the administration's efforts as too modest and too ineffective, as timid and piecemeal. Writing for example in the *Chicago Tribune*, editorialists took aim at the disability program's "excessive generosity" and its skewed incentives, which supposedly contributed to a "waning of the work ethic." "Take the case of a worker with two dependents and with a take-home pay of $8,259 after taxes. Under present law, if he quits work because of, say, a lower back pain, he is entitled to $7,774 a year in Social Security disability benefits—or 94 per cent of his former take-home pay." In two years, the *Tribune* contended, these benefits would increase even more—so much in fact that "only an incorrigible workaholic would want to go back to work."[14]

As both liberal frustration and conservative ire with Carter grew, Ronald Reagan stood poised to be the standard-bearer for Republicans in the 1980 presidential race. Reagan hoped to make the race a referendum on big government liberalism and welfare dependency. The intense lights of the campaign produced glaring (if oversimplified) polarities— bleeding-hearted liberalism versus coldhearted conservatism, compassionate Democrats versus fiscally responsible Republicans, and so on. Caught between these polarities, Carter signaled—in the middle of his campaign—that a reassessment of the disability system was in order. In June 1980 he signed a new law (H.R. 3236, the Social Security Disability Amendments) mandating that the Social Security Administration do more to encourage disabled citizens to return to work. In the president's view, the law was "designed to help disabled beneficiaries return to work by minimizing the risks involved in accepting paid employment." In short, the new incentive offered more carrot than stick—assuring people on disability who doubted they could handle returning to work that they would not risk losing benefits if they tried and failed. They were assured of "automatic reentitlement to benefits" if the return to work failed within a year.[15] Protection in the event of medical mishaps was assured for three years. The rationale behind this policy shift was that the disabled truly wanted to work but needed coaxing. They were not welfare cheats, chiselers, or thieves—all they needed were the right incentives to find their way back into the workforce. Conservatives predictably decried these last-minute reforms as insufficient; as they saw it, the psychology of dependence was a deep cancer demanding much more drastic medicine.

If Carter's therapy seemed timid to Reagan supporters, Carter's followers saw the Right's medicine as draconian and gratuitously painful. Days before the election, Carter asked voters to consider Social Security disability as a bellwether issue, for it revealed Reagan's hard and compassionless heart. In the closing days of the campaign, he recalled Reagan's passionate opposition to Medicare and other social insurance programs. Reagan, he reminded voters, had called these programs "socialist" inventions that preyed on liberty and freedom itself. "Governor Reagan's first major experience in public life was to engage in an active, hard-fought campaign against Medicare," Carter noted. "Governor Reagan worked to convince the American people that Medicare, which protects all of us against medical expenses when we retire or are disabled, was socialism." Looking into strong political headwinds predicting a Reagan victory on Election Day, Carter insisted that those who had built this system would never waver. They supported it because it promoted retirement with dignity not because it bred dependency: "I oppose cutting back basic social security and disability provisions on which most Americans rely . . . It protects almost all of us from disability and provides a hedge against dependency as we grow older . . . Governor Reagan can remember, as I can, when older Americans lived in constant fear of financial disaster, when men and women who had worked hard all their lives had to face a retirement without dignity." In Carter's view, the election was about dignity, decency, and social justice. "I am proud to stand for social security and for decent health care," the president concluded, "and I propose to continue the great fight for social justice in our country." But Carter would not have that chance. A solid majority of American voters—most notably, the Southern Protestants who had supported Carter in 1976—ignored the president's warnings and elected Reagan in a landslide.[16]

Taking office in January 1981 after his victory, Reagan began an artful two-step on the disability question: attacking liberalism with rhetorical vigor and withering humor, while also pointing to Carter's own reforms as precedent for his own Social Security review and cuts. Meanwhile, his HHS secretary expanded the continuing review process and ruled against thousands of people who had come to depend on regular payments. When congressional Democrats denounced the aggressiveness of these disability reviews, Reagan used Carter for cover. Noted the president, "There is the program of social security disability, and . . . in 1980, under the previous administration, a law was passed to try and clean up what was believed to be a gigantic abuse of that program. So, there are things that can be done." But the goal of Reagan's policy went well beyond Carter's attempts to battle fraud and tweak skewed incentives: instead, Reagan proposed to reduce the size of government and the scale of dependency by the hundreds of thousands; to weed out chiselers, frauds, ineligibles, and anyone who could work for a living; to turn to the private sector for answers to all social problems; and, thereby, to promote a

conservative vision of America and its work ethic.[17] A pivotal and punitive chapter in the conservative politics of pain had begun.

Speaking at a press gathering in October 1981, Reagan used a shocking example to portray people on disability as profoundly undeserving
of government support. Defending his Social Security policies before a
group of out-of-town newspaper editors, Reagan explained that his administration was not pursuing major cuts but merely "clearing up some
things on the periphery, such as people getting disability in Social Security that weren't entitled." Putting a troubling face on the problem, he
asked, "Doesn't it sort of strike you as strange that [serial killer] Son of
Sam, serving that seventy-five-year sentence up there for all his murders,
is getting $350 a month from disability, social security, because they say
he's incapable of holding a job? And this is going on all over the country." If any editor in the room had been confused about Reagan's views
on disability claimants, they no longer had an excuse now. Son of Sam
had been arrested in New York City a few years earlier, charged with
several ritual murders that shocked and horrified the nation. As if this
were not clear enough, Reagan offered the editors another example of

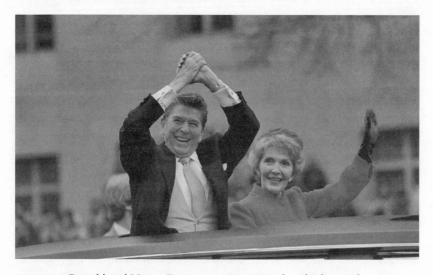

FIGURE 3.1.   Ronald and Nancy Reagan waving triumphantly during the new
president's Inaugural Parade. Washington, D.C. January, 20, 1981.

Image courtesy of the Ronald Reagan Library.

waste, fraud, and disability abuse—again using the criminally insane: "We have people in California that I know of, in mental institutions for the criminally insane, who are drawing regular payments because, due to their mental illness, they had been judged incapable of holding jobs. But now, we're paying their room, board, medical care, and laundry, housing, and yet they're getting that payment."[18] These were not rhetorical accidents but the kind of biting and exaggerated stories Reagan had told for decades, tying the disabled to deeply stigmatized people—to the criminally insane—as representatives of the failure of liberal society. For years his rhetoric had been a minority viewpoint within his own party, but now, speaking for a majority as president and policy maker in chief, Reagan was in a position to act against what he saw as this unconscionable fraud.

The War against Welfare and Learned Helplessness

The Reagan formula framed America's dilemma as a stark choice: on one side, a failed and overliberalized society taken in by subjective complaints of pain and, on the other, a conservative restoration founded on objective criteria for measuring true need. For decades and even centuries, regard for the pain of others and the structure of relief had been an issue for the design of good government and sound civic affairs. Since World War II, the rise of chronic pain had posed a multifaceted challenge with an ideological edge. People in pain came in many forms: soldiers crippled by a series of wars; industrial and service workers coping with work ailments and repetitive labor injuries; the elderly and their ailments, their numbers growing in proportion to the general population. Certainly, liberal social programs like Medicare and Medicaid had encouraged society's increasing sensitivity to the subjective pain of others. Collectively, these trends worried liberals and vexed conservatives alike—from the Eisenhower and Johnson eras through the Nixon and Carter terms.[19] It was Reagan, however, who framed the issues so dramatically, so starkly, and in such partisan terms that pain became a wedge issue and a litmus test for one's views on crime, fraud, and dependency writ large.

Where gate control theory had been intimately linked to liberalizing the pain field and validating subjective pain as true pain in the late 1960s into the 1970s, older theories of pain as psychologically illegitimate (common in 1950s psychiatry) reappeared in the 1970s and 1980s to support and echo rising neoconservative sensibilities. Steven Brena, the Atlanta pain clinic director who had introduced the notion of pain as a learned experience (see chapter 2), found that his theory resonated with an increasingly conservative populace. In his 1978 book, *Chronic Pain: America's Hidden Epidemic,* he wrote that Western society had "gone too far in passing laws granting monetary compensation for escape from work via pain complaints." In his own clinic, he had observed "the wisdom of St. Paul's instructions to work for a living." A life on the dole created "devastating effects of learned sick-behaviors and related feelings of worthlessness" and "trapped [potentially able workers] in a nightmare of welfare lifestyles."[20]

"Chronic pain is often a conditioned socioeconomic disease," Brena wrote in a May 1981 article. "A majority of chronic pain patients show pain behavior in excess of biomedical findings and disability ratings out of proportion to their actual physical impairment." Where President Carter and his HEW secretary Califano had made fraud and abuse a central concern, Reagan's HHS secretary Richard Schweiker elevated these types of questions—the medical proof of pain—to a new level.[21]

For Brena, one mystery of pain was why some people dwelled on their experience while others did not; he used the psychological theory of learned helplessness to explain the disparity. The concept (developed by observing the behavior of animals and people who have no control over their situation or outcomes) proved to be appealing for those worried about the unintended effects of pain relief and even welfare. In situations of chronic distress, Brena asserted, people who fixated on their pain and who had pending disability claims reported higher subjective pains. Even after being medicated, their complaints persisted. By contrast, pain sufferers who did not fixate on their pain and who did not have stakes in the disability system reported lower subjective pain. Simply put, the pain sufferer with no pending disability claim, no spouse on whom to lean for support, and low pain behavior had a better response to medications. This was true for either placebos or analgesics.[22] Though Brena's formulation was not explicitly political, there is little doubt that this view of learned pain and disability resonated with the rising conservative sensibilities of his time.

The migration of theories of learned pain, malingering, and helplessness from social science, the laboratory, and the clinic into political and legal disputes should not surprise us. This movement of theory into politics and policy had long defined how pain knowledge and theory circulated. Certainly, since the 1960s, actors in law, medicine, and policy had been aware of the moral and civic stakes of judging pain. Now, in the 1980s, pain had become an index of the American welfare problem—a problem seemingly tailor made for welfare's critics. As historian Michael Katz observed in 1986, "Nobody likes welfare . . . Conservatives worry that it erodes the work ethic, retards productivity, and rewards the lazy. Liberals view the American welfare state as incomplete, inadequate, and punitive. Poor people, who rely on it, find it degrading, demoralizing, and mean." Prominent voices on the right even ridiculed the notion of compassion as a misguided liberal construct. In the new administration's view, the pain disability question symbolized the fundamental challenge of their time—the need to draw a sharp line separating the fraudulent, criminal, and undeserving from the truly needy. "Malingering may be the Administration's greatest fear in relation to its disability program," commented one observer looking back at the Reagan years, "because the government cannot financially afford to promote, even indirectly, such a practice by granting benefits to those persons not truly disabled."[23] For Reagan, fiscal austerity and cutbacks to federal aid to the poor and disabled would surely bring more pain, but it was a necessary harsh medicine to heal the suffering nation.

When Schweiker, a former Republican senator from Pennsylvania, took charge of HHS, he quickly expanded Carter's continuing review process into a more sweeping purge. The term, used by administration critics, is not unwarranted. By the time his work was done, 1.2 million recipients had been reviewed, with more than 490,000 removed from the rolls. The pace was stunning, prompting charges that the administration was being inhumane. The economic recession that year, combined with the cuts, drove many to extreme acts. Herbert Tuttle was not the only suicide attributed to the cuts in disability. A month later, Harold Lutz (a forty-five-year-old with diabetes and recovering from triple bypass surgery) shot himself as well, after spending a year trying to win Social Security benefits. In the face of such events, however, White House insiders worried not about people but about negative press coverage. Reagan's chief pollster, Richard Wirthin, wrote to Reagan's inner staff—Edwin Meese, James Baker, and Michael Deaver—bemoaning the "negative fallout triggered by President Reagan's 'suggested' Social Security reform package . . . [which had] reinforced some latent fears we know the electorate has carried about the President and more specifically about his economic program."[24]

The purge of the disability rolls produced thousands of legal appeals. Administrative law judges and appeals judges grappled with the legal status of people in subjective pain, as they had for decades since the *Page* case in 1963. The danger on one side was that "incorrect denials can leave deserving claimants, who are often in precarious financial conditions, without a crucial source of income." But the opposing danger was rewarding cheaters, since "erroneous grants of benefits reward liars at public expense, waste resources that could be put to any number of more productive uses, and may ultimately reduce the level of funding available for people who are legitimately disabled." These tensions pitting conservatives against liberals now left the campaign and legislative battlefield and migrated into the courts. In the final analysis, this legal scholar concluded, to avoid the dangers it was best to seek a middle ground; "the public interest is ill-served by either type of mistake."[25]

Increasingly, the Reagan administration's insistence on clamping down on liars and cheats won adherents in court. Law itself was in transition, with legal liberalism besieged, as Laura Kalman noted, by the New Right, by taxpayers' revolts, and by cultural conservatism. The 1970s had given rise to a new style of legal analysis, symbolized by the economics-minded Richard Posner, who insisted that all "people involved with the legal system act as rational maximizers of their satisfactions." The mantra of law and economics declared that the courts should depend less on psychology, sociology, or compassion for its rulings and more on evidence drawn from economics and science. More and more, Social Security disability cases became tests for this conservative outlook, with judges pushed to use objectivity and economics (not subjectivity or theories of compassion) in ruling on the plea for public relief.[26]

In 1981, the very thing that Jimmy Carter and liberal Democrats had warned against was coming to pass—a harsh and challenging new era for the disabled. Despite critical news coverage of its policies and a growing legal backlash, the Reagan administration pressed ahead in 1982, adopting "an 'in house' ruling," called Social Security Ruling 82-58, which "instructed Administration employees to credit only medically substantiated pain allegations." The ruling declared that "there must be an objective basis to support the overall evaluation of impairment severity. It is not sufficient to merely establish a diagnosis or a source for the symptom." By 1982, these reforms had saved $216 million and promised to save $458 million the next year. Congress, however, was beginning to balk. As the *Washington Post* reported, "Many Congressmen say the pain and confusion the reviews have caused isn't what they had in mind when they asked the Social Security Administration in 1980 to improve the monitoring of the disability income program, and its welfare sister, Supplemental Security Income." As the *Post* recounted, the reforms "aimed at weeding out the undeserving . . . have in many cases imposed an unnecessary burden on thousands of disabled people," even those who met the government's strict standards.[27] Many who lost their benefits were forced onto state welfare rolls, shifting the burden of relief to the states. And there was one other casualty of the purge: the bad publicity surrounding the purging of the rolls led to misgivings in the administration about Schweiker. His days on the Reagan team were numbered.

When Margaret Heckler took over leadership of HHS from Schweiker in early 1983, her first challenge was to "soften the image" of the department—acknowledging the ill effects of the disability reforms and admitting errors but also pressing ahead with the Reagan agenda. She confessed that some decisions had produced unnecessary pain and hardship. She promised to put a kinder face on what congressional Democrats and the press regarded as an inhumane public relations disaster. In a June 1983 Op-Ed, Heckler wrote that she "had no idea that the sudden, three-year review of millions of cases we then mandated might result in hardships and heartbreaks for some innocent and worthy disability recipients." In her view, the Reagan reforms were done on a humane basis. They "introduced a face-to-face human contact at the very beginning of the review process and set the stage for a face-to-face hearing at the very first level of appeal—represent[ing] a giant step toward humanizing this program." But the backlash had been harsh, she acknowledged, and "President Reagan felt we needed to do even better. That's why I have just announced additional major reforms of disability review." Heckler declared that the "number of people exempted from the continuing disability investigation process [would be expanded] by 200,000, bringing the total exempted to more than 1 million, or 37 percent of those now on the rolls." Another 135,000 people with "functional psychotic disorders" would be temporarily exempt, and the program would move from "profiling" to random selection in its review process. The new secretary of HHS remained unapologetic about the overall goals, however, noting that fraud was still pervasive and citing a statistic from the Carter administration that claimed that as many as "one-in-five" of the nearly three million people on disability were ineligible. Fraud, she claimed, was costing "two billion taxpayer dollars a year."[28]

Heckler's compassion campaign raised the question of whether Carter had been right all along about the heartlessness of Reagan's social welfare policies. By early 1984, the department had orchestrated a provisional resumption of benefits while waiting for the Congress to write new rules and guidelines that would reconcile court opinions and administration policy. In the meantime, the news media noted that the reforms and backtracking had thrown disability rulings into "a state of legal confusion and administrative chaos." Heckler faced another challenge: how to manage the thousands of appeals and lawsuits from purged claimants that were now winding through federal courts, where many judges had grown hostile and suspicious toward the administration. By some accounts, disability lawsuits now clogged the courts, accounting for 15–20 percent of new filings in some districts.[29]

By 1984, with Reagan heading into a re-election fight, most commentators (even his supporters) admitted that purging the rolls had gone too far. Journalist Charles Lane admitted that "the huge SSDI program must be trimmed—but with a scalpel, not a meat ax. The Reagan administration tried the latter, and it didn't work." Characterizing the administration as "malingerer-hunters," critics on the left insisted that the review of more than one million beneficiaries was excessive. Running to unseat Reagan in 1984, Carter's former vice president Walter Mondale made this issue of fairness a central one—throwing Reagan into the defensive about his commitments to people with disabilities. With Congress still debating disability and the administration's "heartless" approach to people in pain, Heckler acknowledged that Social Security officials "made some mistakes, causing 'hardships and heartbreaks' for disabled people."[30]

In the first presidential debate in October 1984, Mondale took the fight directly to Reagan, forcing the president to defend his lack of sensitivity to people in pain. Recovery from the 1981 economic recession had been achingly slow. Reagan admitted that "there is no way that the recovery is even across the country, just as in the depths of the recession, there were some parts of the country that were worse off, but some that didn't even feel the pain of the recession." But Mondale followed up, insisting that Reagan's policies had also caused much of the pain, particularly to the poor and vulnerable:

> There is no question that the poor are worse off . . . How you can cut school lunches, how you can cut student assistance, how you can cut housing, how you can cut disability benefits, how you can do all of these things and then the people receiving them—for example, the disabled, who have no alternative—how they're going to do better, I don't know. Now, we need a tight budget, but there's no question that this administration has singled out things that affect the most vulnerable in American life, and they're hurting.

Mondale's accusation stung the president who, everyone observed, seemed lethargic in his first face-to-face encounter with Mondale.

Months before the elections, broad swaths of the public seemed to agree with Mondale that Reagan's cuts had hurt the most vulnerable and many who were truly in need. But one exchange between Mondale and debate panelist James Weighart also stung the liberal Democrat, providing insight into pain and privilege at this political juncture. "Mr. Mondale," said Weighart, echoing a kind of detachment from Mondale's commitments, "is it possible that the vast majority of Americans who appear to be prosperous have lost interest in the kinds of programs you're discussing to help those less privileged than they are?"[31] Mondale had no effective response. No matter how true his attack on Reagan had been, Mondale's criticism alone would not alter the direction of the election. The American electorate, whatever its misgivings about the "meat ax" approach to social programs, was pleased that the economy had rebounded from recession; the prosperous were content and not particularly disturbed by the plight of the "have-nots." Moreover, many voters believed the president had rebuilt the nation's standing in the world by confronting the Soviet Union and decrying the ideological bankruptcy of Communism at every turn. They believed, as Reagan optimistically promised, that it was "morning again in America" and considered the administration's harshness as necessary fiscal pain.[32] In November, Reagan was re-elected for four more years in another landslide.

The Power to Judge Suffering

By the time of the Reagan presidency, a robust body of legal literature had accumulated around the proof of pain—with the law as a site where weighing clinical, objective, subjective, psychological, and anatomical pain evidence was amassed and debated. As the public disability system expanded, the legal and social stakes in proving pain and suffering grew. In addition to the judges and lawyers, new professional groups had sprung up to engage with the challenge of assessing pain. Standing alongside the medical profession, one such group, for example, was the National Association of Disability Examiners. An offshoot of the National Rehabilitation Association, they developed a new professional focus—training men and women to arbitrate pain and disability disputes. An expansive system for assessing disability had blossomed—with cadres of government administrators, administrative law judges, disability experts, doctors, and bureaucrats in many sectors assessing pain at a scale never before seen.[33]

In the wake of the Reagan-era purging of the rolls, this legal machinery was thrown into overdrive—grappling with the consequences of conservative spending for the citizen's right to relief. For the administration, using "objective" medical evidence to recalibrate disability became a stalking horse for its political goals of fiscal sobriety and welfare reform. Standing in the middle of these struggles, administrative law judge Alan Goldhammer and Social Security Administration attorney Susan Bloom observed that, prior to Carter's August 1980 regulations, "the federal courts almost uniformly provided that a finding of 'disability' could properly be based upon a showing of severe and incapacitating symptoms alone." Under the Reagan proposal, however, the legal definition of disability "would rest *solely on medical grounds* and would not take into account vague . . . factors, which are so difficult to determine in a consistent manner." Reagan's stance went well beyond proposals from conservative Democrats like Ways and Means Congressional committee

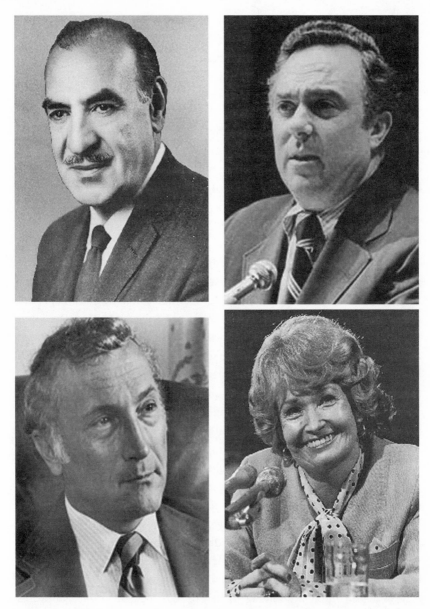

FIGURE 3.2. Four secretaries of the U.S. Department of Health, Education, and Welfare (and later the Department of Health and Human Services) who managed the federal government's policies on pain and disability; *left to right,* Anthony Celebrezze (Kennedy administration), Joseph Califano (Carter), and Richard Schweiker and Margaret Heckler (Reagan). Califano image courtesy of Food and Drug Administration; all others courtesy of the Social Security Administration.

chair J. J. Pickle (Texas), who had supported Carter in his efforts to crack down on fraud. Comparing the administration's proposals to Pickle's in May 1981, a member of Reagan's policy team, Eric Hempel, observed that Pickle's approach to Social Security reform was tough on the pain claim but not tough enough.

> Section 205 [*sic*, 206] of the Pickel [*sic*] bill would make it more difficult to qualify for disability insurance simply by claiming pain or other discomforts . . . [providing that] claimant testimony as to pain and other symptoms shall not alone permit a finding of disability . . . . unless medical signs and findings established by medically accept-able . . . techniques show that there is a medical condition that could reasonably be expected to produce such pain or other symptoms.

To the White House, this "reasonable expectation" was an unwarranted loophole too easily exploited by too-liberal judges of disability. As Hempel noted, "The Administration proposal would tighten disability criteria considerably further by limiting qualification to medical factors alone." Objectivity was thus linked to fiscal restraint. Later, in signing one resulting piece of reform legislation, Reagan insisted that "several billion dollars a year were being spent to support people who were not, in fact, disabled."[34]

In the politics of how pain should be judged and by whom, the resulting lawsuits set up a complicated struggle for power among the executive, legislative, and judicial branches of government. In the 1976 *Miranda* case, the First Circuit Court of Federal Appeals determined that "the Secretary is not at the mercy of every claimant's subjective assertions of pain" when determining eligibility for disability. In the early 1980s, the Reagan administration took the combative position that, just as it could disregard applicants' claims, it could disregard courts with whose findings it disagreed. With the administration's new policy of nonacquiescence, a complicated new political era was unfolding, with the executive branch simultaneously seizing power and devolving responsibility for disability to the "laboratory of the states" (a phrase first used by Justice Louis Brandeis earlier in the century).[35] In this litigious era, plaintiffs turned to the courts for relief, and conservatives (seeking to limit their access to the courts) decried the rising tide of "frivolous lawsuits," as they often had in the past, and called for tort reform.

By 1984, the courts' repeated rulings to restore benefits presented the Reagan administration with a political dilemma—a legal roadblock on its path to establishing a conservative pain standard. Would the administration comply and uphold the liberal rulings on subjective pain made by judges clinging to the *Page* standard on subjective symptoms? Or would they find a way to uphold its principles? Reagan's ardent followers had come to vilify liberal lawyers, advocates, and judges almost as much as welfare "cheats," seeing them as enablers of dependence. In the wake of the 1980 election, one senior justice on the California Supreme Court who knew Reagan's politics well from his years as governor, rightly predicted the political-legal disputes to come: "They will say that the courts 'legislate' rather than 'interpret' the Constitution, and that the courts are 'soft on crime.' These are no more than code words to the effect that the courts have been too vigilant in . . . protecting the disadvantaged and the minorities from direct and indirect exploitation." Indeed, it was Edwin Meese (who had served Governor Reagan as legal affairs secretary and chief of staff and who was now Reagan's chief policy maker) who most insistently and sharply "attacked liberal judges, psychiatrists, and lawyers [for] trying to outwit the criminal justice system." Aside from attacking the so-called liberal activism of judges, Reagan supporters also took aim at the obvious lack of uniformity across these courts—particularly on questions of disability.[36]

The administration's hubris in defying the courts on disability rankled judges and enraged members of Congress. The practice also called Congress back into the fray, with Democrats like Pickle in the House now pushing for new legislation to hold the administration to congressional standards of pain and disability evaluation. At the same time, some state governors balked at the administration's noncompliance with court rulings, siding with the courts—particularly because the cost of coverage now fell back onto the states. Arkansas governor Bill Clinton, for example, directed his state officials to ignore the administration and "to comply with Federal court decisions holding that severe pain by itself could be a disabling condition." Yet Clinton (later ridiculed by conservatives for professing to "feel the pain" of voters) also acknowledged that state officials had "virtually no real power" to affect individual cases.[37] When Arkansas officials tried to keep people on the rolls, they were simply overruled by Social Security officials.

The politicization of pain reached a frenzy in 1984 as the Democratically-controlled House, the Republican-controlled Senate, various states, and the Reagan White House battled one another and as the administration also took fire from plaintiffs, the courts, and state officials. At stake was not only the government's relationship to people with disability claims but the power to judge and govern, that is, which branch of government had the authority to decide these vexing issues of pain and relief. Physicians could only observe as Congress reasserted its authority, debating who was in true pain. Pennsylvania's moderate Republican senator John Heinz insisted that "pain is an extraordinarily complicated medical phenomenon, and it is frequently the case that pain that can be objectively identified cannot be linked to an underlying impairment." Where some lawmakers puzzled over the definition of pain, others, like Louisiana Democratic senator Russell Long (son of the famed populist governor and senator Huey Long), fumed against the courts and the executive branch as well, asserting congressional primacy: "if the regional courts are going to persist in ignoring the policy objectives expressed by Congress and persist in refusing to grant appropriate deference to the duly promulgated regulations of the Secretary, the Congress may be forced to find ways of dealing with this situation." The majority leader of the Senate, Kansas Republican Bob Dole, himself a World War II veteran who lost the use of his right arm in battle, supported the administration's hard-line stance. Accordingly, the final Senate bill continued to place the onus on purged claimants to prove that their condition had not improved. The Senate bill also included language suggesting that some cases could not have regress to the courts, a move that reflected Republican suspicion of the courts and plaintiffs. By contrast, the House called for HHS to give beneficiaries the benefit of the doubt—to presume that an already-disabled person's disability continued unless medical evidence showed otherwise. Just months before the presidential elections, the House, Senate, and White House had reached an impasse.[38]

Pressure on Congress also came from the gathering momentum of Lorraine Polaski's case, which had grown into a major class-action suit. Polaski had received disability benefits since 1979, but her eligibility was terminated in 1983. The Minnesota housewife appealed, contending that the secretary's decision "was not supported by substantial evidence because it improperly discounted her allegations of pain." Moreover, her suit argued that HHS had produced "no evidence to show either that her condition had improved or that the original decision finding her disabled was erroneous." Polaski argued that the secretary had used erroneous standards on pain and medical improvement, "directly and flagrantly" contrary to the law as set out by the Court of Appeals for the Eighth Circuit. Within months, others had joined her suit against the Reagan administration's purge. *Polaski v. Heckler* was affirmed as a class-action suit in Minnesota District Court in April 1984, with one federal judge accusing the department of existing in "a state of lawlessness." As the case headed for the Eighth Circuit Court of Appeals, where it was heard in June, Heckler agreed to temporarily halt reviews. A decision on *Polaski* was expected in December, and so the lawsuit cast a long shadow over election year maneuvering in Congress. As it moved toward higher courts, the case placed increasing pressure on the Congress and the administration to settle their pain dispute through legislation.[39]

On September 20, 1984, Representative Pickle announced a compromise bill "that will bring relief and hope to thousands and thousands of people all across this land who have been inhumanely removed from the rolls." Both parties could claim victory in the remaining month before the election. Insisting that HHS had taken too much latitude in its purge, Congress now asserted its power to guide the courts and the administration. As Eileen Sweeney of the National Senior Citizens Law Center saw it, the compromise agreement "substantially limit[ed] the discretion previously enjoyed by the Secretary of HHS in addressing disability issues." The final disability legislation was a victory for liberals in many regards, except on the question of pain. On the pain question, the compromise legislation punted the contentious epistemological question on subjective pain to an outside commission—mandating that HHS convene an expert group to deliberate, evaluate policies, and recommend changes on the relationship of pain and disability. An expert panel—led by none other than Washington's John Bonica—began its work on April 1, 1985, with a mandate to report its findings to Congress by December 31, 1986.[40]

The pain question at the heart of welfare and disability politics remained unresolved and polarized, but the search for middle ground had begun. At its core, the stakes in this pain debate revolved around wrenching issues of compassion, dignity, and justice before the American electorate. "There is no kindness in finding an individual 'disabled' who really is capable of performing work activity and who would prefer the dignity of being independent of benefit payments," two Social Security administrators concluded in 1984, "if the individual can be led to understand that he can be independent of those." They sympathized to some extent with the administration's tough position, noting that "there is much to say for an approach which largely ignores subjective expressions of pain and dysfunction and relies primarily upon that medical evidence which can be independently verified and assessed as producing a medically legitimate state of incapacity." Ultimately, however, the conservative pain standard would be modified by some combination of congressional action and court ruling. One by-product of the 1984 debate was the rising awareness—among expert disability adjudicators—that subjective pain could neither be dismissed outright nor held up as an intrinsic disability without careful scrutiny.[41] Reagan's executive declarations would have to yield to legislative and judicial judgment.

Legal commentators found several ironies in the 1984 pain and disability compromises, which carefully dissected and redefined how the law should regard people in pain. Congress had won a concession, mandating that subjective pain should not be dismissed outright in disability cases. But, as legal scholar Margaret Rodgers noted, Section 3 of the legislation largely affirmed the administration's position even as it created the first-ever statutory standard for the evaluation of pain, "designed to end the confusion over pain testimony in disability benefits cases by codifying the Administration's existing policy on pain." The law stated that "an individual's statements as to pain or other symptoms shall not alone be conclusive evidence of disability . . . there must be medical signs and findings . . . which show the existence of medical impairment that results from anatomical, physiological, or psychological abnormalities which could reasonably be expected to produce the pain." But signing the bill also represented a concession for the president. Yes, the administration still held the upper hand on precisely how to implement the subjective pain standard at HHS. And the administration had also forced another major concession on plaintiffs' rights—the act limited new class-action litigation over how HHS used, or misused, the medical improvement standard to review cases. However, henceforth, it would be harder for the conservative administration to end benefits in its formerly unilateral, draconian style.[42]

In December, the Eighth Circuit announced its decision in the *Polaski* case, ruling that HHS had wrongly terminated her benefits. The majority (taking the recent pain legislation into careful consideration) saw the debate as part of a troubling conflict between the courts and the Reagan administration: "in 1984 alone, we reversed or remanded to the Secretary because of inadequate consideration of pain in at least thirteen cases, while affirming the Secretary's analysis of pain or other subjective complaints in none." The court victory affirmed the legitimacy of Polaski's subjective pain. "It is hard to envision a more urgent situation," wrote the court. "Claimants who lose or are denied benefits face foreclosure proceedings on their homes, suffer utility cutoffs and find it difficult to purchase food. They go without medication and doctors' care; they lose their medical insurance. They become increasingly anxious, depressed, despairing—all of which aggravates their medical conditions."[43]

With this ruling, the purge era that spanned Reagan's first term appeared to have ended. The settlements and court decisions meant that nearly three hundred thousand people (60 percent of the people previously removed from the Social Security disability rolls) would have their benefits restored. Yet the administration's appeal kept the issue in court years longer. It would take a Supreme Court ruling in 1987 before the Polaski story was complete and HHS was compelled to reopen a final group of eight thousand cases it had refused to hear. By the end of the Reagan era, the courts were forced to wade deep into the politics and governance of pain. The intense dispute between those who would impose a conservative pain standard over a liberal one had been tamed. As one 1987 study noted, "the Polaski standard" along with the congressional compromise had together "better defined the criteria for evaluating pain and thus to have decreased the disagreement between SSA and the federal courts."[44]

The administration's other legacy in the jurisprudence of pain was to appoint to the courts judges sympathetic to its own ideology. By the 1990s, as one administrative law judge noted, the courts had gradually swung to see things through a more conservative lens—preaching the gospel of law and economics, seeking more uniformity, and upholding objective evidence as a standard for judging pain and disability. But they still differed widely on how to "apply the requirement of objective evidence (or what they do to get around it)." Skirmishes continued as Congress continued to fight with the White House and the courts on this topic; through the 1980s and early 1990s the jurisprudence of pain continued to be an ideological battle zone. The legal literature on pain, legal judgment, justice, and disability continued to grow. Writing in 1992 in the *California Western Law Review*, Margaret Rodgers noted that consensus on the pain standard remained uncertain: "the pain standards articulated in [other cases such as] Bunnell, Luna, and other decisions are, by themselves, insufficient to correct the unfairness which currently exists within the disability determination process."[45]

By the end of the Reagan era, the conservative plan to remake government and society had forced the courts to wade deep into the politics of pain. Whether you were a lawyer, a politician, a physician, a pain complainant, or an engaged citizen, your position on the pain question was a good index of your deeper political commitments and passions. No consensus had emerged on the war between liberal and conservative pain standards—only an orchestrated, fragile compromise. One scholar described the era's court rulings, legislative proceedings, administration rules, commission reports, and class-action suits as producing a "decisional quagmire." Indeed, the statutory pain standard produced by Congress in 1984 only threw the controversy back into the courts and back to HHS— where judicial and administrative interpretations continued to reflect the troubling welfare politics of the era.[46] As a result of the Reagan-era battles, the courts now were compelled to referee the debate between conservative and liberal views on pain and to seize a measure of power in the pain disability debates.

Whose Pain Matters? Reagan's Legacy

The angry legal and political battles of 1984, spilling over into the late 1980s, provoked an adjustment in the conservative pain standard—that is, in how the political Right strategically spoke about and used government to manage the pain of others. In the midst of the debate over Reagan's failures of compassion and heading into his re-election, the politics of pain took another turn when the White House began to seize on a new pain discourse to mobilize its avid moralistic followers. The new issue was "fetal pain." The concept was nod to the Moral Majority wing of the party and an important 1980s movement, in which fetal personhood became the rejoinder to the feminist abortion rights advocates. As historian Sara Dubow skillfully noted, the cry of fetal personhood set up a new politics of whose pain mattered. Calling attention to fetal pain bracketed off the experiences of women carrying the fetus, aiming to indict liberalism from yet another angle—criticizing feminism from inside the womb. Where some on the right decried learned helplessness, others claimed to defend innocence and true helplessness. As the senior editor of the *National Review* insisted in a new journal called *Human Life Review* in 1984, "The pain of the aborted fetus is ineligible for the liberal's selective but purposeful 'compassion.'" The antiabortion film *The Silent Scream*, purporting to depict a fetus in pain during an abortion, was produced the same year.[47] With this powerful gesture toward a new kind of pain worthy of relief, the outlines of a new moralistic politics (aimed at another liberal "-ism," feminism) would begin to unfold within the conservative movement.

Addressing a March for Life rally on the fifteenth anniversary of the *Roe v. Wade* Supreme Court case that legalized abortion, Reagan embraced the fetus as the new iconic modal sufferer. Speaking to a gathering of the Religious Right, he said, "We're told about a woman's right to control her own body. But doesn't the unborn child have a higher right, and that is to life, liberty and the pursuit of happiness?" The question, of course, was not merely rhetorical but a political reframing of the question of whose happiness matters more—mother or fetus? Whose pain should take precedence in public policy? Reagan championed the fetus's pain as a pain only the righteous knew, noting "if every member of Congress could see that film [*The Silent Scream*], they would move quickly to end the tragedy of abortion." The president reminded the crowd that "a few years ago, I spoke about the pain that we now know an unborn fetus experiences in the course of an abortion. At the time there was an outcry of enraged criticism and angry denials." In his final year in office, the president insisted that physicians had since proven him right, quoting a letter signed by twenty-four doctors that stated that fetal pain was "firmly established." It was as if the liberal politics of compassion toward disability and pain had been co-opted by the Religious Right. In the same way that the Left had used pain to establish the rights of disabled in the 1960s, the

Right now hoped to use the claim of "medically validated" pain to establish new and sweeping personhood and citizenship claims.[48]

A keen political observer could see how the Republican pain platform was shifting in the late 1980s and early 1990s. In Reagan's second term Secretary Heckler sought to turn the question of pain management in new directions—emphasizing how innovation and private-public partnerships were tackling the problem. This was an effort to reclaim the disability and pain debate and to turn it into a Republican-friendly issue. One step was to marry the cause of disability to Republican themes like innovation—neutralizing the Democrats' claim that they alone spoke for people in pain. In December 1985, for example, Reagan welcomed to the White House "an exciting new partnership between the Government and the private sector . . . the National Initiative on Technology and the Disabled." Among the "devices of liberation" the partnership would promote, he said, was a device called Comp-U-Talk for people incapable of speech. Reagan also described a new way of battling pain: "an implantable device called the human tissue stimulator which shows great promise for controlling chronic pain, like that associated with arthritis, rheumatism, and cancer." The political combat with liberals had been grueling in Reagan's first term; the administration now turned away from the harsh rhetoric, toward co-optation and reframing (creating a rhetoric of pain and relief Republicans could endorse)—a significant theme in the second half of Reagan's presidency.[49]

Like the liberal pain standard before it, the conservative pain standard was not static but evolving—adapting to the charge that Republicans did not care about disability or the vulnerable and finding new ways of demonstrating its own brand of compassion. (Singing from this political playbook written in the late 1980s, George H. W. Bush and his son George W. Bush would both call themselves "compassionate conservatives.") The strategy was a result of the times—a response to a party buffeted by bad press, lawsuits, and political criticism, by the rise of the Religious Right, and also by the advent of new health challenges like AIDS, which, as C. Everett Koop noted, challenged conservatives as well. The new disease "became associated with drug abuse, with sexual promiscuity, and with IV drug paraphernalia, and a huge number of the conservatives in this country said 'they deserve what they got, just ignore them and let them die.' Well, you can't be a doctor and do that; you can't be the Surgeon General and do that."[50] The relentless rise of chronic pain had continued, and the emergence of new health challenges tested conservatism in fresh ways. In response to such developments, tough-minded conservative talk about pain as merely "learned helplessness" rang particularly hollow.

The questions of which—and whose—pain mattered most and how to deal with people in pain continued to be socially and politically divisive. The appearance of baffling pain syndromes complicated matters further, raising anew worries of pain complainers as coddled hysterics. In the case of fibromyalgia and chronic fatigue syndrome (CFS), derisively termed the "yuppie flu" in the press, traditional laboratory evidence was conspicuously lacking. As one journalist noted in the late 1980s, "Whether patients have fallen into the grip of a new, worsening scourge or have merely succumbed to the latest health hysteria is confounding many medical researchers." CFS exemplified one kind of pain, a subjective pain found primarily among middle-class, young, upwardly mobile professionals (yuppies) suddenly afflicted by unexplained aches of unverifiable origin. Like Polaski's pain, CFS sufferers' pain was difficult to objectively validate; their claims were regarded as highly suspicious, especially in determining disability benefits. Women claimants, as Dara Purvis has documented, received particularly tough scrutiny. As one administrative law judge commented in 1991, the problem with these new maladies was that they once again swung wide open the door for subjectivity to re-enter the discussion of pain and relief, with the attendant "potential for manipulation because outward manifestations of pain can easily be contrived by a calculating claimant."[51] The American pain problem, in short, would not subside—it would only evolve with the cultural politics of the times.

Amid the Right's transformations, people in chronic pain found themselves caught up in partisan battles, seeking care amid rising skepticism and facing unsteady judgments in the courts, Congress, and clinics. The Reagan era catalyzed two concerns simultaneously: on the one hand, of excessive indulgence and overtreatment, and, on the other hand, of endemic undertreatment driven by excessive skepticism about people in pain and rising barriers to relief. "It is an irony of our age," noted the *Washington Post*, reporting in 1986 on the findings of the expert National Institutes of Health panel led by John Bonica. There were "millions of Americans in hospitals—late-stage cancer patients, burn victims, accident victims—[who] suffer unnecessary, sometimes agonizing pain." For them, doses of narcotic analgesic were too low, and physicians were stingy with relief.

Outside the clinic, in contrast, were "millions more unhospitalized— the numbers cannot be measured accurately—[who are] dangerously overdosing on painkillers often inappropriately prescribed for their chronic pain from headaches, backaches, pinched nerves and arthritis." Fears of addiction to a growing range of painkilling drugs also shadowed relief at every turn, with opioid drugs administered carefully and patients watched closely for signs of dependence. Methadone continued to be a flash point of therapeutic controversy. Even the doctor's dilemma of relief—whether to treat or not to treat, weighing the unintended costs of relief, drawing the line between the deserving pain sufferers and those unworthy of relief, deciding on liberal relief versus conservative care— reflected the political calculations of the day.

By the late 1980s, both political parties courted pain: both said they defended people in true pain, and both claimed the high ground of compassion. The difference was whose pain (among all the sufferers) mattered and was more real, whose carried the greatest political valence, and whose should sit at center stage in social policy. Some pains were more righteous and warranted greater sympathy than others. In Reagan's worldview, the pain of the taxpayer was true pain; the pain of the disabled or the addict was suspect. The pain of the fetus outranked the alleged pain of the disabled housewife or injured worker as a basis for conservative social policy. The Republican argument did not, therefore, dismiss subjective pain outright but instead used the pain debate to define what Reagan saw as essential differences between conservative and liberal commitments and values. Speaking to religious broadcasters at the launch of his 1984 re-election bid, Reagan defended the unborn by citing their pain. Medicine was on his side, he claimed; for the president alleged that doctors also believed that "when the lives of the unborn are snuffed out, they often feel pain—pain that is long and agonizing." Summarizing the ironies of this new turn in pain politics, one commentator noted, "The reactionary right prefers the selective approach . . . If only a portion of his well-directed fervor against abortion were marshaled against the pain that children feel after they are born . . . he could claim to be authentically pro-life."[52]

Pain Polarized

To say that there was a conservative position and a liberal position on pain in the Reagan years ignores many complexities; it accepts too easily the political binary developed and used by Reagan so effectively as a political bludgeon. Liberals like Carter had, in fact, initiated the disability reforms that Reagan's administration developed into a large-scale tool of welfare reform. In this effort, pain (particularly the subjective pain of people like Polaski) became a symbol for Reagan of the dependence, the learned helplessness, and the growth of government that conservatives so detested. Reagan had taken Carter's moderate policies and turned them to a new purpose. In the process, the war on abuse and fraud became an all-out war on people claiming to be in pain—precisely as Carter had warned in 1980. The revolution was as much about those in pain as it was about erasing a liberal pain standard that held too much sway in society.

But the effort to impose a conservative pain standard provoked a fierce Congressional backlash, heightened tensions with the courts, and produced the kinds of relentless litigation that conservatives also bemoaned. On the surface, the legal dispute was about the status of "subjective" pain, but, underneath, the stakes surrounding the pain standard were incredibly high. At stake—for those purged—were questions of life, health, and death. For liberal Democrats, the dilemma was about placing limits on the Reagan revolution, maintaining society's commitments to compassion, recognizing the legitimacy of disabled citizens, and assigning moral and economic meaning to their suffering. For Republicans, at issue was the future of the welfare state. For the courts, the political question became who had the power to judge, as a brash executive branch claimed an authority to govern it did not deserve. By the end of the 1980s and into the 1990s, the battle over pain had turned the vexing clinical question of pain sufferers into one of the most divisive and polarizing political issues of the time. For people in pain, their politicization at the hands of the Reagan revolution was unquestionably one of the most troubling features of conservatism.

Throughout his eight years in office, Reagan railed against the liberal pain standard. Even when he scaled back the harsh rhetoric of his first years in office (embracing compassion in response to the liberal charges of conservatism's heartlessness), he continued to caricature liberal judges and politicians as laughably gullible. Speaking to Republican governors in 1986, he called for "stage two of our revolution" to focus on "setting aside liberal, Democratic governors, fixed by choice and habit alike in their dependence upon Washington." He insisted that "the proliferation of drugs has been part of a crime epidemic that can be traced to, among other things, liberal judges who are unwilling to get tough with the criminal element in this society." He defended his Supreme Court nominee, the conservative judge Robert Bork, by attacking liberal judges: "Many years ago, when he was serving on the Court," the president quipped, the esteemed Judge Cardozo "received a letter from a member of the public, and it read: 'Dear Judge Cardozo, I read in the newspaper that you are a liberal judge. Will you send me $10, as I'm really very hard up. Sincerely . . . I don't have the name."[53] Laughter at the caricature filled the room. The liberals, everyone understood, were too quick to feel the pain of others and so easily duped by cries of anguish that they would empty their own pockets—and the public purse as well. The caricature had lost none of its power, but Democrats created their own caricature in response: Bork was an "extreme" conservative. In the end, the Bork nomination failed, but these stark polarities would endure.

Whose pain mattered? In a harbinger of the pain politics to come in the 1990s, the man Reagan nominated to be his new HHS secretary (replacing Heckler in 1985), Otis Bowen, found himself personally embroiled in an emerging debate—the line between pain relief and euthanasia at the end of life. A midwestern physician, middle-of-the-road Republican, and popular former Kansas governor, Bowen carried his own pain baggage. Six years earlier, his wife had been dying of cancer. Bowen had administered the powerful but still-controversial and unapproved painkiller, DMSO, to her in her final days. He insisted that he had done nothing illegal, appealing to compassion toward the dying. At the time of his wife's death, Bowen struck a libertarian pose, asking, "Why can't [a] dying person, with severe pain, have easy prescription access to it?" Even though he was Reagan's nominee, critics on the religious right accused him of supporting euthanasia and also of being too weak in his stand against abortion. The case reflected how quickly the political stakes of pain and relief could shift. With the Bowen debate, a new kind of issue loomed on the immediate horizon, with the figure of Jack Kevorkian moving pain politics away from fetal pain to the other end of the life course. In the 1990s, anguish in death would push back against pain at the beginning of life as a new issue for a new decade. And here too, as in so many of the American pain debates of the Reagan years, the courts would decide; people in pain, seeking relief, would plead their case before the highest pain judges in the land—the U.S. Supreme Court.[54]

FOUR

Divided States of Analgesia

....

Stand, I pray thee, upon me, and slay me: for anguish is come upon me.

2 SAMUEL 1:9

W hen Sherry Miller turned to Michigan pathologist Jack Kevorkian for relief in 1992 she was in severe pain and living a life of horrible desperation. Like the other people who turned to Kevorkian for help, Miller had a well-documented trail of suffering and physical demise. Diagnosed with multiple sclerosis in 1983, her body was deteriorating steadily. By 1989, she used a wheelchair; often, her father carried her. When she first wrote to Kevorkian in 1990, he encouraged her to seek treatment for the disease and to consult a psychiatrist. By 1991, she had decided to commit suicide—a decision supported by her family. A year later, Kevorkian consented to help her by rigging up a "suicide machine" very much like the one that Janet Adkins, a fifty-four-year-old Portland, Oregon, woman suffering from Alzheimer's disease, had used to end her life in 1990.[1] For these flagrant acts, Kevorkian found himself castigated by doctors, criticized and mocked by the media as Dr. Death, and charged in legal dramas spanning from 1990 to 1999. The questions at the center of the legal storm were these: Was Kevorkian practicing compassionate pain relief as he alleged, or was he committing murder? And what constitutional rights, if any, would be granted to such acts carried out in the name of pain relief?

Among the people Kevorkian helped to die, all their pains differed. Marjorie Wantz's pain contrasted sharply with Miller's, but she too wrote to Kevorkian for help. Wantz suffered from extreme vaginal pain, for which she had undergone nine or ten surgeries. Unrelieved, she contemplated suicide. Caregivers raised questions about her mental competence, but these concerns had already been put to rest by a psychological examination. Wantz had gone to clinics in Cleveland and Detroit as well as to the Mayo Clinic where she was told nothing could be done beyond the pain pills, four times as strong as morphine, she was taking. When she first approached Kevorkian for help, he suggested other therapeutic options, even pointing Wantz to hypnosis. The mystery of her condition was that it was not due to any discernible degenerative disease—as Kevorkian quoted one of her doctors, "It would have been better off to be cancerous, at least in six months you might be dead." For two years, Wantz asked Kevorkian for help in dying, even attempting unsuccessfully once to shoot herself. She wrote, "No doctor can help me anymore. If God won't come to me, I'm going to God. Can't stand it no longer." For her, the only truly effective form of relief from such anguish would be death.

On October 22, 1991, Sherry Miller and Marjorie Wantz committed suicide, together, in a cabin in Michigan. Of the two of them, only Wantz ended up using Kevorkian's device—Miller's veins were, by this point, too weak. Although Kevorkian was not actually present for their deaths, he had openly assisted them in their planning, going so far as to participate in television interviews on their decision beforehand. Later, when he faced state charges over what was becoming known as physician-assisted suicide (PAS), he explained to juries that his aim was not primarily to help Miller die but to relieve her pain. Kevorkian believed that he was on a mission: "my ultimate aim is to make euthanasia a positive experience." His only crime was to give her the means to carry out that compassionate act of self-relief leading to her death. Hearing his pain defense, jury after jury would acquit him, and a fourth case would be declared a mistrial. Only in 1999, under much different circumstances, when he was not allowed to use the pain defense that served him so well through most of the decade, would Kevorkian be convicted.

The suicide machine Kevorkian had invented was simple enough—it first administered a saline solution, then the push of a button precipitated the injection of pentothal (thiopenthal), which slowly induces coma. Adkins had one minute after pressing that button to change her mind. When she did not, another injection of potassium chloride and a muscle relaxant followed, stopping the heart. Death came six to seven minutes later.[2] While controversy flared over the issue of physicians' roles in helping terminally ill patients end their own lives, the awkward, makeshift setup of Kevorkian's apparatus made it a particularly dangerous flash point for those in the pain field: it was eerily similar to the patient-controlled analgesia devices that pain specialists had championed in the 1980s as empowering patients and putting relief into the hands of sufferers. The major difference between the two was the drugs administered and the finality of Kevorkian's brand of relief; for many critics of PAS, Kevorkian and his machine embodied the excesses of liberal pain relief and a moral problem at the heart of liberalism more generally (the inability to distinguish between compassion and murder).

The Wantz and Miller cases, along with the earlier Adkins suicide, launched Kevorkian's notoriety, but they also opened a new chapter in the politics of pain in America—moving this new question of pain relief alongside the other disability and pain issues that already occupied legislatures and courts (chapter 3). Kevorkian's practice caught legislators off guard. Michigan's existing laws were, in fact, unclear about the legality of what he had done—a fact that compelled the state's political and legal establishment to work furiously on new legislation. As the Michigan legislature moved to ban the practice and as courts weighed the constitutionality of the new state laws passed hastily by legislators, prosecutors charged Kevorkian with a range of violations, including murder. Even while on trial, Kevorkian did not relent. He had assisted in twenty-seven suicides before the trial and would participate in another twenty-eight during the case. More criminal charges followed as the jury trial, which began in 1992, continued through 1996. In the end, Kevorkian was acquitted by a jury swayed by the argument that Wantz, Miller, and Adkins had a right to this kind of relief.

Yet, legal, clinical, and political uncertainties expanded in the wake of these pain controversies. For many physicians, pain relief in terminal illness was routine, but it was also widely known that the medications also lowered blood pressure, reduced respiration, and played a role in hastening death. Kevorkian's controversial work pushed this pain relief work into uncharted legal territory, upsetting both liberal trends in regulated, compassionate care and conservative arguments for restraint with his far-reaching libertarian insistence. The legal implications were sweeping. Was this a "mercy machine," as Kevorkian's supporters called it, or a weapon to commit premeditated murder, as prosecutors insisted?[3] Was this man providing true relief or merely exploiting the ambiguous line between compassion and suicide? Were these women innocent dupes, as prosecutors alleged, or brave, free-willed people who had suffered long enough? The case carried political implications as well. Turning old political alliances upside down, disability activists recoiled from Kevorkian, arguing that legalizing his actions opened the door to devaluing people with disabilities—seeing them as more easily expendable. Physicians (particularly pain specialists) inevitably were drawn into the swirling legal and moral debate on suffering, the limits of compassion, and their professional relations with the law. As Kevorkian's case was debated and John Bonica, the seventy-seven-year-old father of pain medicine, lay dying at the Mayo Clinic in 1994, a new fractious era in American politics was emerging. Social divides ran deep, beginning with the question of whether the doctor was an accomplice to a crime or a compassionate friend to people in pain.

For this generation of aging Americans—particularly for baby boomers now in their 50s and contending with the realities of advancing years, infirmity, and death—the issue of relief at the end of life migrated to the political center. To be sure, the moral question of pain relief's limits had always existed. Walking a tortuous line in the 1950s, for example, Pope Pius XII had reconfirmed the Catholic Church's endorsement of pain relief for the terminally ill "even if they [these measures] hasten death," but he had also condemned the practice of outright euthanasia. Decades later, pain relief pushed these moral boundaries again. Publicly practicing deathbed relief on a scale that would never have been imagined before, Kevorkian became a polarizing figure in an era of fractious, morality-based politics.[4] How the PAS story would play out had sweeping implications— for individuals, for the state, and for the law.

If the 1980s had seen "fetal pain" emerge as a flash point of right-wing political discourse (driven by religious activism, abortion politics, and "fetal personhood" claims), then the 1990s opened another cultural and political front in the American pain wars. Now, as if in answer to the right, activists on the political left focused on pain at the other end of the life course—death. In language that was galling to the Religious Right, activists on the left spoke of compassion, death with dignity, and the "right to die" free from pain. Gradually it became obvious that judges and the courts would decide on PAS and pain relief not on ideological grounds but as a constitutional matter of individual liberty. In this battle, established liberal and conservative positions on the use of federal versus state power would be turned on their head. The PAS movement threw American religious conservatives—who had gained a strong hand in the Republican Party and in Congress—on the defensive. In Oregon, for example, a 1994 public referendum that established PAS as state law compelled many in the Republican Party to rethink its long-standing libertarian views on individual freedom and small government, with conservative religious activists (joined by nonpartisan religious figures) turning to the courts to stop the Oregon law.[5] It was a deep irony that the states' freedom from federal oversight that Reagan had so championed now drew the ire of Republicans in national government. As pain politics refractured along partisan lines, pulled to polar ends of the life course, people living and coping with day-to-day chronic pain could only watch as their fight for relief was defined by a new set of controversies in the American political landscape. By decade's end, the constitutional right to relief, the doctor's role, and the state's rights to regulate relief would arrive at the U.S. Supreme Court.

Doctoring and Liberty across Divided States

That pain relief was political practice was not new, particularly for physicians. As we've seen, decades of litigating pain had placed the courts in a position of power to judge suffering and determine the limits of relief, particularly in disability cases. The 1970s and 1980s had also produced a growing role for federal government agencies from the Federal Drug Administration to Health and Human Services to the Drug Enforcement Administration in regulating, adjudicating, and prosecuting the misuse of pain drugs. An expanded war on drugs raised the stakes for doctors who prescribed narcotics for their patients. The expanded role of the courts, the police, government, and politicians in pain management left many physicians deeply frustrated by the oversight, which (in their view) interfered with the doctor's work of relief.

The election of Bill Clinton as president in 1992, with his strong push for health care reform, created a combative climate for all health issues and drew physicians into a growing political fray. The call for reform ignited an old fight with organized medicine, precipitating a record number of doctors to run for political office. As one 1994 report noted, "Republican Party chairman Haley Barbour says it should be no surprise that doctors are leaping into politics. With the president trying to 'blow up' the current health-care system and replace it with a government system, doctors 'understand the threat.' "[6] But unlike in the 1950s, not all doctors shared the American Medical Association's conservative antigovernment outlook. Many supported the Democratic initiative for single-payer insurance. Still others ran on a libertarian platform that rejected what they interpreted as government interference in health care, including regulatory restrictions on pain treatment and PAS. By the time Kevorkian went on trial, a notable group of physicians had begun crossing the divide between medicine and legislation, pushing from several points of view for reform in the name of people in pain.

Consider, for instance, the actions of Stratton Hill, a Texas pain specialist at Houston's M.D. Anderson Cancer Center. After years of being victimized by what he saw as an unforgiving government oversight of pain medicine, Hill sought a political détente. As he put it, "I'm tired of apologizing for using narcotics to treat patients in pain." Like-minded practitioners had been bringing these concerns to state and federal official for years. (In 1980 and 1984, for example, the U.S. Congress heard and rejected appeals to approve heroin as a painkiller for cancer patients.) Using his professional stature at the state's premier cancer center, Hill approached the state legislature in the late 1980s and advocated for new legislation that would allow him to practice aggressive, compassionate care for his patients without fear of prosecution. The law, he believed, should not threaten doctors as it currently did but should instead protect them from prosecution for acts of compassionate care using strong painkillers. He insisted that there were "many cancer patients in pain, especially those with advanced cancer, [who] are not getting enough opiate narcotics to relieve their suffering." In his view, "cultural anti-drug pressure 'intimidates' doctors into prescribing doses that are too small and short-lasting."[7]

Hill saw that physicians and pain sufferers were caught in a punitive cycle of police and government oversight that led doctors to prescribe conservatively and sufferers to distrust those who might help them. Both groups, he argued, needed protection—doctors practiced in fear of prosecution; people in chronic pain lived in a similar state of fear tinged with constant uncertainty. The pain field (absent training, lacking independent judgment, and deficient in specialty knowledge) had become shaped by a particular legal, political, and regulatory context of care, with "many physicians prescrib[ing] narcotics too cautiously for fear of getting in trouble with regulatory agencies that often believe 'narcotic use is bad, no matter what the reason for their use.' "[8] For Hill, legislation offered the best chance of protecting physicians from prosecution and freeing them to relieve pain without fear.

A large part of the problem, Hill argued, was that "most medical schools do a poor job training doctors to treat chronic pain." Too few physicians understood the true relationship of aggressive relief and drug addiction, having never been educated about the low likelihood of one leading to the other. Most practiced conservatively, cautiously meting out narcotics while fearfully watching over their shoulders at regulatory agencies. Seeking pain relief in this setting, Hill insisted, was disastrous for patients: a person who was "inadequately relieved . . . then becomes a clock-watcher, waiting in eager anticipation for the next dose which at least will give some modicum of additional relief." But, in turn, the often odd behavior of the undertreated clock-watcher provoked suspicion and increased surveillance—a vicious cycle. "The clock-watcher," he noted, "is in jeopardy of being labeled a drug addict by his or her caregivers."[9] In this way, the normal behavior of seeking relief had been turned into an apparent pathology. In Hill's view, the lines between political ideology and pain relief practices had already been completely blurred—a state of affairs that had turned doctors and patients into would-be criminals.

Hill found many Texas legislators (in a state then in the midst of a sweeping party realignment) responsive to his request for political help for embattled doctors. Democrats still wielded power in the Texas legislature, but their traditional grip on power was weakening with each election. Chet Brooks, a Democrat from Pasadena, Texas, sponsored a bill drafted with Hill's involvement that sought to "prohibit hospitals and other . . . facilities from restricting the use of such drugs by suffering patients treated by a doctor with staff privileges." Like-minded Democrats controlled the legislature, and Texas's Republican governor, William Clements (the first Republican elected to the governor's mansion since Reconstruction), shared their view of physicians as victims.[10] Supporting the call for reform was a particular Texas cultural ethos, a libertarian impulse on the left and right that decried regulatory barriers. (The state's Twenty-Second Congressional District had elected, only recently, the libertarian obstetrician Ron Paul to national office.) This perspective cut across party lines. Some officials in the legislature no doubt also had their own searing experiences with the undertreatment of chronic pain.

Thus was formed a medical-political alliance around the notion that pain care had become an innocent casualty in the heated "war on drugs"; the Texas legislation aimed to rescue these casualties from the battle-front. Section 5 of the Texas Intractable Pain Treatment Act (IPTA) spoke clearly to doctors' freedom to practice: "no physician may be subject to disciplinary action by the board for prescribing or administering dangerous drugs or controlled substances in the course of treatment of a person for intractable pain." Pain, for the moment, knew no partisanship. Endorsing this freedom to practice from the national vantage point, the national AMA signed on to the Texas reform as well, publishing "Balancing the Response to Prescription Drug Abuse." As Stratton Hill noted, even though the abuse of prescription drugs was a growing concern, the AMA's James Sammons had stated firmly that "the war on drugs should not be a war on patients."[11]

In assisting passage of the 1989 legislation, Hill crossed into politics to produce a legislative reform model that doctors, patients, and legislators in other states might emulate.[12] The IPTA movement was off to a promising start—defying the liberal or conservative pigeonholes of the 1980s politics of pain relief. But from the outset, it remained unclear just how much of an impact the Texas IPTA would have on the character of care. Conservative care was deeply rooted in the profession, shaped by decades of fear of drug addiction and overmedication. The law, by itself, could do little to remove these underlying reasons that doctors practiced conservatively. Physicians, for example, still lacked basic education on pain care, DEA oversight still continued, and state boards still meted out medical punishment for too-aggressive pain care; one legal development could not alter that trend.

In California, doctors and legislators watched the Texas experiment and followed suit. Legislators on the coast were driven by different political impulses. They too sought a middle road between the two feared extremes of narcotic overmedication and pain undertreatment. But in California it was not doctors who drove reform but politicians, speaking for patients, who took charge of the debate. State Assembly representative Richard Polanco knew the topic well. His wife had suffered with chronic pain and had experienced many difficulties obtaining relief. For him and other California legislators, the threat of undertreatment demanded a legislative response. By the fall of 1990, moderate Republican governor George Deukmejian signed the state's own Intractable Pain Act, which like the Texas law had libertarian overtones and protected physicians from unwarranted intrusion by federal and state regulatory agencies in the treatment of chronic pain with federally controlled substances. But, even after the passage of California's IPTA in 1990, the legislature's concerns about undertreatment persisted.[13]

Still frustrated by the pace of change in 1992, another California state senator, Leroy Greene, organized hearings at the state Capitol in October of that year in response to doctors' continuing complaints that the regulatory climate had not improved. At the Greene hearings, physicians and patients insisted that the law had not altered physicians' prescribing behavior, and they still encountered problems with prescribing and obtaining controlled substances for chronic pain. The state medical board disagreed, maintaining that no such problems existed. Seeking once again to find balance between the extremes of overtreatment and undermedication, California's new Republican governor, Pete Wilson, appointed a former Republican Assembly representative, Dixon Arnett, to head a medical board studying the issues. Encouraged also by Greene, Arnett established a task force that in November 1993 acknowledged what many physicians and patients already knew—that the undertreatment of chronic pain was a much greater problem than the so-called excessive prescribing others had feared.

The fact that identically named intractable pain treatment acts had passed in states with two distinct political traditions, Texas and California, is both revealing and misleading—for pain relief had overlapping yet particular political meanings in the two places. In both states, reform was driven by common concerns among doctors and patients of undertreatment. But in California's pain politics, in contrast to Texas's libertarian suspicion of government oversight, debate was moved by the political

Left. Already by 1991, the drive for pain relief on the West Coast had a more radical edge, foreshadowing a new set of political challenges to come.

For Californians, the undertreatment concern appeared alongside another issue that lacked traction in Texas politics—physician-assisted suicide. Indeed, in 1991, the same year that Republican Pete Wilson succeeded Deukmejian as the state's governor, citizens had gone to the polls to vote on the controversial Proposition 161, Physician Assisted Suicide. Moreover (as in Washington and Oregon but unlike in Texas), California's drive for aggressive relief was also informed by popular pressure in a state where referenda and direct democracy defined the political landscape—practices for which the state had become widely known since the People's Initiative to Limit Property Taxation (tax revolt) in 1978. California's pain politics thus sat far to the political left of Texas's and much closer to Oregon—a state that was, at this moment, also voting on PAS.

In 1991, a coalition of religious groups successfully beat back the California PAS Proposition 161, spending large sums to defeat it by 54 to 46 percent. Ironically, the PAS defeat accentuated the need for compromise pain relief legislation, for, if deadly relief was not politically possible, then surely more moderate relief should be embraced. Even for opponents of physicians helping terminally ill people to die, compassionate care stopping short of euthanasia became all the more urgent to redirect the desperation of people who believed that suicide was their only answer to pain. Reforming pain care was crucial to keeping suicide off the ballot again. So it was that pain relief and PAS connected—with the two seen on the left as conjoined, as part of the fight for compassionate care and dignity in death, and the two seen as distinct on the right, with the reform of pain care understood as a way to short-circuit the popular drive for PAS. After PAS's defeat, the same group that ran the successful campaign against Proposition 161, Cavalier and Associates, now formed the California Pain Management Coalition; it was this group that now worked with Assembly representative Richard Polanco when he introduced a pain relief bill calling for a pain management committee within the attorney general's office to advise doctors on these increasingly complex pain matters.

With pain relief now a multifaceted political, legal, and moral conundrum in California, a March 1994 Los Angeles pain summit was organized with Senator Greene in attendance, along with experts from medicine, nursing, pharmaceutical manufacturing, and law enforcement from all over the country. As in other times, politicians again took up the question of who was in pain and what relief they warranted. Through pain, Californians debated hierarchies of deservedness, the limits of social compassion, and patients' rights. Most observers agreed, for example, that the cancer patient was the most worthy of aggressive relief. The easiest political case was cancer and terminal illness, where almost everyone agreed that, in principle, addiction should never be an impediment to aggressive pain relief. But if the aggressiveness of relief should depend on the gravity of the condition, then who should judge severity? The pain summit's report, released July 1994, focused on the "rights" to be pain free—stating vaguely that patients had the right to be relieved of their pain. The summit report went even further, however, implying a doctor's duty to relieve suffering: "we should create by statute a positive legal duty for physicians to relieve pain." These were not merely semantic distinctions but also legal recommendations. Three years earlier a North Carolina jury had paid close attention to these distinctions, awarding $15 million in damages to the family of a nursing home patient denied opioid medication who then died painfully with prostate cancer. As legal scholar Ben Rich noted, the jury concluded that the "nurse's refusal to administer the opioid analgesics necessary to relieve Mr. James's pain, on the rationale that he would become addicted, constituted a gross departure from acceptable care." In such state settings, the question of relief (granted or denied) was being reframed as a legal question of malpractice, as a moral question of medical duty, and as a political question of patients' rights.[14]

Fearing threats from prosecutors on one side and from undertreated patients on the other, pain doctors faced a dilemma: with whom would they align? In the late 1980s and early 1990s, some charted a more confrontational approach on the policing of relief. While Hill chose political compromise, others, like William Hurwitz, tempted prosecution with his aggressive relief practices. In September 1991 the DEA entered Hurwitz's practice in the District of Columbia and arrested him. Hurwitz had prescribed as much as 500 milligrams a day of oxycodone for a patient suffering with hip-bone deterioration. Where 20 milligrams was the norm, the patient had built up a tolerance over time for the drug. The DEA claimed that such high dosages could only be used recreationally, but pain advocates insisted that people like Hurwitz's patient did not become "high" on the drug—the high dosage was necessary simply for the patient to function normally. Hurwitz saw the legal oversight of pain medicine as a travesty. He wrote later, "I was charged with having prescribed excessive doses of opioid analgesics in the treatment of thirty patients who, it was acknowledged by the Board of Medicine, had conditions causing intractable pain." Along with Hill, he saw himself and his patients as victimized—not only by prosecutors but also by medical boards who had grown timid and sensitive to political pressure—and ignorant of the details of pain relief and addiction. The medical board "hearing might well be characterized as a Kafkaesque inquisition," he insisted. "This was not anything close to an open-minded search for the truth in which legal adversaries present evidence before an impartial finder-of-fact. This Board thought it knew from the outset what constituted proper pain management, and it thought it knew that the high doses of medication I prescribed to many of my patients were illegitimate and without clinical rationale."[15] Doctors in other states across the country faced similar threats. Elsewhere, at New York University, Ronald Blum, the university's chief of oncology faced charges (later dismissed) "by narcotic agents for alleged overprescribing of Diluadid to his cancer patients."[16] Facing such oversight, nurturing a powerful sense of victimization, and feeling abandoned even by their own profession, pain doctors like Hurwitz worked in one of the most politicized and legally contentious realms of medicine.

Hurwitz's anger about miseducation and defensive medicine among his fellow professionals was well founded. National surveys and studies of physicians found widespread confusion among state medical boards over pain and addiction theories—with limited understanding of the differences among concepts like drug tolerance, drug dependence, and drug addiction and with legal self-protection foremost in their minds rather than patient care. Even as late as 2002, a survey of 627 state medical board members across the country found that "while most respondents agreed that the prescribing of opioids for the cancer patient was legal and generally acceptable medical practice, only 12 percent were confident in the legality of prescribing for the patient with chronic non-cancer pain; the majority of respondents (77 percent) would discourage this practice or even investigate it as a violation of law." In other words, the legal and political environment convinced most board members to see themselves as would-be prosecutors rather than defenders of relief. As Hurwitz insisted, in this environment his patients "were treated like addicts and criminals. They were stigmatized, insulted, neglected and abandoned. [They were] betrayed by the whole medical profession with the refrain, 'I would like to help you, but I can't. I don't want to lose my license.'" Doctors, he argued, were not treated any better than patients; "who can blame the doctors, who are themselves the victims of the thuggish drug-control police and the heartless and mindless bureaucrats who serve on boards of medicine[?]"[17] What was a physician to do in this surveillance-intensive context?

In Oregon, emergency room physician John Kitzhaber pursued another course from Hill's in Texas or Hurwitz's in D.C.—running for office, rising to become president of the state senate in 1989, and eventually pushing through the state's controversial and pioneering Oregon Health Plan (focused on rationing) and its Death with Dignity legislation. He also eyed the governorship. It was a strategy Hill would have endorsed. As Hill later wrote, "Physicians should strive to change social attitudes toward pain control with narcotics by enlisting the support of colleagues and, if necessary, by political activism." Physician practice, he believed, was constrained by legal intimidation: "There is a lack of evidence of a clear, direct relationship in the United States between laws and regulations governing drugs and adequacy of pain control. However, anecdotal reports indicate [that there is] implied, and in rare cases, real, intimidation of physicians by drug regulatory agencies and medical licensing boards." What was needed, he believed, was to bring pain statutes into agreement across the states to insure uniformity of care and to remove legal threats to doctors, which continued to be the nemesis of relief: "It is necessary to standardize and define the language in our statutes, especially state statutes, so as to remove the vagueness and ambiguities that intimidate physicians using narcotics for pain control."[18]

Once the doors to legislative action on pain had been opened by doctors like Hill, Kitzhaber, and others, it proved impossible to shut them again. By aligning themselves with elected officials to improve pain medicine, reformers like Hill were betting that the political currents would continue to be on their side. But what if the winds of reform started blowing not in the direction of protecting doctors and liberalizing compassionate care but in the direction of even stiffer oversight and prosecution? What if a more conservative mind-set on pain relief came to prevail in the 1990s? This unanticipated situation is precisely what happened as states and the federal government looked with alarm at Michigan's Jack Kevorkian and at Oregon's 1994 referendum on physician-assisted suicide. These events shattered whatever tenuous détente had been achieved around compassionate pain relief in Texas's and California's IPTA laws.

Like Stratton Hill, Jack Kevorkian refused to apologize for aggressive, compassionate care; but Kevorkian was not a team player like Hill. He sought no political allies and brooked no compromises. A man with a single-minded fascination with death, he felt betrayed by his own profession. By the mid-1990s, Dr. Death and death with dignity took center stage in the American pain debate. In the wake of Kevorkian's actions and, more importantly, with the legal debate unfolding over the Oregon law came a profound challenge to the social norms of pain relief and to the state's and federal government's power to regulate it.[19]

Between Mercy and Murder: Kevorkian's Pain Defense

For many opponents of physician-assisted suicide, morphine administered at the end of life could be nothing more than covert euthanasia; it was, in short, yet another perversion of liberal compassion: murder masquerading as relief. But where was the line between premeditated assisted suicide, bordering on murder, and merciful, liberal compassion? What limits, if any, should society place on self-determination in relief? These were the moral and legal questions put to the Kevorkian jury—questions without clear answers that cast a dark shadow over all patients in pain and practitioners of pain medicine. As the PAS debate entered the courts in the 1990s, it skewed the politics of pain anew; for now opponents tainted pain relief not only as costly and counterproductive but also as the thin end of the wedge leading to moral depravity. Kevorkian stood in for these fears, his trial accentuating the suspicion that all kinds of evil would be conducted under the guise of pain relief. The vagueness of existing statutes, legal precedent, professional guidelines, and popular opinions on matters of such gravity also created legal havoc—driving the question of pain squarely into legislatures and the courts where ques-

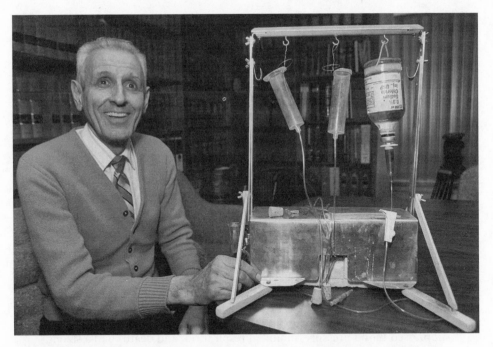

FIGURE 4.1. Dr. Jack Kevorkian poses with his "suicide machine," crossing the politically contentious line between compassionate pain relief, euthanasia, and murder (Michigan, February 6, 1991).

Photo by Richard Sheinwald. Image courtesy of the Associated Press.

tions of morality, murder, compassion, and pain relief would be weighed together.

When Kevorkian invented and first used his suicide machine in 1990, it embodied a brash political statement aimed at his fellow practitioners. He explained that he was "trying to knock the medical profession into accepting its responsibilities, and those responsibilities include assisting their patients with death."[20] On trial, however, he spoke of people's pain, using successfully what became known as the "pain defense." As he saw matters, the medical profession's key defect was its failure to soothe compassionately, particularly people suffering at the end of life. His repeated courtroom defense—that he was only trying to relieve excruciating, interminable pain and that, in the course of doing so, his patients died—made a powerful moral appeal to the sympathy of jurors and judges. In his defense, he consistently and successfully blurred the lines between pain relief and euthanasia; one merged seamlessly into the other.

After the initial dismissal of charges in Adkins's death on grounds that prosecutors failed to show that Kevorkian (and not Adkins) had carried out the acts leading to her death, Kevorkian was retried after the deaths of Wantz and Miller. In these and other acquittals, juries saw the case for PAS in terms of pain relief and the freedom to choose. In privileging pain relief in their decisions, juries voiced a popular sentiment. They accepted that Kevorkian was driven by compassion and concern for pain; he acted as a doctor. As one legal scholar noted, "We take it as obvious that the three prosecutions and acquittals of Dr. Kevorkian fit the classic model of political trials in the Anglo-American tradition where juries, either in the space created by ambiguous legal rules or by exercising their nullifying power, speak powerfully for community sentiment."

Observers highlighted other important features of the case—Kevorkian had become something of a "moral entrepreneur" in the field of assisted suicide.[21] His argument for compassion and pain relief (even if it led to suppressed blood pressure, inhibited respiration, and death) had a strong appeal not only in the courtroom but also in broader society. Here was a new form of relief going well beyond disability benefits for a new era in a society where citizens were living longer than ever, where economic prosperity meant avid consumption of life-sustaining medicines, and yet where degenerative diseases persisted for people in their fifties, sixties, and seventies. Marjorie Wantz, age fifty-eight, was born in 1933. Janet Adkins, age fifty-four, was born in 1936. Sherri Miller was born in 1948; she was forty-three years old. They were a cohort whose birth straddled the Second World War and who constituted the leading edge of the baby boom; they had known the comforts of the postwar, consumer-oriented society. They had been avid consumers of much that American medicine had to offer from surgery to psychiatry; but now they were grappling with the best way to leave this life. It is not too much to say that, for this generation, death with dignity had a powerful appeal not as a giving up on medicine but as a continuation of what many Americans had come to expect regarding citizens' right to relief, personal liberty, and medical and consumer freedom. Kevorkian's pain defense (the notion that pain relief was ethically defensible medical practice even when it precipitated death) was successful with judges and jurors, as it had been perhaps ironically with Pope Pius in the 1950s.

In his defense, Kevorkian drew on an old principle in religion, ethics, and pain relief put to new legal use. The so-called principle of double effect, which had deep origins in Catholic ethics with the writings of Thomas Aquinas and which had been revived with the rise of bioethics, revolved around whether one could engage in evil acts in pursuit of the good. Applied to pain medicine, the principle acknowledged that it was nearly impossible to disentangle the good act of compassionate pain management from the evil of putting another person to death, especially when pain drugs also lowered respiration and possibly hastened death. The concept defined a moral ambiguity at the heart of relief. The question of where compassion becomes killing slowly attained powerful cultural and legal resonance not only in Kevorkian's case but also in many others. In issuing his opinion on Kevorkian's earliest murder charge, Circuit Judge David Breck, for example, saw the long-term excruciating pain of Kevorkian's patients (and his work ending "lives of horrible desperation") as a crucial factor in dismissing charges. In much the same way that gate control theory catalyzed social change in the 1970s or the way theories of learned helplessness shaped disability social policies in the 1980s, so too the theory of pain used in Kevorkian's defense— compassion that led as a consequence to death—became a flash point for controversy. Disentangling the two issues, pain relief and end-of-life care, became a crucial subject for interest groups across a wide political spectrum.[22]

The principle of double effect had dangerous implications for pain professionals, for it fed into PAS opponents' view that the entire field of pain management was a closeted form of Kevorkian-style euthanasia. Opponents now sought to squash any practices even remotely resembling PAS; but others who objected to PAS took another route, realizing that, to undercut the market for Dr. Death's services, they must embrace a more liberal style of pain medicine. In this view, desperate people in pain needed better relief and "safe harbors" for care precisely so that they would not rely on the likes of Kevorkian. Thus did PAS provoke a new round of legislative activity on pain reform, and in the aftermath of Kevorkian's 1996 acquittal, legislators in Michigan "introduced a package of pain management bills aimed at cutting the market for Dr. Jack Kevorkian's services." Similarly, in Florida, as the trial was underway, the legislature took up an intractable pain treatment act that specified that "nothing in this section shall be construed to condone, authorize, or approve mercy killing or euthanasia, and no treatment authorized by this section may be used for such purpose." Florida's IPTA statute was passed in 1995, creating a safe harbor while also cautioning doctors against crossing the line to PAS. The emerging question—now fully engaged in state legislatures and by ethicists, physicians, patients, and the public across the country—was how to comfort the ailing, how to bring peace at the end of life, without allowing doctors to be accomplices to crime.[23]

With systemic undertreatment of pain now well documented, a medical consensus for reform emerged—but what kind of reform? PAS advocates charged that people in pain were turning to suicide because doctors were so fearful of prosecution for practicing compassionate pain relief. Ironically, PAS opponents also mobilized behind this view, coming to see the value of liberalizing pain relief for people in chronic pain. For his part, Kevorkian was not entirely isolated in pushing the boundaries of acceptable legal pain relief. In December 1996, reviewing the details of the case against Dr. Hurwitz, the television program *60 Minutes* illustrated the continuing paradox of relief—people in intractable pain, with inadequate access to pain medicines, choosing suicide as their better option. The *60 Minutes* exposé featured Hurwitz, Hill, and a video taped by Hurwitz's patient the day before he committed suicide. In the video, the patient clearly laid out his calculations, "explaining that he would rather live with pain medication, but couldn't go on living without it." Fear that other doctors might follow Kevorkian's or Hurwitz's example pushed palliation to political center stage, turning the legislators' growing fear of Dr. Death to the pain specialist's advantage. But, even with modest legislative attention to improving pain care, most pain specialists could not avoid being tainted by any association with Kevorkian and his pain defense. In the glare of politics, many specialists were pressed to explain and defend themselves. A New York State task force, for example, concluded in 1994 that there was no good reason to rethink the state's ban on physician-assisted suicide, but it also felt compelled to insist that the "effort to characterize pain relief at end of life as euthanasia is mistaken."[24]

Kevorkian, meanwhile, did himself and the cause of liberalizing relief no favors. As opponents of the Oregon law successfully pushed a repeal of the Death with Dignity law onto the state ballot and as the courts weighed the limits of PAS in several states, the single-minded Kevorkian pushed PAS to an absurd new level—well beyond his ability to defend his actions on the basis of compassion. In September 1998, he would videotape himself administering a lethal injection himself, rather than allowing the patient to do so—once again daring authorities to charge him. The fact that he administered the medicine himself and recorded it changed the stakes; from the legal perspective, he had strengthened the state's case for a murder charge. Further complicating his defense, his license to practice medicine had been revoked eight years earlier. When he went to trial this time, it would be for second-degree murder, and the rules for such a trial gave him no room to invoke the pain defense. The grandstanding doctor also foolishly chose to represent himself in court. Prohibited by the judge from telling the jury the horrible pain and desperation of his patient (details deemed irrelevant to the murder charge), Kevorkian had dramatically increased the likelihood of being convicted on murder charges. In April 1999, a jury found him guilty and sentenced the pathologist to ten to twenty-five years in prison.

By the late 1990s, it was also clear that the political Left was fracturing on the question of PAS, with disability activists lined up solidly against the practice. As early as the late 1980s, disability scholar Paul Longmore had warned, "I don't think it's far-fetched or paranoid to assume that these same suicide rights advocates will use this law to push for significant expansions. They don't just want it for the terminally ill. They have a very broad agenda." On the right as well, the politics of pain was fracturing conservatives—with the religious wing of the Right developing an aggressive belief in the role of the federal government in challenging the state's right to determine the character of relief. As one antiabortion advocate noted, *Roe v. Wade* had opened the way to this new travesty: abortion rights "was a precedent for killing people, and its impact has gone far beyond abortion," said Marie Dietz. "We had warned years ago that euthanasia would be the next step."[25] Thus did the culture wars suggest new alliances around people in pain. With Oregon squarely in their sights, religious conservatives in national government (in Congress and later the White House) would reject their own party's longstanding skepticism regarding federal power in shaping state social policy on these contentious moral questions of the day.

Ultimate Relief: The Supreme Court, Oregon, and Death with Dignity

The PAS debate became to 1990s cultural politics what abortion had been two decades earlier, but where abortion mostly unified right and left against one another, PAS was a more fractious issue within each political party. On this topic, the Religious Right parted company with small government conservatives, and disability rights advocates split from the mainstream Left. For the courts, PAS also became a major test of citizens' constitutional rights, raising new questions similar to the way privacy rights and abortion rights were conjoined.[26] As the courts looked closely at PAS, an entirely new legal and constitutional terrain came into view: Was medically induced death a constitutional right? Was it legally acceptable as a corollary to aggressive relief? Did doctors have a moral obligation or a legal duty to relieve pain? If the line between pain relief and euthanasia was unclear medically, could the law draw the distinction any more clearly? And what level of government should make such relief policies—the Congress, state legislatures, the people of Oregon? These were among the major constitutional questions that now spiraled off from the new practices of pain relief.

Because divisions across the states on pain policies were so profound, a crucial issue before the federal courts concerned not only the individual's right to self-relief but also federalism. Could each state chart its own course in such matters, or should national law claim precedence?[27] Was there such a thing as a constitutional right to pain relief, akin perhaps to the right to privacy that the liberal Burger court had endorsed in *Roe v. Wade*? What began as trials of a few outlandish doctors soon raised the possibility that pain relief might actually be an American right—and such a question could only be ruled upon in the higher courts.

Beyond Kevorkian in Michigan, liberal-leaning West Coast states were having a profound impact on relief politics. In Washington, Oregon, and California, popular democracy movements pushed these three diverse states to establish new rights in flagrant opposition to the federal government—particularly with regard to the use of drugs to bring relief. In 1988 the California-based Americans against Human Suffering attempted (but failed) to place a PAS bill on the ballot—the first attempt in the United States to legalize assisted suicide through a referendum. Four years later, in 1992, California advocates succeeded in getting the initiative (Proposition 161) on the ballot. But that November voters rejected it. Oregon advocates then took up the challenge, putting their own death with dignity law before the voters in 1994. It allowed physicians to prescribe, but not to administer, lethal doses of drugs for patients who had less than six months to live, who had been deemed mentally competent, and who chose death voluntarily in front of witnesses. Also on the ballot in 1994 was a gubernatorial race featuring legislator and physician John Kitzhaber—who had helped establish the Oregon Health Plan—as the leading candidate. His election by a 51 percent vote mirrored the outcome on the PAS referendum (also 51 percent). Kitzhaber stepped into office amid a tidal wave of national interest in PAS and the Oregon law. But, with the law's passage came a strong legal backlash as opponents challenged its constitutionality.[28] The law's implementation would be rocky and now depended on the federal courts.

The 1994 referendum—standing in direct conflict, for example, with federal laws against the misuse of barbiturates—set up a pitched (and still ongoing) battle between the states and the federal government over the control of drug policy and the limits of pain relief. The Oregon law also put physicians and pain sufferers who followed its guidelines at increased risk of federal prosecution. Appeals by opponents of the referendum put the 1994 law on hold, and in 1997 the people of Oregon were compelled to vote a second time on a new PAS referendum. Only a year earlier, California had continued pushing for state sovereignty in such matters, endorsing the use of medical marijuana and passing Proposition 215 (Compassionate Use Act of 1996) "to ensure that seriously ill Californians have the right to obtain and use marijuana" for a variety of ailments including "cancer . . . , AIDS, chronic pain . . . , arthritis, migraine, or any other illness for which marijuana provides relief." A year later, when the people of Oregon approved the PAS referendum a second time (overcoming the remaining legal obstacles), the law finally took effect. These developments crystallized the tension between the state law and federal law. For the DEA, federal law prohibited physicians from prescribing controlled drugs for the purposes of suicide; physicians who practiced PAS risked losing their licenses.[29] Despite the tensions over enforcement and jurisdiction, Oregon pressed ahead with implementing the law—even as the Supreme Court decided to hear a case on PAS coming out of Washington State.

In these divided states of analgesia, while many Americans were transfixed by Michigan's legal circus and the political drama in Oregon, in Washington a physician named Harold Glucksberg launched a lawsuit that would ultimately bring these considerations over who should control relief before the U.S. Supreme Court. Glucksberg had challenged the state's 1979 ban on PAS quietly, arguing that the law was unconstitutional in relation to the Fourteenth Amendment's due process clause. In 1992 a district court agreed with Glucksberg, finding Washington's ban unconstitutional. In March 1994, the case was argued before the U.S. Court of Appeals, Ninth Circuit. Two years later, the court issued an opinion that saw PAS not as a test of liberal compassion per se but as a problem of liberty and due process. The majority found: "Heated though the debate may be, we must determine whether and how the United States Constitution applies to the controversy before us, a controversy that may touch more people more profoundly than any other issue the courts will face in the foreseeable future." The Ninth Circuit found in favor of Dr. Glucksberg, swayed by considerations of self-determination and individual liberty. The justices concluded that "a liberty interest exists in the choice of how and when one dies, and that the provision of the Washington statute banning assisted suicide, as applied to competent, terminally ill adults who wish to hasten their deaths by obtaining medication prescribed by their doctors, violates the Due Process Clause." This was, in the circuit court's view, not an issue for governments but for individuals to decide. "By permitting the individual to exercise the right to choose we are following the constitutional mandate to take such decisions out of the hands of the government, both state and federal, and to put them where they rightly belong, in the hands of the people."[30]

The Circuit court's affirmation of the rights of the people over that of the state was quickly appealed to the U.S. Supreme Court, with the battle lines now drawn between what many saw as moral polarities—liberals embracing compassion and permissiveness toward drugs and the dying on the one hand and religious conservatives' defending of the sanctity of life on the other. Pain politics was also defined by moral perversity. As the Drug Reform Coalition Network saw it, "the enemies in the battle for pain relief [were also] state medical boards and the Drug Enforcement Administration." For this advocacy group—fiercely dedicated to liberalizing drug laws—the *Hurwitz* case, the *Kevorkian* cases, the *Glucksberg* case, and many others were examples of the war on drugs run amok. As they saw the situation, caught in the decades-long moral panic around drugs, people in pain were being offered a shocking choice—limited access to pain medicines yet legal recourse to suicide if the laws backed by the PAS movement succeeded. As one of Hurwitz's patients, a prominent attorney, wrote about the drug wars, "The chilling effect this type of action has on the willingness of *any* physician to provide legitimate treatment for persons with chronic pain cannot be overstated." The irony of PAS from this perspective was that it promised to give patients "the right to unobstructed assisted suicide by the federal courts, but no right to a decent quality of life by any as-yet recognized body of law."[31]

As the *Glucksberg* case moved forward, physicians and state boards heard increasing criticism about their profound lack of knowledge about pain and its proper management; indeed, for some observers, medicine's own failure to think carefully about compassionate care had opened the way to these desperate measures. This was Kevorkian's argument. Feeling abandoned by a profession that did not "feel their pain," patients had turned to him. Stung by these criticisms, state medical boards became aggressive policy makers in the Kevorkian era. In October 1996, the California State Board of Pharmacy, for example, became the first such board to issue regulations detailing the proper use of opiates in pain management. A year later, all of the state medical boards convened nationally to write new rules on pain management. The guidelines sought to help doctors navigate the politically charged terrain, to help them "comply with acceptable pain management standards and . . . help DEA and other regulators determine whether such treatment is appropriate under the circumstances." At the same time, the guidelines tried to "help ensure patient access to needed controlled substances for pain management." It was precisely in this context that researcher David Joranson, a pain policy specialist in Wisconsin, commented that the increasing trend toward pain doctors working with legislators on pain legislation (starting with Hill in Texas in 1989) had turned out to be a double-edged sword. Physicians were not seizing control; rather, they were ceding authority on pain to activists, elected officials, and the courts. "Opening the door to legislative action on medical issues requires careful consideration," David Joranson noted. "This process is political and complex, and its outcomes are difficult to foresee."[32] But in truth, however, the pain debate had sat firmly in the realm of politics and law for some time, with physicians constantly struggling for relevance in the debate over liberal relief and conservative care.

Now the question of pain and ultimate relief was in the courts. How would the Supreme Court's nine justices rule on Dr. Glucksberg and, by extension, the practice of physician-assisted suicide? The court took up both the *Glucksberg* case alongside another from New York, *Vacco v. Quill*, where physician Timothy Quill and two other physicians had charged that New York's ban on PAS was inconsistent with the state's legal recognition of the right to refuse life-saving treatment.[33] How would it reconcile the lower courts' diverse viewpoints? In *Compassion in Dying v. Washington*, the Ninth Circuit had ruled that "compassion is a proper, desirable, even necessary component of judicial character; but [it is] . . . certainly not the sole law of human existence. Unrestrained by other virtues . . . it leads to catastrophe. Justice, prudence, and fortitude are necessary too." Ohio's Supreme Court had ruled in 1996 that physician assisted suicide was not a crime. In Florida, one court found that a privacy provision in the state constitution gave individuals the right to physician-assisted suicide. But the Florida State Supreme Court had overturned that ruling, finding that the state's constitution gave no such right. In Michigan, meanwhile, the courts and legislature were still feverishly grappling with Kevorkian's disconcerting work. Oregonians were in limbo, preparing to vote a second time on PAS. And now the nine Supreme Court justices were to reconcile these conflicts and to decide on the constitutional questions of pain and ultimate relief for all Americans.[34]

In many ways, the justices were a microcosm of the shifting political fault lines and tilt toward conservatism that had come to define American society by the 1990s. They were led by the arch-conservative William Rehnquist, who had been appointed to the liberal Burger court by President Nixon. For years, Rehnquist was in the minority, but, as the political currents shifted and gave conservatives power in Washington, the balance of the court had swung. The court tilted decidedly in Rehnquist's direction with President Reagan's appointment of Sandra Day O'Connor in 1981, who was increasingly seen as the conservative swing vote on a host of hot-button issues—affirmative action, abortion rights, discrimination law, and so on. Around the time of O'Connor's appointment, one astute author observed that "during the early days of the New Deal, it was the liberals who made the sharpest attacks on the courts and the conservatives who were the judiciary's strongest defenders." Then later the "conservatives and the right wing found the Warren Supreme Court an anathema," and now with O'Connor's nomination it is the liberals' turn again to be alarmed.[35] With Rehnquist's ascendance to chief justice in 1986 (nominated by Reagan), his court now left liberals anxious about how it would rule on affirmative action, voting rights, state's rights, federal powers, and the reach of government to safeguard the health and welfare of its citizens.

As the PAS and pain debates entered the high courts, the issue complicated and confused the lines between conservatism and liberalism. For one thing, PAS energized libertarian elements on both the left and the right, groups often at odds with Catholics and Protestants in their own parties. For many on the left and right, the strong libertarian and states' rights claims underpinning PAS were shockingly at odds with their liberal and conservative moral commitments. Perhaps the most notably political shift born of the PAS debate was this: classically conservative beliefs about states' freedom from government and individual self-determination—beliefs once at the heart of 1970s and 1980s neoconservatism—now seemed to align with liberals in Oregon, California, and left-leaning states. Liberals held up PAS proudly as a state's rights issue. But here, religious conservatives parted company with older conservative ideals. As historian Daniel Rodgers said of the late twentieth century's "age of fracture," here was a new political climate distinct from the 1960s, 1970s, and even the 1980s, in which one party's "arguments poached on parallel debates around them, reworking their claims and concepts . . . for new occasions."[36] If political advantage could be gained for PAS and medical marijuana, for example, liberal Oregonians and Californians happily championed states' rights (an old conservative appeal in the eras of big liberal government). In these ways, the PAS debate in the courts revealed the subtle remaking of political positions—as liberals embraced Oregon's right to legislate compassionate care, while religious conservatives looked to federal law to stop this trend toward liberty and free expression. The PAS cases showed how difficult it was to fix pain relief neatly with the political labels—liberal, conservative, libertarian.

The Supreme Court justices easily, almost casually, dismissed the issue of whether a person had a constitutional "right to die"; all nine justices agreed that the U.S. Constitution granted no such right. But the question of a right to be pain free at the end of life took much more effort to tease apart. Pain relief at the end of life sat precariously in the gray zone of liberty. No justice wanted to endorse pain relief if it were merely a ruse for allowing covert euthanasia, but no justice wished for people to suffer because of a heartless denial of care. On this topic, the court took its guide from an amicus brief filed by the AMA laying out pain theory and the double effect principle. The AMA stood firmly against PAS as inconsistent with the duties, ethics, and core principles of medicine, but the association hedged on the matter of aggressive pain management near the end of life. Drawing on the same principle used by Jack Kevorkian, the AMA told the court, "The recognition that physicians should provide patients pain medication sufficient to ease their pain, even where that may serve to hasten death, is *vital* to ensuring that no patient suffer from physical pain."[37] The justices of the Supreme Court accepted this logic and followed suit, using the double effect principle to demarcate the middle ground of righteous medicine.

Rehnquist—who had suffered severe back pain for years and who (in the 1970s) had become addicted to a sedative and hypnotic drug Placidyl—wrote the majority opinion on the *Glucksberg* case, with Scalia, Kennedy, and Thomas concurring. All were on the Court's right, having been nominated between 1986 and 1991 by Republican presidents (Ronald Reagan and his successor George H. W. Bush), yet their views did not necessarily echo conservative ideology. The court's remaining justices (Breyer, Ginsburg, Souter, and Stevens), who except for Souter and Stevens had been appointed by Democratic presidents, also agreed that no constitutional right to PAS existed. But the two blocs differed on the rationale and thus wrote separate concurrent opinions. Meanwhile, in addition to siding with the majority, O'Connor—the court's quintessential swing justice—wanted her own independent say. So although she signed on to Rehnquist's statement, O'Connor wrote her own opinion—joined now by Ginsburg and Breyer. More than any of the opinions, it would be hers that received attention, for it seemed to indicate where the middle of the court stood on this question of pain relief as a constitutional right and how the court might rule in the future should the PAS issue come before it again.[38]

Echoing an individual liberty and states' rights outlook championed by small-government conservatives, O'Connor quoted from her earlier opinion in the case of Nancy Cruzan, which had established the right of competent persons to control when their own life support was terminated. There, she noted that "the . . . challenging task of crafting appropriate procedures for safeguarding . . . liberty interests is entrusted to the 'laboratory' of the States . . . in the first instance." This statement suggested that, while the court denied individuals a constitutional "right" to physician-assisted suicide, it would not impede Oregon from creating one at the state level. Accepting the AMA's principle of double effect, she also wrote definitively, "There is no dispute that dying patients in Washington and New York can obtain palliative care, even when doing so would hasten their deaths." The ruling was read as a statement—as close as the courts had ever come—acknowledging, if not a right to die, then a right to relief at the end of life. As one legal observer noted, "Justices Breyer and O'Connor [and Ginsburg] . . . are saying in effect (and quite possibly this view has the support of a majority of the Court) that if a state were to prohibit the administration of pain relief desperately needed by a patient if and when the increased dosage of medication is highly likely to bring about death, they would want to revisit the law of death and dying and consider whether such a restriction on pain relief is constitutionally permissible."[39]

But the effort to rewrite the laws on death, dying, and pain would not end with the court's 1997 *Glucksberg* ruling, nor would politicizing pain in the Congress and states subside; the stakes were far too high for that. Ruling before Oregonians had a chance to vote again on PAS in November 1997, the Supreme Court invited debate on the topic to continue—which it did. That year, nine states considered legislation banning assisted suicide; eleven introduced bills authorizing it. The high court wished to see these battles play out. When the dust settled in the states, Oregon stood alone; no other state had joined in legalizing PAS. The court preferred this approach—to let the people of the states decide the parameters of pain relief. Emboldened now by the court, states also took up an array of pain bills, with pain as a continuing proxy for the cultural battles on the left and right.[40]

When Oregon's Death with Dignity law went into effect, a new era of lawful relief had opened—albeit in one small corner of the nation and only for a small subset of patients on the fringes of the large population of people in chronic pain. With a critical eye on Oregon, the Republican-controlled U.S. Congress struck back. Having dramatically seized control of the House in the 1994 midterm elections and still swinging hard to the right, national Republicans responded to the court by taking quick action on its own national PAS ban. First was federal funding. A bill signed into law by President Clinton, the Assisted Suicide Funding Restriction Act of 1997, barred the use of federal funds—including Medicare and Medicaid—for assisted suicide. Clinton, the same man who famously told Americans "I feel your pain," sought the middle ground of compassion, observing that the bill "will allow the federal government to speak with a clear voice in opposing these practices." Signing the law, he endorsed the view that "to endorse assisted suicide would set us on a disturbing and perhaps dangerous path." The act passed the House overwhelmingly on a vote of 398-16 and the Senate vote was unanimous.[41]

But there was apparently very little that opponents of Oregon's law could do to stop assisted suicides from going forward there, for following the state's November 1997 vote (in which 60 percent voted to uphold the results of the 1994 election), PAS as a form of relief became legal. The law had survived many political and legal challenges. It had been enjoined by a federal trial judge, but that ruling was overturned on appeal. In November, when the Supreme Court refused to consider the last appeal by its opponents, PAS became Oregon law. At that moment, the Clinton administration announced that (despite the president's objection to the practice) the federal government would not interfere. The law—once and for all—would be a matter of state jurisdiction. In 1998, fifteen terminally ill Oregonians used the new right to commit suicide with physician assistance.

But the battle over relief only seemed to have ended in Oregon's favor; in fact, it was still not over for the Republican-controlled Congress. Each of the first fifteen Oregonians to exercise the right granted by the PAS law used barbiturates in their deaths—drugs that were federally controlled substances. Here (in this inherent tension between state and federal law over drug policy) the Republican Right in Congress found yet another opportunity to attack. Senator Orrin Hatch (R-Utah), Representative Henry Hyde (R-Illinois), and other conservatives promised more federal legislation to undo what Oregon had done. The legal apparatus of federal drug regulation (built up since passage of the U.S. Controlled Substances Act and establishment of the DEA in the early 1970s under Nixon) gave them one last opportunity to exercise control over what they saw as a morally suspect rogue state.

Pain and the Right's Turn toward Intrusive Government

For small-government conservatives (who had long decried government's heavy-handed involvement in the doctor-patient relationship and who championed individual freedom and states' rights), the Oregon law challenged their commitments to weak federal government. For four months in 1998 (from June through September), antiabortion Republican representative Henry Hyde and his colleague in the Senate, Don Nickles, built a legislative case against Oregon's law. The two introduced the Lethal Drug Abuse Prevention Act that took direct aim at Oregon by seeking to use federal power to limit doctors' ability to prescribe. The bill would strengthen federal law so that it clearly prohibited physicians in Oregon (or any state) from dispensing or distributing a controlled substance for the purpose of causing, or assisting in causing, the suicide, or euthanasia, of any individual.

Every political observer could see the proposed act for what it was—an attack on Oregon motivated by those who believed that religion should be more, not less, vociferous in the protection for life. Swayed by this powerful view in the party, conservatives in Congress championed the notion that federal powers must be used whenever Christian religious norms were threatened. As one right-to-life group said to its members in a mailing, "The Lethal Drug Abuse Prevention Act of 1998 . . . would reverse the outrageous decision of Attorney General Reno that *federally controlled* drugs can be used to assist suicide and euthanasia in states like Oregon where the practice has been legalized. This is our chance to help stop euthanasia before it becomes imbedded in American medicine and culture." California Democratic representative Pete Stark, in contrast, responded with a plea for small government: "If we've learned anything from the managed care debate, it is that the American public wants medical decisions made by doctors and their patients, not health plan or government bureaucrats . . . We are here because the Christian right is pushing this issue as yet another part of their wish list."[42] There was, of course, deep political irony in this moment—for the pain debate (and its proximate connections to other hot-button issues such as abortion, fetal pain, and the right to life for the Religious Right) had completely flipped the party's long-standing views on states' rights and federal power.

As Hyde and Nickles led the charge for the heavy exercise of federal power aimed at overturning Oregon's Death with Dignity Act, the AMA—traditionally aligned with Republicans and averse to government intervention into medical practice—was forced again to choose sides. Ultimately, they opposed the 1998 act as an unwarranted intervention in medical practice. By the end of the year, this bill was dead, with no clear majority in Congress willing to support it. Yet, the Right did not relent. The next year, another attack on Oregon's liberal relief law would rise from the ashes of the Hyde-Nickles defeat.

In early 1999 (a year that saw Republicans boldly impeach and try President Clinton in the House and Senate), middle-of-the-road legislators answered the Hyde-Nickles pain bill with their own pain legislation. Oregon's own Senator Ron Wyden and Representative Darlene Hooley, Democrats both, introduced the Conquering of Pain Act of 1999 into the U.S. Senate and House as a rejoinder to the Religious Right's proposal. Their bill sought to amend the Public Health Service Act to respond to another pain problem—the ongoing public health crisis of undertreated pain.

That same June, Nickles and Hyde answered with another effort from the right, offering a repackaging of their previous bill—now craftily entitled the Pain Relief Promotion Act. In co-opting the language of relief that Democrats Wyden and Hooley had embraced in their own bill and modifying their goals, they hoped to win the support of the AMA, which they did. The new Hyde-Nickles bill sought to amend the Controlled Substances Act so as to authorize the DEA to determine and regulate such standards as "legitimate medical purpose" and to examine a physician's "intent" when prescribing pain medicines (opioids). In its language at least, the legislation sought to seize the middle ground, aiming both to promote pain management and palliative care in the name of compassion while also empowering the DEA to block all efforts at the state level to legalize physician-assisted suicide. As a spokesperson for the pro-life activities of the Conference of Catholic Bishops told the Hyde committee, "It has certainly never been true since 1984, when the Controlled Substances Act was amended by Congress, that this Federal act slavishly follows what States may view as a practitioner's ability to handle federally regulated drugs."[43] The legislators' intent was clear: to use the federal powers of the DEA to make Oregon's Death with Dignity legislation unworkable. The bill passed the House in a 271-156 vote but, like Wyden and Hooley's bill, it went no further in the Senate.

The Clinton White House and many states opposed the Hyde-Nickles bill, seeing tragic irony that a bill named for promoting compassionate pain relief actually endorsed heavy-handed federal intrusion into medical practice, overruled state policy makers, and threatened to limit access to pain relief nationwide. Arguing against the bill, Democrats turned old Republican states' rights arguments to their own advantage. The Pain Relief Promotion Act also drew opposition from many state medical associations; they parted company with the national AMA, which lent its tentative support to the legislation despite the group's professed allegiance to small government and the inviolate doctor-patient relationship. Even physicians in states like North Carolina, long sympathetic to the states' rights appeal, voiced concern about the Hyde-Nickles bill. The Texas Medical Association (in the state where Stratton Hill had first won protection for doctors and sufferers) opposed it too, concerned that its own state policies would be threatened by federal powers. As Texas's libertarian-leaning Republican representative Ron Paul concluded in opposing the bill, "I am strongly pro-life . . . But I believe the approach here is a legislative slippery slope. What we are doing is applying this same principle of *Roe v. Wade* by nationalizing law and, therefore, doing the wrong thing . . . If we can come here in the Congress and decide that the Oregon law is bad, what says we cannot go to Texas and get rid of the Texas law that protects life and prohibits euthanasia[?]"[44]

Critical coverage of the Hyde-Nickles bill in the press and the medical literature soon followed, portraying the legislation as a vast overreach, a federal power grab by religious zealots, and a veiled attack on people's ability to control their own pain. The accusation would become, in many ways, the theme for Republican congressional politics in the mid-1990s. The *Journal of the American Medical Association* published a critical article labeling the Pain Relief Promotion Acts of 1999 a serious threat to palliative care. The *Washington Post* editorial page called it a "bad bill on dying." Other criticisms followed, with some support—for example from the *American Medical News*. Doctors testified before congressional committees and sent letters, both pro and con, highlighting that the profession no longer spoke with one voice—that of the AMA.[45] The tense situation was precisely what David Joranson had warned would happen when pain specialists, already working in a politically, morally, and scientifically contentious field, invited legislators for help with reform. The outcome of the marriage was difficult to predict and impossible to control.

Who had the right to judge pain? Who should define the terms of relief? These remained simultaneously clinical, political, and legal questions—the terms of the debate shifting with the political winds in D.C., Oregon, Florida, Texas, and elsewhere. Oregon's governor, John Kitzhaber, labeled Congress "medical meddlers" for dictating to the people of Oregon. Oregon senator Ron Wyden stood up for his state's right to choose, waging a successful filibuster against the Hyde-Nickles bill—even though Wyden had voted twice (as a private citizen) in Oregon against the PAS measure. The congressional battle—mobilizing and fracturing voters on the left and the religious right—continued right through the tumultuous 2000 election year, pitting Vice President Al Gore against Texas governor George W. Bush. Faced with such professional skepticism and public ridicule about the party's claims of compassion (and ultimately with Nickles outmaneuvered by Wyden), the "pain relief" bill died a long slow death in the Senate.[46]

Despite the political ironies, legal defeats, and internal contradictions in its position, the conservative attempt to impose a new pain standard on state and medical policy still would not relent. With Bush's election, the Right sensed another opening. Into 2001, with the Republicans poised to control Congress and the White House, the Religious Right tried again to legislate pain and end-of-life care—swinging between political grandstanding and serious reform. In addition to its ceaseless attempts to pass some version of the Pain Relief Promotion Act, another interventionist moment arrived with the case of Terri Schiavo in Florida. From the heights of the Senate and the House, Republicans took up the cause of the Florida woman declared to be brain dead. She was languishing in a persistent vegetative state. Her husband had decided to withdraw life support, but her parents and right-to-life activists in Florida and around the nation rallied to defend her—holding on to whatever slim evidence of brain activity they could find. At one point, Senate majority leader Bill Frist, himself a physician, stood on the floor to claim that Terri was indeed alive. Much of the discussion revolved around the question, does Terri Schiavo feel pain? In the eyes of medical colleagues and much of the public, Frist (and the entire Republican caucus) had crossed a line. He now stood accused by his medical colleagues of doing what no physician should ever do—making a diagnosis while standing a great distance from the patient, having never personally investigated the case. Moreover, such conservatives now embraced and extended a long-standing liberal concern for the pain of others to such an extent that they stood accused not only of exaggerating the pain of others but also of inventing pains that did not actually exist. The Republican claim that it was liberals who believed in large and obtrusive government would be hard to sustain in this environment.

Oregon, however, remained a galling concern. Bush's attorney general, John Ashcroft, a former senator and a devout Christian conservative from Missouri, now used the powers of the Department of Justice to target the state—issuing an interpretive rule in late 2001 stating that the federal Controlled Substance Act prevented the use of the drugs Oregon had allowed with its Death with Dignity law. Ashcroft was effectively insisting that the Justice Department was well within its powers (those granted by the Controlled Substances Act) to decide how physicians should use any such substance—from a Schedule 5 cough suppressant like codeine to Schedule 1 drugs like marijuana and LSD and every type of drug in between. It would take years, and several steps through the federal courts, before the Supreme Court would rule on this bold claim to federal power. In its 2006 decision on *Gonzales v. Oregon*, the Supreme Court—in what one observer saw as "a classic states' rights ruling"— rejected Ashcroft's overreaching attempt to tell the states what kind of compassion they could display.[47] This would be the right's final attack on Oregon. As it had in *Glucksberg*, the Supreme Court declined to establish

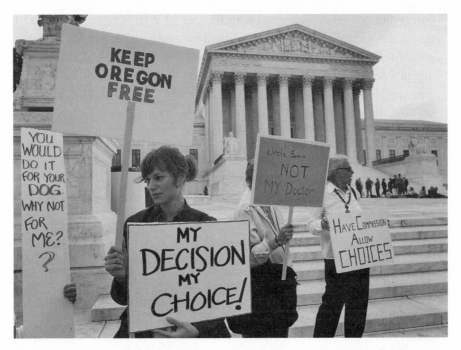

FIGURE 4.2. Protesters outside the U.S. Supreme Court, awaiting its ruling on the constitutionality of Oregon's Death with Dignity Act in 2005.

Photo by Charles Dharapak. Image courtesy of the Associated Press.

a nationwide constitutional right to die, but it did uphold the state's right to create the means for a physician to assist in a dignified death.

Courting Compassion

When these vexed questions of pain relief arrived yet again at the U.S. Supreme Court, the nine justices were ruling on far more than pain; they were deciding fundamental legal, moral, political, and philosophical questions that had long been refracted through the question of pain, compassion, and relief. In taking up *Gonzalez v. Oregon*, the court considered yet again whether Americans had a fundamental right to pain relief, whether the Constitution granted citizens a right to die when their anguish proved too much, whether doctors had the capacity to judge such matters and to administer a calming, lethal dose of medicine, whether federal laws superseded state law on these questions, and whether these questions of pain and relief were within the scope of issues articulated in the U.S. Constitution or the Controlled Substances Act. Again, the court would rule in Oregon's favor—declaring against the attorney general's overreaching interpretation of the controlled substances statute. In this ruling, the court—and particularly the "swing justice" Sandra Day O'Connor— would strive for the center between the political Left and Right, seeking to articulate a policy on the unsteady middle ground.

How would pain be governed? The question of who was in true pain, whose pain matters most in society, and what should be done for people in pain rippled across the country and merged with the increasingly partisan and morally charged political landscape. This was not entirely new. As previous chapters showed, the path by which pain management moved into the high court had been paved by the litigious climate of the 1980s, by the Reagan-era disability debates, and by muted concerns about fetal pain. But in the 1990s, doctors (some brash, others cautious) courted relief legislation. Stratton Hill had led the way, inviting the Texas legislature to protect doctors who cared aggressively for people in pain. Harold Glucksberg presented another model of how the politics of pain medicine itself turned doctors into political actors, as did John Kitzhaber, who crossed completely from medicine into the Oregon legislature and the governor's office. Where Hill and these others sought legislative support, Jack Kevorkian stood apart—flamboyantly goading lawmakers, judges, and medical boards to rewrite the rules of relief. Meanwhile, the people of Oregon created another lasting pathway to reform built on the notion that majority rule and direct democracy could best manage the people's pain.

As pain politics fractured along multiple lines (not only by party but also by state and region), the search for compromise that Stratton Hill had begun became deeply polarized, and it was left to the courts to try to repair the breach. If liberal compassion was winning victories, it was also producing deep skepticism about excesses of relief. As was true in the contentious Reagan years with the administration's battles against disability-related pain as unworthy of benefits, the courts continued to be the place where these conflicting ideologies of pain and compassionate relief played out. Doctors, empowered to administer relief, could never truly control this pain debate, but they continued to provide much of the pain theory that supported judgments on relief. In America, the question of who was in pain and what relief they needed had long since become a matter for voters, politicians, lawyers, and judges to decide. In the final analysis, pain was a legal concern, and the high court in the 1990s deferred to the states—allowing a divided state of analgesia to become the law of the land.

Although the courts could settle individual pain battles, including the running dispute between the Bush administration and Oregon, in the state's favor, they had no power to repair the breach in pain politics. As a stage in the history of pain and U.S. political history, the fractured state of analgesia revealed how (from abortion to death with dignity) the cultural politics of the 1990s split and transformed Democrats, but more so Republicans, along ideological lines. The question of Oregon's right to govern its own people's pain (in life and in death) threw the Religious Right into a pitched fervor; a shocking inversion of the party's states' rights position followed. The Right could support states' rights as long as that state's views of people in pain lined up with its own. Attorney General Ashcroft, the Bush administration, and the Republican Congress continued to see the Oregon law as expressing an excessively liberal view of pain and pain relief. For them, end-of-life pains warranted no such relief. The pains that best made policy, in their view, were the pains of the fetus and the pain of Terri Schiavo. Ironically, on this last point, the Religious Right found support from disability rights activists—who had been opponents in the days of Reagan's attack on disability rights.

The debates over PAS and access to pain relief highlighted just how much the Religious Right had come to influence the conservative movement in the late 1980s and into the 1990s. Their dominance was achieved at the expense of moderates, small-government conservatives, and libertarians like Texas representative and physician Ron Paul, who believed, for example, that heroin should be legalized.[48] PAS had unsettled religious members of the party—Catholics, evangelical Protestants, and some Jewish leaders—who looked to Washington for a strong response. Meanwhile, the AMA (which traditionally leaned right in its politics and usually fiercely opposed government oversight of health care) responded meekly to the shocking round of government intervention into health care—coming not from liberal officials but from its traditional allies on the right. In court, the medical group deferred to higher authorities on the question of relief. After years of political and judicial battles and whatever their misgivings about PAS, no doubt some AMA leaders were relieved when the Supreme Court endorsed the principle of double effect, giving doctors latitude in determining where pain relief merged into euthanasia.

Conservatism might have strayed far from its old strictures on activist government, but conservative justices like O'Connor would not follow the Ashcroft Justice Department's reading of pain relief law. Her views on the laboratory of the states echoed principles articulated by Reagan, who had appointed her to the court in the 1980s. If Republicans now endorsed the aggressive use of federal power and limits to state laws on pain relief (all in service of legislation to protect those "in pain"), she could not follow. For Republicans of an earlier generation, this was an assertion of power they once considered to be a quintessentially liberal pathology. As these new problems of pain relief arrived at the high court in the 1990s, the justices well understood that freedom from pain was a complex civic question—encompassing citizens' quests for death with dignity, freedom from chronic pain, self-determination, and constitutional rights of life and liberty.[49]

In this 1990s politics of pain, here was a final irony: for many people living and coping with chronic pain (people who were neither dying nor yet to be born), the era's stark polarization of the pain debate focusing on "fetal pain" on one hand or "death with dignity" on the other distracted attention from their own struggle. The politics of pain had not only polarized but also warped the landscape of pain care, further complicating their own hopes for relief.[50]

FIVE

OxyContin Unleashed

....

A good man will seek to take the pain out of things. A foolish man will not even notice it, except in himself . . .

WILLIAM SAROYAN, "THE HUMAN COMEDY"

The revelation in 2003 that conservative provocateur Rush Limbaugh had maintained a secret addiction to the painkiller Oxy-Contin carried a deep political irony. This arch critic of liberalism, social indulgence, and big government's coddling, a man who extended Reagan's ideas and who had wailed against President Clinton's "I feel your pain" rhetoric, had treated his own pain liberally and to excess. Many commentators at the time remarked on Limbaugh's political hypocrisy, casting him as a conservative double standard. Limbaugh had once said about drug users, "Go out and find the ones who are getting away with it, convict them and send them up the river."[1] On its face, the Limbaugh episode was a puzzling contradiction. If excessive "bleeding heart" liberal compassion had produced a crisis of dependency and learned helplessness, then what are we to make of the conservative provocateur's long-term addiction to the most famous painkiller of his day? His story conjoins the personal and political in the same way that the saga of many other people in pain had done (Rosie Page, Lorraine Polaski, and so on). Like their travail, his was a testament to the times in which he lived—to the growing gap of relief between the privileged and the poor, and to the post-Reagan years and the world conservative deregulation had created. The surge of painkilling drugs into the market since the 1980s (encouraged by both Reagan-era conservative deregulation and continuing liberalization) had both relieved and damaged society, and by the early years of the new century a new liberal-conservative consensus began to emerge around the need for market surveillance. Limbaugh was a poster image for these developments; so too was OxyContin.

The late twentieth-century pharmaceutical market expanded by taking advantage of many features of the American political landscape, exploiting both liberal and conservative pain policies. Private industry promised relief in ways conservatives loved, through direct-to-consumer advertising (DTCA) of drugs; to libertarians, drugs promised better access through the rise of Internet pharmacies; and to liberals, lowering the barriers to regulation promised effective remedies for the under-treated.[2] Limbaugh's addiction shed light on the exuberant drug market that regulatory reform had produced; but OxyContin's rise also forced both liberals and conservatives to look closely at the world they had made—a marketplace that claimed to solve Americans' problems far more efficiently and completely than government programs ever could, but one that also had the capacity for great harm. Seen in this light, the Limbaugh case is not a paradoxical story but a coming-to-fruition narrative.

By the turn of the twenty-first century, the forces of liberalized access to relief (through medical marijuana and physician-assisted suicide) and the forces of neoconservative deregulation (weakening FDA oversight of industry) had opened the door to innovation in the pain market. Combined, these forces unleashed a new world of relief symbolized by drugs like Bextra, Vioxx, Celebrex, and OxyContin. OxyContin seemed ideally suited for the era—it was an old drug, identical to the Percodan of the 1950s, but now in a time-release formulation for people in too much of a hurry for repeated medication. It also appealed to cancer physicians wary of opioids in end-of-life care. The drugs promised relief without addiction. But, like other business booms of these decades, the drug bubble was also susceptible to profound busts; and many of the era's new pain-killers experienced shattering failures as well as success (measured in pills prescribed, revenues and stock prices, but also in side effects, deaths, and fraud prosecutions).[3] By 2010, few of the players involved in the pain-relief markets—patients, doctors, drug manufacturers, and regulators—had escaped the controversies that defined the OxyContin era or the policing and increased political scrutiny that marked these times. Limbaugh was just one of many casualties.

In the early years of the pain drug boom—a time that coincided with the introduction of DTCA—people like Limbaugh became avid shoppers. This flowering of consumerism was precisely the kind of development that free-market conservatives had long championed, but it also produced new patterns of excessive consumption. In the OxyContin era, market diversion—the illicit resale of prescription drugs—became the new face of addiction. Limbaugh was accused of the crime of "doctor shopping." Of course, Americans had long shopped for doctors in the medical marketplace. In the 1980s, the term "doctor shopping" referred not to a consumer crime but to a right—the patient's right to shop for medical care in a market increasingly controlled by insurance companies and health management organizations. The criminalization of doctor shopping was thus a new legal development of the late 1980s and 1990s—a response to emerging consumer and industry excesses. By the time Rush Limbaugh turned himself into Florida authorities, "doctor shopping" referred to the now-illegal diversion of prescription drugs into the black market and the process by which patients fraudulently moved from physician to physician to circumvent controls on the quantities of prescriptions available to individual consumers. Ironically, doctor-shopping laws were one of the legal mechanisms developed by state governments to respond to the deregulated market and to excessive relief. The rise of such laws signaled that the age of deregulation and liberalization had run its course, and a new era of government surveillance had arrived—embraced by politicians on the left and right, across the ideological spectrum.

As in times past, the debate over who was the person in pain reflected, converged with, and shaped adjacent political disputes. Was Rush Limbaugh a victim of a drug being investigated as addictive by Congress and the FDA, as his lawyers stressed in court—a misled consumer in need of sympathy and enhanced protection? Or was he a perpetrator of fraud—a criminal who used complaints of pain to find illegal forms of relief? Or was he in true pain, desperately trying to evade the restrictive and fearful cadre of doctors, police, and bureaucrats society had set up to dole out stingy relief? A close analysis suggests that Limbaugh's Oxy-Contin case contained all of these features; but, more important, his case was a parable of pain and relief in the deregulated, probusiness environ-

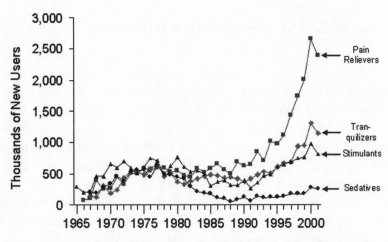

FIGURE 5.1.   A 2002 National Household Survey on drug use documenting the sharp upsurge in U.S. consumption of pain relievers.

Reprinted from Pilar Kraman, *Prescription Drug Diversion* (Lexington, KY: Council of State Governments, April 2004).

ment created by both conservatism and liberalism. In finding OxyContin, Limbaugh had encountered a world partially of his own creation—a new American pain dilemma.

In this new world, the gap between people privileged with too much relief and those coping with too little had grown. Drugstores in poor neighborhoods were loath to stock painkillers for fear of break-ins and robbery, leaving local patients traveling longer distances for medications. Increasing evidence suggested that ethnic minorities had lower access to analgesic care in hospitals as compared with whites. Meanwhile, Oxy-Contin, which had quickly earned a reputation as "hillbilly heroin" because of its prevalent use in rural America, now gained a reputation as the prescription drug of choice among upscale abusers.[4] Social disparities bedeviled caregivers in end-of-life cancer relief. While some Americans were receiving too much relief—often through criminal means—other people were suffering with few remedies in sight. Where did Limbaugh stand on this spectrum of overmedication and undertreatment? This was the political question unleashed by OxyContin and confronting liberals and conservatives alike.

Boom and Bust: Deregulation and Its Discontents

For much of the century, the questions of how to regulate the marketplace for relief and whether well-being was best served by the market or by government broke along political and economic lines. At times, liberal politicians like Estes Kefauver (shocked by drug scandals, aggressive marketing, and side effects) have tilted heavily toward regulating the industry; at other times, market-oriented conservatives in the Bush, Reagan, and even Clinton years leaned toward deregulation. The question of drug regulation hinged on the question of whom to trust—whether industry's claims about pain and relief were honest or venal and whether consumers could use potent drugs appropriately.

In the eyes of the drug industry, its type of pain relief was a market good. Pain medicines were also the sector's financial lifeblood. Fast relief, a seemingly enduring American consumer ideal, was tied to such products as the blockbuster tranquilizer Miltown in the 1950s, new analgesics in the 1960s and 1970s, and a vast array of other nonopioids in the 1980s, 1990s, and through today. In the 1990s, Americans were told (as they had been in previous eras) that they didn't have time for pain and that products like Vioxx and OxyContin offered new kinds of fast-acting or long-term relief. Since the 1950s, "fast relief" has been a dominant advertising motif. Less heralded has been the accompanying parade of side effects, dependence, abuse, and other recurring regulatory, policing, and political headaches that came in the shadow of such promises. In many of these cases, early claims of superior pharmacological relief gave way to concern and reassessment, opening the door to regulatory debate; but new painkillers were always around the corner, and the cycle would begin again.

By the time that ibuprofen, the first of a new family of powerful nonsteroidal anti-inflammatory arthritis and pain drugs, appeared on American drugstore shelves in the 1970s and 1980s, its success came amid a new antiregulatory business environment in which such drugs would thrive. With the election of Ronald Reagan in 1980, the decade became fertile political soil for painkillers. Deregulation in all sectors of the economy had become the new watchword. The age of consumer protection that followed the thalidomide scandal in the early 1960s was giving way to a new era that cast the Food and Drug Administration regulatory process as squelching the market, shackling innovation, and standing in the way of true relief. In the decade that followed, pharmaceutical regulatory policies aimed to open the floodgates of innovation, cut "bureaucratic red tape" in drug approval, open television marketing to drug companies, and speed the flow of products from drug maker to consumer. But these policies raised an old question: Was the pain patient victimized more by the savvy marketing, or was the person in pain being victimized by the red tape of government regulation?

Reagan-era policies opened the doors to expedited FDA drug approval in the 1980s, but the question persisted as to whether an industry unfettered by regulation was truly a gift to consumers or a curse to the gullible. In this argument (one of many catalyzed by the conservative revolution), Reagan was on the side of business—even wondering aloud after the 1980 election whether "the 1962 [post-thalidomide] reforms that required drugs to be proven effective as well as safe should be scrapped."[5] In his 1985 State of the Union address, Reagan insisted that "we stand on the threshold of a greater ability to produce more, do more, and be more. Our economy . . . is getting younger and stronger; it doesn't need rest and supervision, it needs new challenge, greater freedom. And that word—freedom—is the key to the Second American Revolution we mean to bring about." For free-market conservatives, as they came to be known, freedom meant freedom from government regulation of business, including drug companies. It also meant consumer freedom because of a faster, easier pathway for experimental drugs through FDA approval and on to the market. The administration consolidated regulatory policy under Health and Human Services secretary Richard Schweiker and shelved new rules put forward by the Carter administration for keeping close track of adverse drug reactions, defective medical devices, subpar infant formula, and so on.[6] Across government, the administration limited the authority of regulatory agencies, pushed for faster drug approval, and (under pressure from AIDS activists) began to see itself as a handmaiden of the drug innovation process—helping speed much-needed relief to market rather than standing in the way.

In the wake of deregulation, drug successes and drug scandals soon followed. In Reagan's first term, the arthritis drug Oraflex became the first canary in the coal mine—a test case framing a liberal-conservative debate on the market's virtues and its damaging effects. Market analysts saw the arthritis pain field as "ripe for a breakthrough" and predicted that the 1980s would produce a drug to attack bone loss as well as pain. At stake was the relief of 6.5 million Americans with rheumatoid arthritis and almost thirty million with osteoarthritis. As the *New York Times* reported, "Some of the growth [in the arthritis market] is attributed to the aging population. Another factor is the switch of aspirin users to prescription drugs; which cost more but can deliver the needed dosage in fewer pills and are easier on the stomach." Industry analysts put the potential market at $700 million annually, with annual growth potential of up to 20 percent.[7]

To feed and nurture demand, the major drug companies, including Pfizer, Eli Lilly, and Bristol Myers, turned to senior pain specialists to learn more about the pain patient—honing in on the pain market. Who were they? Were they elderly men or middle-aged housewives? Were they stock traders, advertising executives? And what kind of pains did they suffer? Reporting on one survey, pain pioneer John Bonica described pain consumers as "people who sit around watching television most of the time . . . Tension headaches are very common for them." The sedentary lifestyle associated with major industrial nations gave rise to more pain. His study also found that women experienced more pain than men and that "headaches are a malady of the middle class, affecting people mostly in the $15,000–$50,000 annual income range."[8] Pain was everywhere, but unevenly distributed. Stock traders reported feeling less pain than "average Americans," while advertising executives and people who worked at "computer video-display terminals" reported higher than average rates of headaches.

Tailoring new products to different consumer needs, companies hoped to gain a market share against Upjohn's Motrin, the blockbuster that had previously commanded the pain market. In 1981, sales of Motrin alone had totaled $1.9 billion, with profits of $181 million for Upjohn. Eli Lilly's Oraflex was another exciting new entry in this lucrative race for pain profits and rapid relief. The product entered the market to much acclaim, but it sent the company on what one business reporter called "some wild rides up and down." Within four months of approval by the FDA in April 1982, Oraflex became one of Lilly's most popular drugs, with sixty-four thousand prescriptions filled. Sales reached $708 million in the first half of the year, with net income of $228 million. Some patients reported remarkable improvements in pain and mobility.[9]

The Expanding Market *1982 projected market share, based on $717 million total sales of prescription drugs*

Manufacturer	Antiarthritic Drug	Market Share
Upjohn	Motrin	25.8
Syntex	Naprosyn	20.9
Merck	Clinoril	16.7
Merck	Indocin	12.6
Eli Lilly	Nalfon	5.6
Pfizer	Feldene	5.6
Johnson and Johnson	Tolectin	5.0
Warner Lambert	Meclomen	4.3
Eli Lilly	Oraflex	2.8
SmithKline	Ridaura	0.7

Source: Figures from "The Boom in Arthritis Drugs," *New York Times*, April 23, 1982, D1.

But with such booms came troubling busts. When a British regulatory body linked Oraflex to sixty-one deaths there and eleven deaths in the United States since its American distribution four months earlier, the story rapidly pivoted from a parable of the market's virtues to a tale of its perils. In July 1982, the company learned of reports of twelve deaths, twenty-three cases of jaundice, and reports of severe liver and kidney problems among those on the drug; that same month, it warned physicians to reduce dosages. Pressure built as consumer activist Ralph Nader's Public Citizen Health Research Group (and other groups) filed a federal suit in Washington, D.C., requesting court intervention to halt the drug's sale. HHS Secretary Schweiker (who was then at the center of the administration's battle to remove claimants from the government's Social Security disability rolls) was compelled to act. The drug, he noted, was off the market and would stay off until the FDA conducted its own assessment; by June, eight deaths in the United States apparently linked to Oraflex were being investigated. By August, Eli Lilly announced the suspension of worldwide sales of the drug, as the number of U.S. and U.K. deaths rose to seventy-two, as uncertainty over the product's safety reigned, and as stock prices fell from $60 to $53 per share.[10]

The unleashed pain market would be vulnerable to such swings throughout the 1980s and into the 1990s. Oraflex's misfortune was a stark turnaround for such a promising product; commentators read the story of the drug's withdrawal from the market as an early warning of the perils of Reagan-era deregulation. Eli Lilly insisted that it had done nothing wrong, but the case seemed tailor made to stand in as a referendum on Reagan-era policies. As Reagan's political focus had shifted to various efforts to speed drug approval (including allowing nontraditional DTCA), critics zeroed in on whether these policies were to blame for the Oraflex debacle. Pressured by these events, Schweiker backed away (but only slightly) from HSS's earlier proposal to speed up new drug applications "out of fear that it may have inadequately reviewed the anti-arthritis drug Oraflex."[11] Greater caution seemed warranted. Where free-market conservatives saw these up and downs (in earnings, profits, and losses) as the market doing its intended work, producing winners and losers, critics of the administration's policies saw market excesses and consumer exploitation—measuring the drug market, for example, by lives lost.

Critics of the Reagan administration pointed to another problem highlighted by the Oraflex debacle—selective prosecution by the administration of the nation's drug offenders. While the Justice Department was taking an ever-harder line against illegal drug users, it failed to hold industry executives accountable for the deaths produced by their own bad drugs. In August 1985, Eli Lilly pled guilty to misdemeanor charges in the Oraflex case, admitting that it had mislabeled the drug and had failed to inform the FDA about adverse reactions. But under a plea bargain agreement with the Justice Department, the company was fined only $25,000. A former chief medical officer (a British citizen who had since left the United States) pled no contest to similar charges, paying a $15,000 fine. Critics of the administration charged that Justice Department lawyers had recommended prosecution for three of the company's officers (who apparently knew of overseas deaths tied to Oraflex but had failed to disclose them during the U.S. approval processes), but that senior Justice officials overruled its own lawyers. As Democratic representative and chair of the House Judiciary Subcommittee on Criminal Justice John Conyers saw it, this was one of the ironies of conservative governance. Overstating the deaths, he bemoaned the fact that "on the one hand, street criminals are prosecuted to the fullest extent of the law.

On the other hand corporate officials who may be responsible for the death and injury of hundreds of thousands of people are merely slapped on the wrist."[12] As critics on the political left saw it, the Justice Department was picking winners and losers in the pain economy. For the next two decades, these ironies of policing and the pain market would multiply.

Congressional Democrats charged that the Justice Department was too lenient in its refusal to pursue a trial in the Oraflex affair, a symbol of a coddling approach to the industry as well as a reflection of the Department's fear of losing at trial (a charge Justice officials denied). Democrats in Congress continued to attack the administration on this point well into Reagan's second term, with investigations and reports accusing not only the Justice department but the FDA as well of failure to protect the public health, failure to act on known side effects, and evasion of oversight in the name of speeding overseas drugs into the U.S. market. Though this debate started with painkillers (Johnson and Johnson's Zomax met a similar fate), the story continued with other drugs, like Hoecht's antidepressant, Merital. The FDA had become a drug promotion unit more than a consumer protection agency, the argument went, and skeptical Democratic lawmakers insisted on "the agency's need to enhance the public's protection from dangerous and unproven medicines."[13]

Under the George H. W. Bush presidency in the late 1980s and early 1990s, the FDA began a slow shift toward remedying some of the damage wrought by deregulation. Yet market infatuations with "revolutionary" painkillers, followed by fallout from the disclosure of drug side-effects, remained common. In 1989 under Bush, for example, the FDA approved Toradol as a nonnarcotic pain reliever. Its maker, Syntex Corporation, announced that it would market the drug for the treatment of postoperative pain, a market then dominated by narcotics. Toradol's promise was simple—it was not an opioid, and numerous medical journals embraced the drug's promise over the next two years. By 1992 and 1993 (the end of Bush's term and the beginning of the Clinton administration), however, widening use of Toradol had produced significant health concerns, principally about its link to kidney damage and hemorrhages. As with Oraflex before it, Toradol sales declined. So did Syntex's stock, but the problem was not limited to Toradol. Another Syntex pain reliever, Naprosyn, once hailed as an "anti-arthritis wonder drug" in the

1970s, had come under increasing scrutiny by the FDA over the integrity of its animal testing and over the drug's safety. Both drugs were shadowed by skepticism about inflated claims, damaged by competition from new products like ibuprofen, and undermined by the 1993 expiration of their patents. The clinical reports on Toradol grew worse between 1995 and 1998, validating the drug's effectiveness while stressing the elevated dangers of gastrointestinal bleeding.[14]

The opening of the pain market to unbridled competition, in other words, fostered its own ironies, political struggles, and risks for consumers. Drugs like Oraflex, Syntex, and Toradol (and later Vioxx and Oxy-Contin) mixed high risk with high relief, thus adding uncertainty to the pain medicine field; eventually, their booms and busts began to turn the tables on deregulatory zeal. Yet, for industry, the imagined profits of pain were more than worth the risks of recurring scandals and litigation costs. Investors hoped that every new drug would follow the path not of Oraflex and Toradol but of Motrin (ibuprofen). Available by prescription since 1974, ibuprofen gave "competitors financial aches," won praise as a "popular choice for easing pain and swelling of arthritis," and was (in 1984) about to be approved for over-the-counter sales projected at $1.3 billion. The makers of Tylenol took to the courts, filing suit to forestall and even rescind the FDA's approval for over-the-counter sales. As another drug company executive noted, it was "an arrogant and unconscionable effort" to maintain their own market share.[15] The desperate legal maneuver was unsuccessful.

By the mid-1990s, these cycles of success and failure raised many questions about the need for vigilance—continuing physician vigilance, FDA surveillance, consumer alertness, and sustained policing and prosecution of the aggressive industry. As in so many other areas of the Reagan revolution, the courts played a powerful and prominent role in adjudicating these pain disputes. Plaintiffs and lawsuits came in many varieties—some taking on the companies for product liability, others charging the administration with wrongdoing, and sometimes the companies themselves engaging in legal battles for market supremacy. Another front in the legal battle was over whether consumers, harmed by the products they had used, had been adequately warned of the risks. As one *Wall Street Journal* writer noted, the system of consumer information in the United States had produced an odd situation in which "the average U.S. consumer typically receives less information on prescription drugs than the average Italian or Mexican." [16] For anyone looking to the market for relief, new forms of vigilance would become vital.

Within a decade of Reagan-era reforms, the age of deregulation had spawned a new period of pain drug lawsuits; jury awards for pain, suffering, and death; and investigations of both industry and FDA practices. In this context, Eli Lilly would be called to account for the damage Oraflex had produced, but it could also boast that "a Federal grand jury which investigated the Oraflex issue for fourteen months made no charge that Lilly withheld any information prior to U.S. approval . . . or that Lilly intentionally violated any law," noting that any mistakes were totally inadvertent. In other legal settings, however, consumers wronged by pain drugs found redress. In November 1983, for example, a man whose eighty-one-year-old mother, Lola Jones, of Phoenix, Alabama, had died after taking Oraflex for a month, won a $6 million award in federal court. The plaintiff alleged that the media campaign had convinced Mrs. Jones that the drug was a cure for her arthritis. After the verdict, Jones's lawyer noted, "We're a little disappointed in the dollar figure, but we made our point. It was a good win." [17]

Winning some cases by jury trial, settling others, and losing some, Eli Lilly (and other companies that played the high-stakes pain game) now also sought their own form of relief—calling for Congress to pass tort reform legislation and provide the industry with legal protections from "frivolous lawsuits." Probusiness congressional Republicans, in another bow to the industry and the market, had found a new reform issue in the 1980s—calling for measures to limit "excessive" jury awards and to stem the tide of such lawsuits. (The industry had won a major victory in 1986 when Congress passed—and Reagan signed—the National Childhood Vaccine Injury Act, a law creating a special court to regularize awards to people claiming injury and removing the litigation threat that drug makers and vaccine manufacturers claimed was crippling the industry.) [18]

The Problem of the Liberated Shopper

By the first year of George H. W. Bush's presidency, the effects of deregulation were, at best, double edged. Faster drug approvals, for example, had won unlikely followers on the left. Writing in 1989, physician George Annas asserted that the combination of AIDS activism and deregulation "threatened to transform the U.S. Food and Drug Administration (FDA) from a consumer protection agency into a medical technology promotion agency." But the promise of faster access to drugs was also becoming a dangerous roll of the dice for consumers. Democrats blamed deregulation for scandals in the savings-and-loan industry, and, as for the drug industry, even staff reporters for the business-friendly *Wall Street Journal* observed in 1989 that the FDA was engaging with the drug industry more as a partner than as a regulator and, as a result, "lurching from one crisis to another" and becoming party to industry malfeasance. "Three FDA employees already have pleaded guilty to taking illegal gratuities from generic-drug makers," noted the *Journal.* "Two generics companies have admitted duping the agency with falsified data. And the FDA has found manufacturing and record-keeping problems at nearly all of the twelve generic-drug makers it has investigated so far."[19] The revelations—an indictment of deregulation—were also a shift in the liberal-conservative debate. Where the Reagan years had so powerfully vilified government as the consumer's bane, now it seemed that the character and trustworthiness of American drug firms (and their close relationship with the regulators) was endangering the health and well-being of consumers.

With lowered barriers to relief, new drug products flourished and consumption rose; but so too did a new problem: drug diversion. Although diversion is often linked to prescribing physicians, it was also a product of deregulation—a natural outgrowth, an unintended derivative, of the boom market. As early as 1990, Democratic representative Pete Stark (California) characterized pharmaceutical companies and careless physicians as no better than drug pushers, with patients as their victims. He pointed, for example, to "one New Mexico doctor who was responsible for 28 percent of all Valium prescribed to Medicaid recipients in the state" as one example of abuse.[20] Other commentators noted that, with the rise of such commodities in the pain market, the diversion of prescription drugs onto the black market now arose as a major law enforcement concern. One among many concerns was the misuse of over-the-counter medications such as Sudafed (valued on the black market for its ingredient pseudoephedrine in the manufacture of methamphetamine).

Policymakers' attention turned slowly away from the primary users for whom the drug was marketed to secondhand markets—and the processes by which prescription drugs were, increasingly, being resold, repurposed, and remarketed.

In the politics of pain relief, guileful consumers (more than industry) were often blamed for skewing these pathways through which drugs traveled; to address this behavior, government surveillance was compelled to expand. Interviewed in 1994, one Connecticut enforcement official noted that "prescription drug abuse doesn't get the same attention that illegal drugs get. And yet we conservatively estimate that this accounts for 30 percent of the nation's drug abuse." This new problem required that investigators develop new knowledge and tools, including (according to this same investigator) "how the legal distribution systems are set up, who has access to drugs, and how the records are kept at hospitals, clinics, long-term care facilities and pharmacies." Investigators also cast a suspicious eye on professionals, needing to know more about the ways in which doctors, nurses, and pharmacists (whose rates of chemical dependence were much higher than in the general population) diverted drugs. But one of the most common ways of diverting drugs from legal distribution channels was through the phenomenon that came to be known as doctor shopping. "A patient will present to a physician difficult-to-diagnose ailments such as severe back or muscular pain that are typically treated with a pain killer. After receiving the prescription, the patient will repeat the performance for three or four more physicians." Another surveillance concern of the 1990s became the blurred line between drug companies and drug pushers. Yet other developments also blurred these lines, most notably when California passed its medical marijuana laws in the mid-1990s and the DEA under Clinton promised harsh enforcement action against dealers as well as against "doctors who help to provide otherwise illegal drugs" to their patients.[21]

Unsettling the market in other ways, the avenues by which people in pain learned about prescription drugs and how they navigated the new drug economy had changed dramatically in the 1980s and 1990s with DTCA. Although it was not allowed across the board until 1996 with the Clinton administration, the direct marketing concept had emerged from Reagan-era promarket philosophy. In the 1980s, companies like Upjohn had gingerly tested the waters of DTCA by urging patients to "talk to your doctor" about treatments for specific conditions; after a short moratorium by FDA, more liberal DTCA regulations of the early 1990s allowed full-throated advertisements. Now, the pharmaceutical industry put information about specific drugs—Claritin, Prozac, and other new products—directly before buyers in the name of consumer empowerment, provided that the ads also mentioned side effects. Savvy campaigns became a new advertising reality, unsettling doctor-patient communication as the primary way people learned about prescription drugs. Medical groups like the AMA expressed caution about the implications of turning Madison Avenue loose to sell drugs, as did politicians and public health officials.[22] Was this truly the consumer empowerment free market conservatives wanted? Or was the FDA now enabling consumer exploitation as many critics feared?

News stories with titles such as "Maybe You're Sick. Maybe We Can Help," announced the arrival of DTCA, offering an array of products (often for ailments that consumers did not know existed). This shifting balance of drug marketing and therapeutic information had sweeping implications for consumer drug use and for questions of safety and liability. The rise of limited DTCA was based on the belief that the informed consumer was an empowered consumer and that better health would stem from this trend. At the same time, however, it was also clear that DTCA exposed patients to risks. As one scholar noted, "A major concern is whether consumers actually gain correct information from advertising. Initial studies by the FDA suggested that test subjects recalled potential benefits of advertised products more often than risk information." Another looming concern for manufacturers was whether the ads exposed the companies to liability if they were deemed, later, not to have warned consumers adequately of the risks. At the same time, the aggressive rise of DTCA spawned its own legal battles—as "manufacturers—in the face of increasing price competition—[began] taking one another to court over marketing aimed at physicians, pharmacists and other health professionals."[23]

It was into this competitive and unstable market created by deregulation that OxyContin appeared. The chemically active ingredient in OxyContin was not new. Instead, Purdue Pharma, the creator of the drug, had reformulated oxycodone (better known as Percodan) as a time-release capsule that would deliver relief in stages rather than all at once. Percodan had been immensely popular as a painkiller upon its introduction in the 1950s, but its manufacturer, Endo, came under fire in the early 1960s for misrepresenting the drug's addictive properties. The result of government inquiries and industry criticism was stricter prescription-only controls and a greater reluctance to prescribe the drug.[24] Percodan remained on the market, however, subject to the strict oversight that characterized the "war on drugs." (In the 1970 Controlled Substances Act, oxycodone was classified as a Schedule 2 substance—with a high potential for abuse—alongside cocaine, morphine, and methadone.) Some three decades after Percodan's high promise had crashed to the ground, oxycodone was back; the new and repackaged time-release brand won approval from the FDA in 1998. It appeared alongside the dozens of other leading painkilling performers—Celebrex, the first Cox-2 inhibitor and painkiller for arthritis patients; Vioxx, the second Cox-2 inhibitor on the market; and many other products. OxyContin promised better, faster, time-released, controlled relief with no addictive downside; it was a free-market dream. And, because the drug appealed to those who would liberalize pain medicine and end-of-life care, it found an avid market with cancer physicians seeking to give patients reliable relief without the fear of morphine-related addiction.

Between 1996 and 2000, OxyContin prescriptions climbed from less than three hundred thousand to nearly six million, with annual sales skyrocketing from under $50 million to over $1 billion in 2000. Florida ranked fourth in the nation for per capita OxyContin consumption, behind West Virginia, Maine, and Alaska. As some physicians saw it, the rising focus on end-of-life care drove the trend—one Fairfax, Virginia, physician commented, "If Grandma is placed on morphine, it's like 'Oh, my God.' But if Grandma comes home placed on OxyContin—that's OK." By 2001, the drug's sales accounted for 80 percent of the company's revenue. As one reviewer noted in 2003, "If the drug had remained limited to patients with the most severe pain, the story would probably be different, but advocates for pain treatment minimized the danger of addiction and recommended prescribing OxyContin for milder and chronic pains."[25]

A controlled release pill had strong consumer appeal—it lasted longer, called for fewer repeat doses, and depended less on the user's remembering to take their medicine. The time-release mechanism claimed to be a near-perfect safeguard against addiction. One study argued that "around-the-clock controlled-release oxycodone therapy seemed to be effective and safe" and was accompanied with few side effects—reducing "the interference of pain with mood, sleep, and enjoyment of life."[26] The theory that controlled release inevitably reduced addiction was flawed in many ways, not least because physicians, drug promoters, and drug enforcers failed to take into account the inventiveness of consumers who, in time, would discover that crushing the pill, rather than swallowing it whole, released the full dose of the drug immediately. For drug companies, this argument served a broader goal—feeding their argument that conniving consumers, not the drug itself or improper marketing, were to blame for abuse.

Within a few years of OxyContin's appearance, problems with diversion and abuse appeared; and although OxyContin's abusers were diverse, a caricature of the drug as "hillbilly heroin," came to life. Thus while in 2002, "a rash of armed robberies in suburban Boston" prompted one pharmacy to discontinue OxyContin sales, many stories followed abuse in Appalachia, where the drug was portrayed as a symptom of a broader economic and social problem. The *Cincinnati Inquirer*, for example, characterized the poor region as "ground zero for abuse of a revolutionary narcotic pain medicine" and noted in a headline: "OxyContin Abuse Said Likely to Spread—Appalachian Economy Tied to Painkiller Abuse." In such accounts, the desire for excessive relief was explained by the declining mining industry, the rural economic depression, men's desires for relief amid economic and social turmoil, and doctors blurring the line between compassionate care and drug dealing. The media profile meshed neatly with another emerging rural epidemic—the rise of methamphetamine as a symbol of economic and social decline across rural America. As for OxyContin, arrests in 2001 and poignant stories of addiction attracted the interest of regional and national legislatures.[27] In Florida, as one commentator later put it, the anti-OxyContin story took a new turn. The state was battling the economic declines characteristic of northern states, but it also had a large elderly population where the goals of killing pain for chronic illness and at the end of life had pressing immediacy.

Trying to avoid the stigma of pushing an abused drug, Purdue Pharma characterized the OxyContin fears of 2001 as a "media frenzy" and shrewdly sought to rebrand its product—not as an abused drug but as a remedy for America's undertreated sufferers of pain. Politicians sought the middle ground. Late that year, for example, a congressional committee called the main players to testify on OxyContin. The committee's chair praised Purdue Pharma for a drug that had "brought relief to many Americans" but also blamed the drug for producing "hooked" teenagers, murder, suicide, pharmacy robberies, "big spikes in crime . . . and entire neighborhoods being overtaken either by users or drug dealers." In a Congress prone to drug panics, the chair of the committee speculated that this could well be "the next crack cocaine." In its response, Purdue Pharma sat squarely in the corner of liberalizing relief—calling attention to its advocacy for the undertreated. Writing at the dawn of the OxyContin controversy, J. David Haddox, the senior medical director of Purdue Pharma, defended the company, noting "as an academician, I can say no other company has done more to increase the understanding of pain . . . The media frenzy about OxyContin abuse is interfering with good pain management. In fighting drug abuse, we must not limit patients' access to strong analgesics to . . . preserve quality of life." The company bemoaned the rising barriers for effective pain relief made worse by media hysteria and lack of medical education. "Thirty two percent of anesthesiology residents felt unprepared to manage chronic pain," and only one of the 125 accredited U.S. medical schools offered pain management as a separate course. Physicians, in short, were still woefully undereducated in how to treat pain. Yet they often believed that their patients were poor judges of their own experience—prone to exaggerate the scope and severity of their pain. These exaggerated clinical fears were, a company document argued, one of the main barriers to effective relief.[28]

But claims of OxyContin's dangers went well beyond addiction and the black market; the drug was increasingly gaining a lethal reputation. As one source noted, "In 2001 and 2002, more people died from overdoses of prescription pain medications oxycodone and hydrocodone, such as the brand drugs Vicodin and Lortab, than die from heroin." But with OxyContin producing revenues for Purdue Pharma on the scale of $1.5 billion in 2002 alone, the company decided that the best strategy for its bottom line was to litigate every claim of product liability. It also effectively pointed to others (doctors, patients) as the cause of any problems with OxyContin. In Florida, where Rush Limbaugh would be charged in 2003, 328 deaths were attributed to heroin, but three times as many, 957, were blamed on oxycodone/hydrocodone. In the years leading up to the Limbaugh story, then, Americans were already engaged in an extensive reassessment of OxyContin and its promoters. A new regulatory dilemma emerged. The question was whether regulators would focus on untreated pain and uneducated doctors as many pain relief advocates (and the company) wished or on inflated marketing claims, excessive consumption, and physicians duped by unscrupulous drug companies (as industry critics hoped).[29]

The Rise of Surveillance

As cases of OxyContin abuse mounted, Purdue Pharma's marketing practices worried liberals and conservatives alike—producing strange political bedfellows who slowly embraced the goal of enhanced market surveillance. Physicians who advocated liberal relief aligned with the profit-seeking industry and relief-seeking patients on one side, and conservatives who were usually steady allies of the drug industry and skeptics of government oversight aligned with liberal regulators on the other. Physician-assisted suicide had already begun to split conservatives; for many on the religious right, painkillers unacceptably blurred the lines between pain relief and covert euthanasia (see chapter 4). In this context, state legislatures had written pain statutes to define a clear and sharp line between standards of acceptable compassionate care and illegal "mercy killings." Florida's Republican-controlled legislature passed just such a measure in 1994. With the arrival of OxyContin as an alternative to morphine, legislators on the right were already primed to move toward aggressive oversight and surveillance.

While surveillance took several forms, physicians were frequently targeted first. Florida, Virginia, and other states became the sites of high-profile convictions of doctors involved in running so-called pill mills that offered excessive pain prescriptions. In 2001, Florida doctor James Graves was sentenced to sixty-three years in federal prison—convicted of manslaughter for overdosing patients on OxyContin. As one libertarian critic of the Graves case saw it, OxyContin had ushered in the surveillance society—it was "the first time in U.S. history that a physician was found guilty of manslaughter for prescribing self-administered medication that led to a patient's death." As Ronald Libby (writing in coordination with the libertarian Cato Institute) saw it, the atmosphere in Florida was particularly ominous—with "media-induced hysteria" driven by a series of articles in the *Orlando Sentinel* by reporter Doris Bloodsworth.[30] Purdue Pharma executives agreed.

But, with Limbaugh's case, the media narrative pivoted to a more diverse array of users, constructing stories of pain and relief among the middle class. The *New York Post* characterized Limbaugh as one among a new class of "upscale junkies" who were able to shop for drugs more widely, whether by hiring others to do the purchasing or by using the new phenomenon of online pharmacies to satisfy their needs. Other reports focused on the "college-age kids" and individuals once "comfortably middle class" who, in the grip of OxyContin, had crossed the line "from party guy to junkie low life." One Vermont newspaper presented oxycodone usage as "migrating out of Appalachia to areas such as Columbus, Ohio and Fort Lauderdale, Fla."—a rural plague upon "suburban neighborhoods." Seen in this light, the suburbs and those who lived in them could be seen as victims (rather than as perpetrators) of crime. Limbaugh himself emphasized his virtues even as he confessed to his loyal listeners that "over the past several years, I have tried to break my dependence on pain pills and, in fact, twice checked myself into medical facilities in an attempt to do so." On the right, there was praise for his "refreshing honesty"; the Left responded with scorn for his hypocrisy mixed with hope that he might become less self-righteous and critical of others. But, as one author noted in Florida's *St. Petersburg Times*, "Beyond the damage Limbaugh has done to his highly burnished conservative credentials, his sensational fall has added to the woes of another group: those in chronic pain who rely on OxyContin to relieve their torment. This kind of adverse publicity will only make it harder for patients to get access to the pain medication they need."[31]

Other observers on the left, meanwhile, had been blaming Reagan-era policies for almost a decade for causing these new epidemics; Limbaugh's case did little to change their rhetoric. To Democratic representative Henry Waxman, the rise of OxyContin addiction gave liberal, proregulation Democrats an opening to highlight just how unaware Republican administrations had been about drug marketing, diversion, and industry malfeasance. Waxman, the powerful member on the House Committee on Government Reform, insisted that the George W. Bush administration had been purposefully lax in its oversight of the pharmaceutical industry. As a report prepared by House Democrats for Waxman observed, "In 1999 and 2000, the last two years of the Clinton administration, FDA sent an average of ninety-five enforcement letters per year to drug manufacturers for false and misleading advertisements. The number of enforcement letters sent by the Bush Administration in 2003 is 75 percent below the average level of the last two years of the Clinton Administration."[32]

To Waxman, the problems with OxyContin illustrated how right-wing policies had harmed public health, and its rise revealed the life-and-death difference between the Clinton and George W. Bush administrations' approaches to private sector drug surveillance. The Bush administration DEA had waited three months after Purdue Pharma launched its OxyContin ads to issue weak warnings to the company about its fraudulent claims. A Democratic committee reporting to Waxman observed that "the OxyContin delay stands in stark contrast to the actions of the Clinton Administration. In May 2000, the Clinton Administration cited Purdue Pharma for advertisements that overstated the effectiveness of the drug and presented a misleading safety profile. This citation came only one week after the ads initially ran."[33]

The irony of "reform" in an era when Republicans controlled so many branches of government at both federal and state levels—the White House, both houses of Congress (from 2000 to 2006), many governorships and state legislatures, while making inroads with judicial appointments as well—was that legislation tilted not toward keeping drugs off the market but toward various kinds of market monitoring and postmarket surveillance. The industry's answer to market excesses leaned toward more monitoring of consumption rather than stronger safety or marketing regulations. In 2004, the FDA announced industry-approved initiatives, such as putting "tiny radio antennas on the labels of millions of medicine bottles to combat counterfeiting and fraud." "It's basically a bar code that barks," one industry researcher told the *New York Times*—one that could "make supply chains more efficient and more secure." As the chief security officer for Purdue Pharma commented, "We get calls once a week from state troopers saying they got a guy with one of our bottles." Indeed, Purdue itself played a role in focusing attention on users rather than on the company. In Florida, facing an investigation of its sales practices by the state's Democratic attorney general Bob Butterworth, the company struck a compromise with the term-limited Butterworth in late 2001. As one commentator noted, "Purdue pledged $2-million for software to run a drug prescription tracking system for the state. In turn, Butterworth agreed to end his inquiry."[34]

Other critics, meanwhile, pointed out that tracing pill bottles back through the supply chain would not be enough to stop the OxyContin epidemic. The pain relief economy was far more extensive than this; many players in this pain relief economy (consumers, physicians, drug companies, and pharmacists) had powerful incentives to promote consumption regardless of the social costs. In 2013, the Walgreen's pharmacy chain confirmed that, at the height of public concerns about OxyContin, its officials created a bonus program (a perverse incentive plan) to reward pharmacists who sold more, not less, oxycodone. They were encouraged to look the other way even if customers were "red flagged" as possible abusers. How effective could surveillance be when the perverse incentive to promote OxyContin stretched throughout, and to some extent defined, the political economy from manufacturers, prescribers, regulators, dispensers, and users?[35]

By late 2003, nearly three hundred state and federal lawsuits (including a number of class-action suits) had been launched against OxyContin and Purdue Pharma, but at least one legal commentator—in part defending the industry—argued that most were not brought by law-abiding citizens duped into addiction but by existing drug abusers who happened to find OxyContin as their new drug of choice. In this telling, OxyContin had not created addicts; rather, addicts had besmirched the reputation of a virtuous pain reliever. Who then were these people who blamed the drug for their addiction? Were they deceitful frauds? But another question in the legal debate was the identity of Purdue Pharma. Were they a legitimate company concerned about pain and offering true relief or a deceitful drug trafficker? A new theory of "negligent marketing" threw Purdue onto the defensive: it had been recognized for the first time by the courts in 1999, relating to the sale and manufacture of firearms, and now was being deployed in court against drug makers. But, as the company's defenders argued, Purdue could not be held responsible for diversion and the pre-existing black market. One such claim in Virginia, the case of *McCauley v. Purdue Pharma*, failed precisely because the plaintiff could not prove causation. Particularly revealing of the reach of painkillers in this era was the finding in such cases that, as one legal observer noted, "it appeared that the plaintiffs were already addicted to pain medication long before their physicians first prescribed OxyContin."[36]

The years 2004 and 2005 would be contentious for the painkiller market with government re-energized to fight the industry. Early in the decade, a number of state governors, regardless of politics and ideology, had begun to push back against the pharmaceutical industry's high pricing as a way to restrain ballooning Medicaid expenses. By 2001, a variety of state initiatives, ranging from laws protecting low-income residents to multistate purchasing coalitions, were driving down the price of big sellers like the antiarthritis drug Vioxx. The same year, West Virginia tried a new tactic in cost reduction when it sued Purdue Pharma to recover $30 million in costs associated with overprescribing. As with the lawsuits from individuals, the grounds were negligent marketing. In late 2004, Purdue and the state settled—with the company paying a relatively small settlement of $10 million to pay for continuing education programs for doctors, law enforcement prevention programs, and drug rehabilitation initiatives.[37]

The pain relief market of the 1980s and 1990s continued to work its magic, with booms followed by more spectacular busts. Just when faith in OxyContin was declining, another high-flying pain drug crashed even more dramatically than Purdue Pharma's blockbuster. This time, it was Merck, announcing that its celebrated arthritis drug Vioxx would be removed from the market following disclosures that it increased risk of heart ailments and assertions that the company had kept this information from regulators, doctors, and patients. The Vioxx story deepened the tale of fraud and deceit, pointing more directly at the heart of the industry. It soon became a parable of a new type of corporate malfeasance that imperiled the system of capitalism itself. In 2004, the Bush administration's Justice Department and the Securities and Exchange Commission (SEC) both announced investigations of Merck, with the SEC presumably concerned with whether the company had misled not only the public but also its stockholders about the safety of Vioxx.[38]

Lawsuits against the company followed, and, repeating the trend already established in the OxyContin cases, state governments turned their attention to Merck. Even the conservative Congress and George W. Bush White House could not avoid launching intense regulatory measures. Alongside other corporate scandals like the Enron debacle in 2001 (where the brash Texas energy company had been propped up by elaborate accounting fraud), public attention turned toward cleaning up the malfeasance that seemed pervasive in industries that had been cut loose from regulatory oversight. The maker of Vioxx's competitor drug, Celebrex, decided to press on in the face of similar allegations, electing to weather the storm of inevitable lawsuits and regulatory scrutiny. In the wake of these disclosures, large managed-care organizations like Kaiser Permanente reassessed the appeal of other pain drugs—deciding against dispensing other controversial products like Pfizer's Bextra.[39]

In a sense, this was the free market at work as its advocates intended, for with regulatory barriers lowered only time and widespread use would disclose the true utility of the various drugs circulating in the pain economy; in the meantime as drugs surged through the system, the market produced record profits, considerable relief, and (ironically) much pain. From 1998 to 2005, the number of serious adverse events from prescription drugs climbed from roughly thirty-five thousand to eighty-nine thousand, with oxycodone leading the way. In this light, Rush Limbaugh was lucky; he was part of a much larger group of people who were "merely" addicted. In OxyContin consumption, the United States stood far apart from any other nation. A 2008 UN report observed that 90 percent of the global consumption of pain medicines occurred in Europe and North America but that "in 2007, the United States accounted for over 99 percent of global consumption of hydrocodone and 83 percent of global consumption of oxycodone."[40] As with so many of the drug stories of the decade, the U.S. stood alone—not in the degree of pain in the body politic but in its unquenchable appetite for relief.

The Vioxx crash was financially spectacular—far more calamitous for Merck than OxyContin's case had been for Purdue Pharma, and it tipped the scales decidedly toward government oversight. Even so, the two busts had been similarly damaging to the public health. Facing charges in federal court from the Department of Justice, in 2007 Purdue Pharma and its former executives (the president, medical director, and top lawyer) pleaded guilty to misleading doctors and patients when they claimed the drug was less likely to be abused than other similar drugs (such as Percocet). Purdue Pharma paid a $600 million fine, and the three executives paid a collective $34.5 million in penalties for their part in the deceit: they had known that time-release OxyContin was not safe. Later that same year (and three years after removing its own pain drug, Vioxx), Merck agreed to pay close to $5 billion dollars to settle more than twenty-five thousand lawsuits relating to its promises of relief. (Pfizer followed in 2008 with an $894 million settlement of all lawsuits relating to its withdrawn painkiller, Bextra, and arthritis drug, Celebrex.) Some industry critics believed, however, that all this action was too mild and too late. For them, the fines and legal fees paled in comparison to the profits OxyContin and Vioxx had generated—and would not be a deterrent to other flagrant market booms and busts. During the six years of alleged wrongdoing, OxyContin had generated between $1 billion and $2 billion in revenues per year for the firm; Vioxx had generated an estimated $11.2 billion in total sales between 1999 and 2004.[41]

Until the middle of the decade, the FDA had exercised little postmarket influence once drugs were approved. The agency did not have much power to compel changes in advertising, and probusiness administrations saw little need for aggressive FDA oversight. The best it could do, given its mandate, was to haggle with drug companies to change drug labeling to warn physicians of a drug's downsides. Even as the OxyContin and Vioxx scandals played out, the U.S. Senate voted by a massive majority (ninety-three to one) to establish a surveillance system to track adverse effects of prescription drugs and to enhance the FDA's power to warn the public. Senator Charles Grassley (R-Iowa) turned out to be one of the fiercest critics of the industry, taking relentless aim at the complicity of academics, pain relief advocates, and government in endorsing painkillers. The FDA was in an all-too-cozy relationship with drug makers. "Public safety is at stake," he wrote following an Institute of Medicine (IOM) report on the topic, "along with the credibility of our nation's drug-safety agency . . . Vioxx was like a dead canary in the coal mine, a warning that worse may yet come. Today there's no question left that we need to strengthen post-market surveillance in order to improve drug safety and save lives."[42]

At the same time that the pain relief market expanded, the Iraq war produced two new twists in pain and policy—introducing into politics the question of imposing pain on others for a "greater good"(torture) and shining a spotlight on the anguish of injured soldiers and their need for relief. The rise of torture as public policy (with revelations about brutal treatment of Iraqi detainees by American soldiers at Abu Ghraib prison and administration memos outlining the use of waterboarding—simulated drowning—to extract information) was shockingly new in public debate; the administration's stance increasingly painting the Right as all too willing to inflict pain for the greater welfare of the American public. Characterizations of Bush's vice president, Dick Cheney, as the "Master of Pain" and "Vice President of Torture" for his grim defense of "harsh interrogations" and of Bush as the "King of Pain" became common media fare—for Democrats in Congress and liberals opposed to the war, and also for many Republicans who denounced the administration's positions as alien to American values.[43] The second by-product of the Iraq war, thousands of soldiers in pain from injuries from improvised explosive devices, was a new but also familiar challenge in American political history. The war produced mourning about the soldier's sacrifice and the need for support at home.[44] By the end of the decade, the Iraq experience merged back into the OxyContin era as army experts and senators voiced concern about the dramatic increase in narcotic pain-relief prescriptions for injured troops, jumping from thirty thousand a month to fifty thousand since the war began and becoming "the most abused drug in the military."[45]

With the damage produced by the booms and busts of the pain market stretching so broadly, the embrace of drug surveillance crossed party lines. Senator Grassley called on President Bush to help support these reforms, but he also wrote scathingly to the FDA commissioner that its own personnel were disenchanted that the FDA "has lost its way and 'sold out' to the industries it is charged to regulate." Speaking for Democrats, Senator Edward Kennedy also called for increased market scrutiny—in the case of Vioxx, he pointed out, it took fourteen months for the FDA to get the company to change the drug's label. "Companies routinely promise to conduct studies that are never even started, much less completed," he noted, and they encountered no penalties for doing so.[46] Senators had come together on the need for surveillance. They hoped that a public database of clinical trials conducted by drug companies would produce a transparency about the pain and suffering, as well as benefits, of the ongoing OxyContin era.

The American Dilemma: Overmedicated and Undertreated

If Rush Limbaugh represented one face of the American problem (over-treated pain), there were also many people struggling with undertreated pain. "It is an irony of our age," the *Washington Post* had commented in 1986, in words that rang true decades later. Cancer patients, burn victims, and accident victims were not being adequately relieved, while others were overdosing on painkillers prescribed for a growing array of chronic pains. These striking polarities in pain care came to define the American landscape, reflecting the ironies of a consumer society. For every savvy consumer like Limbaugh who craftily navigated the system to obtain pain relief, there were many others who tried and failed or who came under clinical and legal scrutiny and never obtained the relief they sought. Race, age, and economics defined this pain divide. Patients in low-income neighborhoods found that their pharmacies did not stock strong pain medicines for fear of being robbed. Meanwhile, doctors remained reluctant to prescribe pain medication for chronic disease, fearing drug dependency in patients and wary of professional accusations of fostering addiction leveled against them by medical boards and drug enforcement officials. In the case of sickle-cell disease, as one practitioner admitted, "Physicians sometimes think that patients with sickle-cell anemia and pain compatible with crisis are drug-seeking or responding to other psychosocial factors."[47] Such caregivers practiced medicine under a heavy cloud of suspicion and extended that cloud of suspicion to pain patients.

The pain of minorities (or urban inner-city pain, as it was often conceived) was cast in a different light than suburban pain; researchers characterized minority pain as undertreated—a portrait several studies in the 1990s solidified. In March 1994, emergency physician Knox Todd discovered a striking phenomenon in the annals of pain and relief—that all people's pains were not relieved equally. Based on a study in an emergency room in Los Angeles, Todd determined that white patients being treated for long bone fractures (a highly painful condition) were dosed more liberally than Latino patients with similarly severe fractures. "This disparity in analgesic practice could not be explained by patient characteristics (including sex, language use, and insurance status), severity of injury, or physician characteristics (including ethnicity, sex, or specialty)," wrote the authors. Were caregivers to blame or the patients themselves? The authors could only speculate about what accounted for the gap in relief. "We postulated that the disparity in pain management might arise at two stages of the encounter between patient and physician—pain assessment and analgesic ordering." One possibility was that physicians assess pain differently in Latinos and whites, "either because patients express pain differently or because physicians interpret such expressions differently." Another possibility was that physicians assessed pain in the two groups similarly "but simply choose to address pain less aggressively in the former group." The studies offered no definitive answers—only possibilities—but the clear outcome was less relief. A year later in Atlanta, the authors found similar disparities in pain relief—now across black-white ethnic lines.[48]

By the late 1990s, other studies found that pain relief echoed other forms of social discrimination; patients who received treatment at outpatient cancer clinics serving minorities were three times more likely to be undermedicated with analgesics than patients in other settings. Researchers could only speculate about the origins of such disparities, listing the possibilities: "inadequate prescribing of analgesics for minority patients may result from many factors, including concern about potential drug abuse in minority patients, fewer resources with which to pay for analgesics, greater difficulty in accessing care and in filling prescriptions, and greater difficulty for the physician in assessing pain in minority patients because of differences in language and cultural background."[49] Reforming such a system that produced hidden, rather than explicit and articulated, forms of discrimination (including both overtreatment and undertreatment) was a perplexing problem, akin to the battle against what critics called "institutional racism."

Gender differences in pain assessment were also obvious. According to one influential scholar, women were more likely to be sedated for pain. Discussing her findings at a 1997 Capitol Hill breakfast briefing on pain management (sponsored by Iowa Democratic senator Tom Harkin and hosted by the pharmaceutical company Bristol Myers-Squibb), Christine Miaskowski, professor of nursing at the University of California, Berkeley, noted that pain's undertreatment was a "major public health problem." In some contexts, women seemed to receive dramatically better pain relief. A few years later, Miaskowski's studies found an even more complex gender story in pain: women were more likely to complain about pain, were less stoic, and were also less accurate in reporting their pain than men. Women were more expressive in describing their pain, she argued, yet they were also better at coping with pain than men. Men were less likely to be sedated for pain, but they were more likely to receive pain medications like OxyContin. The findings, of course, echoed and informed broader gender stereotypes—or as a 2003 article on pain in *Good Housekeeping* noted, pain followed a "clear gender gap." Women were "more inclined than men to describe their symptoms emotionally, they [were] also more likely to have their problems downplayed by doctors . . . or dismissed as purely psychological."[50]

That pain should have a gender and racial politics is not a new observation; the meanings assigned to anguish, complaint, and identity had always been a perplexing question in culture and politics. As historian Martin Pernick has noted, at the birth of modern anesthesia in the 1840s, a vibrant discussion flourished about pain, race, gender, and difference. The well-to-do, women, and Anglo-Saxons were said to have a higher sensitivity to pain, while Native Americans, the poor, and blacks were characterized as constitutionally less sensitive to pain.[51] For Mark Zborowski, writing in 1969, pain expression told the story of different ethnic groups—Anglo-American stoicism, Jewish suspicion and complaint, and so on. For Reagan in the 1980s, disability pain in those seeking government support was deeply suspect; "fetal pain" was real. These attitudes toward the pain of others evolved with the political milieu, informed by prevailing attitudes and by a broader politics of belonging and citizenship. In the 1990s, the new question was how these issues of identity could drive overtreatment for some and undertreatment for others. The answer was that minority people in pain and women in pain (depending on their context) were subject to an extra level of surveillance, because to provide pain relief was still, as it was in the nineteenth century, an act of policing boundaries of acceptable behavior and identity.

Disparities in pain relief thus shed light on a fragmented society where the undertreated and the overmedicated were both microcosms of a growing trend in American society where the gap between the poor and wealthy had grown; gaps in pain and relief merely reflected the social divide. This political atmosphere explains how undertreatment (and the image of physicians as denying of care) became a hot-button issue for some, as HMOs and private insurers came under withering criticism for their efforts to limit access to care, while overmedication vexed others. Disparities existed in many places—in the Los Angeles and Atlanta emergency rooms, in chronic cancer care in Wisconsin, in the sickle-cell disease clinics of New York City, and also at the local pharmacy. "We Don't Carry That" ran the title of one study in the *New England Journal of Medicine*; it pointed to yet another problem, "the failure of pharmacies in nonwhite neighborhoods to stock opioid analgesics."[52] Researchers in the 1990s saw these racial disparities in relief, but they were ill equipped at the time to see that these differences between the haves and have-nots had deep origins in the social, political, and economic relationships of the time.

The undertreated (their numbers, their alleged character, their deservedness) inspired political wrangling and new alliances, as drug companies strategically sided with them. The marriage of patients in need and drug company self-interest had become a regular part of the political landscape since the 1980s. Activists groups such as the Drug Reform Coalition Network insisted that the undertreatment of chronic pain was "one of the saddest and least noticed consequences of the war on drugs," with the problem stemming from physician ignorance and fear on one hand and law enforcement threats on the other. For them, "the enemies in the battle for pain relief [were] state medical boards and the Drug Enforcement Administration." They had allies in government, singing from the same script. Presenting the case at the 1997 Capitol Hill meeting sponsored by Senator Harkin and paid for by Bristol Myers-Squibb, all could agree with the spokesperson for the National Institute of Nursing Research who saw the problem as far reaching. "In 1987, 90 million Americans were living with chronic conditions, with direct health care costs of $272 billion annually." By 1995, the number had risen to 99 million. The cost of relief ran to $479 billion annually and was expected to grow. By 2030, it was estimated that 148 million people would have chronic conditions, with an annual cost of $798 billion. Here was another by-product of the OxyContin era, as elected officials from the left, pain reformers, and industry agreed that "pain is our nation's silent public health crisis" and that physician prosecution and "legal myths" about pain relief undermined patient care.[53]

Advocates for liberal relief charged that many of the undertreated were becoming pseudoaddicts, a new term expressing their frustration with the perverse effect of a surveillance-oriented drug policy. The Reagan years had brought renewed attention to illegal drugs, with heightened prosecutions of drug offenders, the "crack" cocaine scare, and a new push for mandatory minimum sentences—all of which cast a shadow over the pain market and pain drug consumers. Coined in 1989 by pain specialists D. E. Weissman and J. D. Haddox, "pseudoaddiction" described the behavior of a patient in real chronic pain whose pain was not adequately relieved with the prescribed opiate analgesic regimen. Chronic undertreatment forced the person to try to procure more medication. "In such cases," experts who adopted the term noted, "the drug-seeking behavior ceases once pain is well controlled." Advocates for pain reform used the term to highlight the failure (indeed, the counterproductive failure) of the war on drugs. The behaviors of patients who were not adequately relieved by their prescriptions could easily be confused with that of drug addicts. As this new theory of pain behavior suggested, not all drug-seeking behavior was criminal or suspicious, and moreover denial of pain relief actually *created* the criminal behaviors.[54]

Amid such obvious overmedication and troubling undertreatment, Americans grappled with where and how to intervene in such a broken relief system—how to do surveillance while showing compassion. One avenue (the law-and-order approach) embraced aggressive federal and state prosecutions of "pill mills" (a new term in the late 1990s associated with rogue doctors, new pain-management clinics, and online pharmacies allegedly pursuing profits through excessive prescription writing) and fraudulent users. Another route (the bureaucratic path) involved new hospital regulations, pushed by organizations like the Joint Commission on Accreditation of Healthcare Organizations (JCAHO) to promote better pain monitoring.[55] Yet another pathway (the surveillance approach) involved enacting prescription drug surveillance systems in state law enforcement to monitor and identify doctor shopping before it became a problem. As some reformers saw it, a fourth reform, industry regulation, involved stricter regulatory control and prosecution of deceitful pharmaceutical marketing and advertising practices. Yet others advocating a more libertarian approach pointed to the problem of untreated pain, the lack of options for many people, and the need for more, rather than fewer, pain remedies. For them, California's medical marijuana law was the model to follow—encouraging "compassionate" relief for people with HIV, wasting diseases, and other painful conditions. But for those critiquing American consumerism, the public's overreliance on pills for all their ailments had become not a solution but the new problem.

The Cost of Doing Business

In 2003, Limbaugh's lawyers asked the judge in his case to see the radio star as a victim twice over; it was an unlikely legal argument for the conservative provocateur, but it accurately captured the tenor of the times. His lawyers claimed that Limbaugh had been victimized, in this instance by a drug that had been falsely offered to physicians as safe and nonaddictive. He was a victim, that is, of the boom and bust market in painkillers that accompanied his rise to fame. Second, his lawyers alleged that— once charged—he was now victimized again, this time by excessive state surveillance and enhanced police powers as prosecutors seized his medical records in Florida (a regional locus of pill mills) and California. These actions, his lawyers said, amounted to a violation of privacy by state governments that had grown too enamored of surveillance at the cost of doctors' and patients' rights. In December 2003, the Florida judge dismissed Limbaugh's privacy argument, but his attorneys appealed and the costly debate over state power moved up the judicial chain.[56] With the political clout, media platform, and financial resources to defend himself (using these libertarian claims), Limbaugh's court battles increasingly focused not on his pain or right to relief but on intrusive government power and its expansive surveillance.

The debate on pain medication, including Limbaugh's case, reflected a broader debate in the 1990s and 2000s on regulation and deregulation, market freedom and government control. The OxyContin promise distilled many ideals of the era into one drug: the promise of fast relief without dependence; the promise of a return to an active lifestyle with pain suppressed without deficits in functioning; the promise of few, if any, side effects; the promise of liberal end-of-life care without opioids; and the promise to remedy enduring gaps in access to care among underserved populations. But pharmaceutical companies' claims of fast relief, like conservatives' claim that markets function as elixirs for social pain, proved to be deeply flawed and dangerous to the body politic. Pain medication was not just a sideshow in the era's political theater, it was a major site for political maneuvering and policy formation—and OxyContin powerfully revealed not only the problem of pain relief but many of the social tensions and anxieties that defined the 1990s.

OxyContin grew out of conservative market policies, but the product also grew out of liberalized relief, riding the desire to extend relief to the chronically undertreated. Although blame for overmedication was obviously shared among doctors, patients, and pharmaceutical companies, it is clear that companies like Purdue Pharma had *especially* taken advantage of the political environment created by both liberals and conservatives.[57] Only later, in 2010, would it be disclosed that Purdue had funded the pain awareness groups who had lobbied aggressively for the undertreated, supporting such organizations as the American Pain Society and others pushing for reform. By 2012, advocates for liberal pain relief admitted that they had been so keen on the mission of pain reform that they had not looked skeptically enough at the company's claims. A leader of the reform effort, Russell Portnoy, who had been a prominent adviser to the FDA in OxyContin's early years, was also a paid speaker for Purdue Pharma and many other companies with pain drugs to sell. Ten years later, the breadth of those payments to liberal pain relief groups became much more clear.

In a scathing letter to the American Pain Foundation, the American Academy of Pain Medicine, and other reform groups, Senators Max Baucus (conservative Democrat from Montana) and Charles Grassley (moderate Republican from Iowa) laid responsibility for OxyContin at the feet of liberal advocacy groups as well. The painkillers actually killed "more people than heroin and cocaine combined," they alleged. They denounced "extensive ties between [drug] companies that manufacture and market opioids and non-profit organizations such as the American Pain Foundation, the American Academy of Pain Medicine, the Federation of State Medical Boards, the University of Wisconsin Pain and Policy Study Group, and the Joint Commission"—all of which depended on pharmaceutical industry subsidies. Using industry funds, such groups had produced thinly researched "guides for patients, journalists, and policymakers" that played down the risks and exaggerated drug benefits.[58]

Just after the Limbaugh OxyContin story appeared in 2003, the columnist Clarence Page noted that Limbaugh's views on drugs had evolved. Page hoped that, in the wake of his long-term abuse, Limbaugh might become a "powerful voice . . . on behalf of other non-violent drug abusers who could benefit from treatment instead of incarceration." "He could make a very good conservative argument," said the columnist. But this hope was, of course, a liberal's dream. Portraying himself as a victim in court, Limbaugh struck a defiant pose on the air. He was unapologetic, politically combative, and partisan when he announced his addiction: "The Democrats still cannot defeat me in the arena of political ideas," he said. "And so now they're trying to do so in the court of public opinion and the legal system. And since I'm not running for office . . . they're going to seek the occasion of this event in my life to see, to find out if they can do any damage."[59]

Three years later, out of rehab and back on his radio show, he put the case simply, refusing to dwell on his pain or his victimization by OxyContin: "I had a problem. I admitted it. I went and dealt with it. I have been clean from the painkillers for almost two years and eight months."[60] However his lawyers presented his case in court, on air he spoke from the old conservative script. Unlike the liberals he caricatured, his pain was real; unlike other addicts, his dependence was merely an unfortunate inconvenience; his recovery was never in doubt; and his defense of his privacy rights from government surveillance was firm, made possible by his wealth. Yet for all this, and beyond the stoic posturing, Limbaugh knew he would remain a symbol of the OxyContin era—an era that both conservatives like him and liberals had helped bring about.

Theaters of Compassion

People in pain have been stock figures in American political theater. As the scholar Javier Moscoso has noted, "The uses of pain
have nothing to do with truth, but rather with drama."[1] Illustrating the
point, the 1966 American film *The Fortune Cookie* placed actor Jack
Lemmon at the center of his era's pain pageant. Lemmon played a sports
cameraman who had been knocked down accidentally by a player during
a professional football game. Though only dazed, he was convinced to
fake severe injuries by his unscrupulous lawyer and brother-in-law, played
by Walter Matthau. He sued the team to win a settlement for his injury,
pain, and suffering. The comedy revolves around the plaintiff's fraud, the
lawyer's greed, the gullibility of doctors, the football player's sense of responsibility, and the attempts by insurance company investigators to un-
cover the scam. In the theatrics of *The Fortune Cookie*, the answers are
satisfyingly clear to the omniscient viewers, and so are the stakes. When
Lemmon lies in bed in a full neck brace watching a television program,
he hears the words Abraham Lincoln says to him (and us), "If you once
forfeit the confidence of your fellow citizens, you can never regain their
respect and esteem." All the more satisfying is Lemmon's decision, at the
end of the film, to embrace virtue and reveal himself as a fraud. With
humor and determination, he redeemed himself fully. Would that distinguishing true pain from fraud were always this simple.

When Reagan came to power in the early 1980s, this overdrawn the-
atrical image of the person in pain became newly embedded in public
policy. As anthropologist Talal Asad has noted, "The modern nation as an
imagined community is always mediated through constructed images."[2]
In Reagan's time, the person claiming fraudulently to be in pain was one

such constructed persona. The disabled person in chronic pain became a symbol of much that was wrong with liberalism—its gullibility, its support for government dependence, and its embrace of welfare at the cost of hard work. The preceding pages have told the story of how these problems of pain and social welfare came to define American political theater and (perhaps more important) how the courts came to play a central role in judging pain. The book shows how and why these questions of compassion and government made good theater and good politics and how they endured as fundamental conflicts that still define the American political landscape. The problem of pain touched intimately on the problem of how the people of the country were bound together.

The questions of which kinds of pain are real, which warrant sympathy, and whose plight is deemed illegitimate have provoked constant political spectacle in the many decades before Reagan and since. Today, these remain powerful moral and political questions at the heart of American government. What to do about pain that doesn't go away but lingers, especially in a prosperous nation where hard work, frequent injury, and aging are all common? Does pain caused by chronic disease warrant special consideration, long-term attention, and ongoing relief? Whose pains should we, as a society, be willing to carry for a lifetime and at whose expense? When is pain and relief merely a fraud?

Beyond pitting liberals against conservatives, the question of pain (as I have argued here) also refined the very meaning of "conservative" and "liberal" as keywords in the American political vocabulary. "Political words take their meaning from the tasks to which their users bend them," Daniel Rodgers has observed.[3] What it means to be liberal or conservative became ideologically solidified around the problem of pain. From the years immediately following World War II until today, the political Right railed consistently against certain kinds of pain, seeing public relief in particular as a symptom of a weak, coddled, and dependent society. As liberal government expanded to address the needs of people professing to be in pain, so too did conservative ire grow. For the political Left, just as consistently, compassion toward the pain of others—the disabled soldier, society's elders, those injured at work, or people suffering from debilitating disease—underpinned an expansive view of government and a comprehensive ideology of what society owes to its citizens. Positions on pain did not always align with party ideology, but for Republicans and

Democrats, these seemingly simple questions—how much pain do you feel? and what kind of relief do you need?—slowly became ideological and policy minefields.

The Reagan era more than any other time solidified partisanship around people in pain. In the relentless political messaging of Reagan-era conservatives, people with pain and disability who made special claims on the government were a problem created by liberals; indeed a gullible belief in subjective pain as real pain defined liberalism itself. This skepticism had simmered for decades (articulated by the AMA's Louis Orr and many others). Pain, especially the coddling of people claiming to be in pain, was a Trojan horse bent on destroying the nation. But in Reagan's time as president, this argument became a potent part of the Right's script; it has continued to define Republican politics for generations since. Thus could the president make the shocking case that the face of disability in 1980s America was that of a serial killer, Son of Sam, who (while imprisoned for committing horrific crimes) continued drawing generous disability benefits. The accusation, made in a meeting with newspaper editors, was scathing; and these renderings of whose pain mattered left an enduring mark on American politics—creating a stark, if caricatured, portrait of how liberals think and how conservatives respond to people's complaints. The power of this pain discourse explains why, years later, Bill Clinton's off-the-cuff "I feel your pain" comment was greeted on the right with such scorn and yet also why it had such positive resonance for those who believe in liberal compassion. The 1992 presidential candidate's words had touched a sensitive political nerve for both the Right and the Left.

But it is too simple to accept as truth the binaries that Reagan-era Republicans enshrined—that liberals believed that all subjective pains were real and that conservatives embraced cold objectivity on the pain question. Nor is it useful to see the liberal pain standard and the conservative case against learned helplessness as mirror images of one another or as opposing discourses in the political world. In truth, in the politics of pain, liberalism, and conservatism often blended into and depended upon one another—the disability entitlement (SSDI), for example, had been established by liberals in Congress, embraced by some moderate conservatives, and endorsed by the Republican Eisenhower. Decades later both conservatives and liberals, including the Democrat Carter, attempted to scale it back. At the political edges, however, the Right and Left often drew the starkest battle lines, often becoming inflamed and fractured around whose pain mattered, whose claims to suffering warranted relief, and what kind of pain relief (market based or governmental) should prevail.

People in pain, sadly, have carried two types of burdens—first, the onus of their own pain, and, second, the burden of being props in this political theater which saw actors assign conflicting meanings to their experiences. The theatrics surrounding pain did not stop with mere rhetoric or ideology but, as we have seen, crept into policymaking, touching fundamentally on matters of governance and power. In the eyes of the AMA, the veteran's complaint could never be just about his bodily injuries (no matter how severe); such complaints were inevitably bound up with his claims on the government, claims that the doctors' lobby saw as a threat to them and to free enterprise in general. The ensuing disputes over pain and disability drew in other actors concerned with governance and power: Congress, disability activists, lawyers, physicians, and increasingly a wide array of judges. The rise of pain also gave rise to merchants and managers of relief, and the preceding pages reveal the ways in which political calculations informed how anesthesiologists like John Bonica, surgeons, drug companies, and physicians like Harold Glucksberg and Jack Kevorkian defined their place in the pain relief economy. Pain (as an experience and as a symbol) also gradually and systematically became a social and legal problem, with the courts drawn into a heated process of evaluating and giving definition to the nature of peoples' pains. To this day, the argument over whose pain should matter (pain at the end of life, "fetal pain," chronic pain) remains a legal quagmire.

In the decades since the Reagan era, one notable trend has been the broadening uses of pain in political argument, with the emergence of end-of-life pain as a vehicle for a new politics of compassionate relief and the rise of fetal pain on the Religious Right. With the assertion that fetuses feel pain, the Right readjusted its ideological position on pain in America to signal rhetorical "compassion" in their conservatism while also narrowing their sympathies. While largely dismissing disability pain in ways similar to the iconic Reagan and while also looking skeptically on end-of-life pain relief as an opening for physician-assisted suicide, the Right pushed "fetal pain" to the political forefront. The move refracted women's experiences in pregnancy and claim of abortion rights through another lens: the imagined experience of the fetus. In 2007, Kansas Republican senator Sam Brownback (and Republican New Jersey representative Chris Smith) sponsored the Unborn Child Pain Awareness Act. The hope, as discussed by historian Sara Dubow, was that this type of pain (which they attached to fetal innocence) would help to establish personhood for the fetus, to gain traction in the law and to mobilize public sentiment for the campaign against legal abortion.[4] That this political invention was unsupported by neurological science did not matter; pain was too valuable a political prop to leave to scientific experts. The Brownback-Smith bill died in committee but won 120 cosponsors in the House and 29 in the Senate.[5] In the cultural symbolism of pain, liberals had their own portrait of the deserving person in pain in the same era—building on physician-assisted suicide and end-of-life compassion in the 1990s, many successfully enacted, state by state, measures accepting marijuana as pain relief for people with a wide range of ailments. As the New Jersey Compassionate Use Medical Marijuana Act of 2010 stated, for example, "Compassion dictates a distinction be made between medical and non-medical uses of marijuana . . . to alleviate suffering from debilitating medical conditions."[6]

Since the 1990s, then, the political theatrics of pain continued to fragment along partisan political lines, and these maneuvers have also moved into the states, continuing a debate over federalism and the distribution of powers. The states have been flexing their political muscles, seeking to write their own laws of compassion while the federal government has sought to influence pain policies from afar. In this new politics of pain, an underlying liberal trend prevails. More states that lean Left and libertarian, from California, Washington, and Colorado to New Jersey have embraced compassionate medical marijuana legislation (in the name of chronic and end-of-life pain relief); by contrast, only a handful of those right-leaning states (like Georgia and Kentucky) proposed and passed so-called Pain-Capable Unborn Child Protection Acts to ensure that pregnant women seeking abortions were told about "fetal pain." The battle is far from over. In the divided states of analgesia, the political theatrics of relief tilts decidedly toward liberalized compassion for persons living with pain, with a much more modest attempt to trump abortion rights by recognizing and validating pain in persons yet to be.

In this political drama scientists and physicians have been important actors on the stage—but their pronouncements on pain have, by and large, been conflicted, and they have played second fiddle to ideologues and lawmakers orchestrating pain policy. Medical theories about why some people cry when hurt and others face pain with grim stoicism, why some seek help and others soldier on alone, have often followed (rather than led) society's cultural arguments. The common 1950s belief that the pain was a sign of the maladjusted personality is a case in point, supporting cultural skepticism about disability and relief. The rise of the gate control theory in the 1960s and 1970s, however, both followed and led. It echoed new thinking about the legitimacy of subjective pain as real pain, but it also provided a powerful rationale for therapeutic experimentation and helped usher in a decade of openness to new kinds of relief from patient-controlled analgesia to acupuncture and electrical nerve stimulation. The theory of learned helplessness that arose in turn in the 1980s had a more modest scientific appeal, but it (like so many theories of pain) gave a thin veneer of legitimacy to policy—in this case, the politically charged conservative claim that relief too easily obtained bred intractable dependence. As disputes over pain and relief migrated to the courts, it should not surprise us that medical theories of subjective pain and objective measurement figured prominently in court rulings. By the end of the twentieth century, other theories like the double effect of painkillers at the end of life were crucial for judges in accepting and ruling on the complexities of physician-assisted suicide. In more recent times, another theory about people in pain (pseudoaddiction, the notion that a restrictive system tending toward the denial of pain care could make even honest sufferers behave furtively in seeking relief) sought to reframe the pain debate and light the fire of reform. In the history of pain management (carried out as a political and medical craft), such medical and scientific theories never stood completely apart from politics—and the evolution of pain theories has been particularly fraught because they exist in such close dialogue with political ideologies and legal theories of relief.

The courts share medicine's fundamental concern with relief—that is, the legal granting of compensation to make injured parties whole again. This was the kind of relief Jack Lemmon's character in *The Fortune Cookie* was seeking. The battle for relief, in the legal rather than the clinical or political context, had its own theatrics—a cast of characters (wronged plaintiffs, defendants, expert witnesses who were often doctors, dramatic claims of harms done, and requests for reparations). The theatrics of pain in the legal arena also had its own evidentiary logic and political implications. As this book argues, it was in the law that pain relief expanded most dramatically as an issue; it was the courts that grappled persistently with the question of pain's measurement and proper relief in relation to fundamental questions of rights—from individual rights to disability relief in the 1960s *Page v. Celebrezze* and 1980s *Polaski v. Heckler* cases, to the right to die without pain in the 1990s, to the right of the federal government to limits the state's powers on such questions in 2006 *Oregon v. Gonzalez*, to the right to relief through medical marijuana playing out today, and to the claim of fetal rights. These questions of pain and relief might start in the sick person's body or in a medical clinic, but increasingly it would be judges in high courts (John Brown in the 1950s and Sandra Day O'Connor in the 1990s) who played a powerful role in determining which medical theories of pain should be applied to the nation's laws of compassion.

If pain and relief often fractured Americans along partisan lines, compassion could also bring political opponents together—sometimes in unlikely ways.[7] Hundreds of pages into the controversial Affordable Care Act (ACA), decried as "Obamacare" by its Republican critics, sits a provision on pain (Section 4305) that calls for advancing research and treatment on pain care.[8] Its inclusion would seem to be on a continuum with liberal lawmaking, with the Left's enduring commitment to compassionately relieving the pain of others.

A closer look reveals that the provision had bipartisan roots, just like the Eisenhower SSDI law that preceded it by a half century. In this case, the provision in Obamacare dated back to George W. Bush's presidency, during which he promised to add compassion to conservatism. Even as the Left and Right fractured around fetal and end-of-life pain, some lawmakers sought compromises. In 2003, Representative Mike Rogers, a Michigan Republican, introduced a bill for a "national pain-care policy," which California Democratic representative Lois Capps later cosponsored in 2007. The bill called for spending $26 million to tackle a handful of problems: to educate practitioners about pain care, to reduce barriers to treatment for underserved groups, to support a national conference to re-evaluate pain management, and to pay for a public-awareness campaign. With an estimated fifty million adults suffering frequent and often disabling chronic pain from low back ailments, migraines, fibromyalgia, cancer, and other conditions, $26 million was a paltry amount. By contrast, that same year President Bush vetoed a bipartisan bill calling for an additional $35 billion for expanding health care to four million poor children; he had wanted a few billion dollars less in a program that already cost tens of billions annually.[9] By comparison, $26 million was a minuscule sum, but in the politics of pain it was a grand gesture—for Rogers and Capps agreed that doctors were poorly educated on the topic of pain care, that undertreatment of pain was a particularly egregious problem for minority and poor populations, that some kind of pain summit of experts was needed, and that a modestly funded public campaign (akin to AIDS awareness) would move the nation's health forward. Born in the shadow of the continuing culture wars over pain, the provision sought the middle ground, yet it too would become a stage prop in the continuing American morality play about citizenship, belonging, and government recognition.[10]

It would take the turnover of presidential administrations and the Democratic takeover of Congress, but in March 2009 (weeks after President Obama's inauguration), the bipartisan Capps-Rogers bill finally passed the House of Representatives. An era of compromise around compassion had apparently returned. There were signs that the Senate might seriously consider the reform when, in early 2009, Senator Orrin Hatch (a Utah Republican who had been part of both the fetal pain and death with dignity pain debates) teamed with liberal senator Christopher Dodd, a Connecticut Democrat, to sponsor the pain bill in the Senate. Hatch announced that he hoped the funding would address inadequate professional training, support a "public-awareness campaign highlighting pain as a serious public-health issue," and "create a comprehensive framework for addressing coordinated research" and greater training capacity of health-care providers. Opting against polarizing pain, Hatch spoke instead of cancer sufferers who "should not have to spend their final days in pain." With such backing, prospects for reform in the Senate looked good.

But when President Obama declared his commitment for more sweeping health care legislation, he transformed the fate of the pain provision.

As happened so many times before, people in pain watched as their particular complaints (arthritis care, low back pain, undertreatment, skeptical caregivers, poorly educated physicians, legal surveillance) became swept into and defined by the broader political controversies of the time. Even with the Capps-Rogers bill inserted into the Democratic health-care reform package, Representative Rogers declared his opposition to the entire measure. He returned to the old songbook, portraying liberal compassion as a charade of selective punishment, a dose of pain for the majority driven by the misguided promise of relief for those in need: "Abraham Lincoln said, 'You can't make a weak man strong by making a strong man weak.' And so what we've decided to do today is to abandon the very principles of America and say . . . we're going to punish the 85 percent of Americans who have earned healthcare benefits . . . to cover the 15 percent that don't have it."[11]

Once folded into the ACA, the promise of pain reform narrowed, its transformation bearing a lesson about how fiscal concerns have often underpinned the Right's criticism of pain reform. The criticism had been lobbed by the AMA for decades: Who shall pay for people in pain, how much would their care cost, and (perhaps most important) would the private pain economy somehow be hurt by these public commitments? As the yearlong political drama over Obamacare stretched from 2009 into 2010, with serious debate comingling with silly accusations that the legislation would result in federal "death panels," the dollars authorized in the Capps-Rogers House bill evaporated—stripped out as a concession to the fiscal concerns of Democrats wary of the stinging conservative critique of expansive liberal government. Gone was the funding for a campaign to inform the public of the high toll of pain across an aging population. There would be no public service announcement telling people of their pain treatment options—messages that perhaps would have competed on the airwaves with commercials for the latest arthritis drug. The provisions for more robust physician education died as well. The problems of the person in pain dwindled in importance next to the sweeping challenges of extending insurance to nearly forty million uninsured. With no funds allocated in the revised Section 4305, all that remained of the original Capps-Rogers bill was a modest requirement to form a commission and a provision for the Institute of Medicine to convene a conference to increase recognition of the problem, evaluate current pain practices, identify barriers to treatment, and establish an agenda for action. In short, those in power and at center stage in Congress asked a chorus of experts to study the problem—to read from their own now-familiar script. The National Institutes of Health stepped in to fund the IOM study. Perhaps not surprisingly, given the scale of the ACA legislation, the broader reform agenda had sidetracked the cause of pain reform. Relief on this front, in other words, was deferred.

As requested by the ACA law, the resulting IOM study, "Relieving Pain in America: A Blueprint for Transforming Prevention, Care, Education, and Research," was published on cue in 2011 and repeated many familiar concerns: doctors were poorly educated on the topic, public awareness about pain lagged, and politics and misguided concerns about addiction shaped how many doctors thought about the topic. Faced with chronic pain sufferers, the study noted, doctors' "reactions ranged from care and compassion to judgmental opinions that lacked compassion and sometimes devolved into blaming"[12] As the leaders of the study noted, meeting the challenges posed by pain in America "will require a cultural transformation in the way pain is perceived and managed on both the personal and societal levels."[13] Published in the midst of a deep economic downturn and continuing partisanship (with cries for repealing the ACA and overturning it in the courts still resonant), the call for cultural change on pain relief had little traction. The theatrics of pain had moved on, with legislators now making political hay around the nation's widespread "economic pain."[14]

For anyone now familiar with the drama—the twisting history and politics of pain in America—the notion that we have a cultural problem understanding other people's pain will not be surprising. The problem, I argue, though it often becomes manifest in medicine, begins in the human condition (aging, infirmity, and the realities of hardship) and quickly becomes complicated by the way the nation's social, legal, and political institutions conceptualize this condition. In 1987, amid that era's controversies over purging the disability rolls, Congress had called for another IOM study ("Pain and Disability: Clinical, Behavioral, and Public Policy Perspectives"). Those expert results, like the 2011 findings, had also called for improved education for the country's doctors, nurses, and caregivers. But the 1987 report also saw failures in government, calling for the secretary of Health and Human Services to "take the lead in ensuring that a broad research initiative on pain and disability is undertaken within HHS and in cooperation with other federal agencies."[15] Nothing was done along those lines to educate the administrators and bureaucrats charged with managing the machinery of relief. Yet, the authors of the 1987 study rightly understood that the need for education could never be confined to medicine; enlightened thinking on pain and relief remains sorely needed in government, politics, and law.

A fundamental, vexing problem ripples through the history and politics of pain: Who should have the power to judge suffering—the patient or the doctor, the state or the federal government, the judge or the politician, the bureaucrat or the ideologue, the surgeon or the pharmacist? Who can detect true pain when they see it? Which of us knows whose pain is real and whose is being exaggerated or faked for so-called secondary gain? The pages above have shown how and why the skepticism about pain as fraud has shadowed sufferers, and they have also shown why questions about the nature of pain have had no easy resolution in the theater of politics and society. The question of pain has been politically, economically, culturally, and legally contentious over the past seventy years and will continue to be so. But just as contentious has been the issue of who has standing to judge and to speak for and about pain in America. One enduring aspect of this political theater is how much people in pain have had to fight to be heard amid the battles waged over them and on their behalf.

Pain, in this sense, does not belong exclusively to those who suffer; it also belongs to those who observe suffering. Here again, the insights of Talal Asad on pain prove helpful when he observes, "The ability to live sanely after a traumatic experience of pain is always dependent on the responses of others."[16] Surely, pain fraud exists, and there will always be skeptics who insist that too many people fit the caricature of the Jack Lemmon figure in *The Fortune Cookie*. But there is no need to add to the scrutiny of sufferers as deceitful; there is enough of that already. Instead I have focused on a broader world of deceit, false claims, fraud, and posturing. Pain fraud includes the artful quacks and drug makers throughout history, promising fast relief while fomenting anguish and dependence—a deceit worth examining. Another is the posturing of health and legal experts who theorize about the pain of others, their shifting theories often supported by sparse education, misplaced fears, and ideology. The poor state of medical education on pain is no fraud, but surely it requires skeptical attention and reform. Then there are the slippery and sometimes deceitful political claims about people in pain made in the name of liberalism and conservatism; this has been my focus. Instead of indulging in more skepticism about people in pain, this book provides deeper insight into those who judge—attention to their political motives, their hypocrisies, their claims of compassion, their attempts to implement meaningful relief, their agendas for the nation, and why they so often turn the pain of others into political theater. It is good to look critically and closely at those who would judge because they, like every sufferer, also live in a world defined by both virtue and fraud.

Acknowledgments

....

I owe a great debt to many people who have provided challenging encouragement over the years and to many institutions supporting the research behind this work. The project was first conceptualized during my days on the faculty in social medicine at the School of Medicine and in the Department of History at the University of North Carolina at Chapel Hill; it grew in scope when I joined Rutgers' Department of History and the Institute for Health, Health Care Policy and Aging Research; and expanded yet again during my years at Princeton—straddling the History Department, the Program in the History of Science, and the Woodrow Wilson School of Public and International Affairs. At all those places (and in other places too numerous to list), this project benefited from astute comments from friends, insightful readings by colleagues, and constructive discussions with many students.

Two major grants played a critical role in supporting the research behind this work and also in supporting a sustained cross-disciplinary community of scholars in which to develop its potential. When the James S. McDonnell Foundation awarded me the Centennial Fellowship in the history of science (a multiyear grant to support a wide range of work on the cultural politics of the biomedical sciences), I envisioned a book on pain as the last in a long line of studies stemming from the generous ten years of support. Having arrived here, I gratefully acknowledge the support of Susan Fitzpatrick, John Breuer, and others at the foundation. Second, the Robert Wood Johnson Foundation Investigator Award in Health Policy Research provided another important grant in support of this project, along with regular interaction with a brilliant policy-engaged community of scholars and administrative support that knows no match from Lynn

Rogut and Cynthia Church. For their comments and insights in the RWJ setting, thanks go to Alvin Tarlov, Rosemary Stevens, Paul Cleary, and especially to David Mechanic, whose leadership and breadth of knowledge (as well as his involvement in pain policy) set a very high standard.

For their feedback and encouragement in many other settings, thanks to Julie Livingston, David Mechanic, Peter Guarnaccia, Ann Jurecic, Mark Schlesinger, Gerald Grob, James Livingston, Uri Eisenzweig, Michael McVaugh, Kenneth Ludmerer, Walton Schalick, W. Bruce Fye, Mia Bay, Kevin Kruse, John Burnham, Steve Conn, Katya Guenther, Kevin Kruse, Barbara Grosz, Charles Rosenberg, Joseph Fins, Carla Nappi, Max Weiss, William Jordan, Christina Paxson, Paul Starr, Julian Zelizer, Ben Rich, Elizabeth Armstrong, Emily Thompson, Marni Sandweiss, Bengt Sandin, Claude Steele, Nancy King, Larry Churchill, Barry Saunders, Alexander Rothman, Kendrick Prewitt, Gail Henderson, Sue Estroff, John Kasson, Joy Kasson, Jonathan Oberlander, Don Madison, Allan Horwitz, Joanna Kempner, David Rosner, Jane Ballantyne, Knox Todd, Chris Feudtner, Dan Segal, Susan Schweik, Susan Lindee, Mark Sullivan, Mitchell Max, David Asch, Robert Aronowitz, Jonathan Kahn, Alan Richardson, Jooyoung Lee, Karen Sue Taussig, David Jones, Jonathan Metzl, Robert Brain, Joel Howell, Jennifer Gunn, Susan Jones, Jeffrey Brosco, Ken Goodman, Martin Pernick, Howard Markel, Holly Smith, Peter Guarnaccia, David Barton Smith, Vincent Kopp, Justin Lorts, Louise Russell, Stephen Pemberton, Mark Rodwin, James DuBois, Robert Proctor, Londa Schiebinger, Helena Hansen, Sam Roberts, Jack Lesch, Catherine Lee, Holly Smith, Leslie Gerwin, Kim Scheppele, Lisa Miller, Sean Wilentz, Janet Currie, Anne Case, Angus Deaton, and Rosemarie Garland-Thomson.

For close reading of the manuscript (or portions of it), thanks to Catherine Lee, Elizabeth Chiarello, Dan Rodgers, Hendrik Hartog, Philip Nord, Sarah Milov, Dov Grosghal, Angela Creager, Graham Burnett, Michael Gordin, Erika Milam, Miranda Waggoner, Elizabeth Armstrong, Bridget Gurtler, Nancy Hirschmann, Rogers Smith, Beth Linker, Alison Isenberg, Hannah-Louise Clark, Edna Bonhomme, Shakti Jaising, Anantha Sudhakar, Wangui Muigai, Catherine Abou-Nemeh, and Evan Hepler-Smith. Thanks also to all of the students in the Program in History of Science at Princeton and fellows in the 2006–2007 class at the Center for Advanced Study in the Behavioral Sciences, whose collective insights on individual chapters helped move the book to a new level.

I owe a special word of gratitude to my wonderful editor at Johns Hopkins University Press, Jacqueline Wehmueller, who saw the value of the project early on, commented on it carefully, and, with characteristic patience, enthusiasm, and insight, helped me to develop it. The work also benefited from the brilliant copyediting and smart commentary of Audra Wolfe and Carrie Watterson.

A number of former students provided research insights, participated in many discussions on the history of pain, helped plan conferences, and gave feedback well beyond what the term "research assistant" conveys. They became key interlocutors over time. Heartfelt thanks to Joseph Gabriel, Rachel McLaughlin, Moshe Usadi, Rachel Watkins, Michelle Rotunda, Stephani Pfeiffer, Curt Cardwell, Dora Vargha, Bridget Gurtler, Justin Lorts, Jane Park, Carolina Giraldo, Dominique Padurano, Richard Mizelle, Greg Swedberg, William Gordon Jr., and Michal Shapiro.

For especially incisive comments and constructive suggestions on the entire manuscript, I want to thank Jonathan Levy, Hannah-Louise Clark, Daniel Rodgers, Hendrik Hartog, Audra Wolfe, Jacqueline Wehmueller, Dov Grosghal, Elizabeth Chiarello, Catherine Lee, Alison Isenberg, and Stephen Pemberton.

My sincere appreciation goes to the archivists who provided important guidance and access to the historical record of pain and politics—at the UCLA Biomedical Library in Los Angeles, particularly Russell Johnson and Teresa Johnson; at the National Archives and Records Administration in College Park, Maryland; at the Dwight D. Eisenhower Library in Abilene, Kansas; at the Ronald Reagan Library in Loma Linda, California; and at the Seeley G. Mudd Library at Princeton University.

Finally, a few words of appreciation to my family who have encouraged, nurtured, and humored my passion for history and writing for many years—to my brother and sister-in-law, Christopher Wailoo and Alisa Lasater, from whom I've learned a thing or two about compassion; to my parents, Bert and Lynette Wailoo, who have always taught me the value of hard work, independence, and looking to the past for inspiration and support; to my historian friend and partner in all things, Alison Isenberg, for dexterous insights too numerous to mention; and to Myla and Elliot Wailoo, and the littlest ones, Anthony and Andrew Wailoo, for giving us all bright reasons to look ahead.

Notes

Introduction: Between Liberal Relief and Conservative Care

1. On his way to the Democratic nomination for president in 1992, the Arkansas governor said "I feel your pain" when confronted by a man with AIDS, making the candidate the object of commentary and ridicule. "Heckler Stirs Clinton Anger: Excerpts from the Exchange," New York Times (March 28, 1992): 9. As one journalist noted years later, when Clinton uttered those words "he may have set himself up for years of razzing and mockery." Natalie Angier, "Yet Another Sex Difference Found: Gaining Relief from a Painkiller," *New York Times*, October 30, 1996, C12; for "I'm not here . . .", Alison Powell and Leigh Denny, "The Toughest Love," *Guardian*, May 14, 1999, A13; "best illustration . . . ," Limbaugh's 1996 television discussion of Clinton can be seen at: Rush Limbaugh, "Bill Clinton Fakes Crying at Ron Brown's Funeral," YouTube video, posted by blogologist on January 22, 2008, www.youtube.com/watch?v=lf8TOGrq8Bo; "just keep in mind . . . ," David Remnick, "Day of the Dittohead," *Washington Post*, February 20, 1994, C1.

2. For "easy to parody . . . ," see E. J. Dionne Jr., ". . . Playing Defense," Washington Post, August 26, 1996, A13; for "the left is so fond . . . ," see John A. Beard, letter, "Thanks to Liberals, 'Civil Rights' has lost its meaning," *Washington Times*, February 11, 1994, A22; for "whiners . . . ," see Paul Taylor, "Makes Me Wanna Whine," Washington Post, August 27, 1995, C1.

3. Ronald Reagan, inauguration address, January 20, 1981, YouTube video, posted by C-SPAN on January 14, 2009, www.youtube.com/watch?v=hpPt7xG x4Xo.

4. The study therefore contributes to the diverse and rich scholarship in disability studies. See for example Paul K. Longmore and Lauri Umansky, *The New Disability History: American Perspectives* (New York: NYU Press, 2001); Rosemarie Garland Thomson, *Extraordinary Bodies* (New York: Columbia University

Press, 1997); and Ruth O'Brien, *Crippled Justice: The History of Modern Disability Policy in the Workplace* (Chicago: University of Chicago Press, 2001).

5. In recent years, scholars in political studies have turned increasing attention to the role of emotions—compassion, fear, anger, disgust—in the cultural politics of citizenship and governance. See for example, Paul Hoggett and Simon Thompson, eds., *Politics and the Emotions: The Affective Turn in Contemporary Political Studies* (London: Continuum, 2012). See also Sara Ahmed, *The Cultural Politics of Emotion* (Edinburgh: Edinburgh University Press, 2004), esp. "The Contingency of Pain." On compassion, see Martha Nussbaum, "Compassion: The Basic Social Emotion," *Social Philosophy and Policy* 13 (1996): 27–58; and Maureen Whitebook, "Compassion as a Political Virtue," *Political Studies* 50 (2002): 529–44. For "it is not dependency . . . ," see A. Cooper and J. Lousada, *Borderline Welfare: Feeling and Fear of Feeling in Modern Welfare* (London: Karnac, 2005). See also Tim Darington, "The Therapeutic Fantasy: Self-Love and Quick Wins," in *Politics and the Emotions: The Affective Turn in Contemporary Political Studies*, ed. Paul Hoggett and Simon Thompson (New York: Continuum, 2012).

6. The literature on liberalism and conservatism in the United States has explored not only the tensions between New Deal liberalism and the rise of neoconservatism but also documented internal tensions in these political commitments—the tensions between, for example, New Deal liberals and southern liberals in the 1940s and 1950s and the internal fracture lines among conservatives on questions of taxes, Communism, race, and so on. Laura Kalman represents another valuable line of analysis—looking closely at the ways liberalism and conservatism coexisted in politics and the ways in which the law became a site for battles over the future of liberal and conservative American society. See Laura Kalman, *Right Star Rising: A New Politics, 1974–1980* (New York: Norton, 2010); and Laura Kalman, *The Strange Career of Legal Liberalism* (New Haven, CT: Yale University Press, 1996). Other valuable works on liberalism and conservatism, to which this study owes great debt, include the following: Bruce Schulman, *The Seventies: The Great Shift in American Culture, Society, and Politics* (New York: Da Capo, 2001); Gil Troy and Vincent J. Cannato, eds., *Living in the Eighties* (New York: Oxford, 2009); W. Elliot Brownlee and Hugh Davis Graham, eds., *The Reagan Presidency: Pragmatic Conservatism and Its Legacies* (Lawrence: Kansas University Press, 2003); Meg Jacobs and Julian Zelizer, *Conservatives in Power: The Reagan Years, 1981–1980; A Brief History with Documents* (New York: Bedford, 2011); Lisa McGirr, *Suburban Warriors: The Origins of the New Right* (Princeton, NJ: Princeton University Press, 2001); Annelise Orleck, *Storming Caesar's Palace: How Black Mothers Fought Their Own War*

on *Poverty* (Boston: Beacon Press, 2005); Brian Balogh, "Making Pluralism 'Great': Beyond a Recycled History of the Great Society," in *The Great Society and the High Tide of Liberalism,* ed. Sidney M. Milkis and Jeromse M. Mileur (Amherst: University of Massachusetts Press, 2005).

7. Transcript of the hearing on Rush Limbaugh's medical records, Palm Beach County, Florida Case No. CA 03 13316, December 23, 2003, www.freere public.com/focus/f-news/1046161/posts.

8. The literature on pain's history (cutting across medicine, social science, humanities, law, and political scholarship) is extensive. See for example Elaine Scarry, *The Body in Pain: The Making and Unmaking of the World* (New York: Oxford University Press, 1987); David Morris, *The Culture of Pain* (Berkeley: University of California Press, 1993); Isabelle Baszanger, *Inventing Pain Medicine: From the Laboratory to the Clinic* (New Brunswick: Rutgers University Press, 1998); Javier Moscoso, *Pain: A Cultural History* (New York: Palgrave, 2012); Esther Cohen, *The Modulated Scream: Pain in Late Medieval Culture* (Chicago: University of Chicago Press, 2010); and numerous other works. To date, none of this scholarship has examined the politics of pain in the way this book intends—that is, by considering the ways in which seemingly separate cultural, biological, social science, legal, and administrative views on pain have intersected and informed one another. Nor have any of these works sought, as this book does, to show how the topic of pain and proper relief underpins American political debates. One particularly thoughtful analysis is Jean E. Jackson, "Stigma, Liminality, and Chronic Pain: Mind-Body Borderlands," *American Ethnologist* 32 (2005): 332–53. On social suffering, see also Arthur Kleinman, Veena Das, and Margaret Lock, eds., *Social Suffering* (Berkeley: University of California Press, 1997) As these authors noted, "Chronic pain syndromes highlight the fault lines in society . . . [Pain] has an anomalous status in biomedicine . . . baffling to clinicians and academic physicians." See also Lous Heshusius, *Inside Chronic Pain: An Intimate and Critical Account* (Ithaca, NY: Cornell University Press, 2009); Jean E. Jackson, *Camp Pain: Talking with Chronic Pain Patients* (Philadelphia: University of Pennsylvania Press, 2000); and Susan Greenhalgh, *Under the Medical Gaze: Facts and Fictions of Chronic Pain* (Berkeley: University of California, 2001).

9. Sylvia Nasar and Alison Leigh Cowan, "A Wall St. Star's Agonizing Confession," *New York Times,* April 3, 1994, 66.

10. Shizuko Y. Fagerhaugh and Anselm Strauss, *Politics of Pain Management: Staff-Patient Interaction* (Menlo Park, CA: Addison-Wesley, 1977), iv.

11. Martha Nussbaum, "Compassion: The Basic Human Emotion," *Social Philosophy* and Policy 13 (December 1996): 28.

12. Edmund Burke, "On the Sublime and Beautiful," in *On Taste, On the Sublime and Beautiful, Reflections on the French Revolution, and A Letter to a Noble Lord* (New York: Cosimo, 2009), 114.

13. John Stuart Mill, *Utilitarianism*, 2nd ed. (London: Longman, Green, Longman, Roberts, and Green, 1864), 17.

Chapter One: The Trojan Horse of Pain

1. Louis M. Orr, "To Socialize Medicine and Socialism by Way of the Veterans Administration," *Journal of the American Medical Association* 162 (October 27, 1956): 860–65.

2. Lt. Col. Henry K. Beecher, "Pain in Men Wounded in Battle," *Annals of Surgery* 123 (January 1946): 96–105.

3. Ibid.

4. For "it was inevitable . . . ," see *Annual Report: Administrator of Veterans Affairs, 1963* (Washington, D.C.: General Printing Office, 1963), 61; Marshall Andrews, "Veterans Put Big Burden on President," *Washington Post*, January 20, 1949, C13.

5. Barbara Welke, *Law and the Borders of Belonging in the Long Nineteenth Century United States* (New York: Cambridge University Press, 2010).

6. "Proper care or our uniformed citizens and appreciation of [their] past service . . . are part of our accepted governmental responsibilities." Dwight D. Eisenhower, State of the Union address, February 2, 1953, *Public Papers of the Presidents: Dwight D. Eisenhower* (Washington, D.C.: United States Government Printing Office, 1954), 12:33; for an authoritative history of SSDI, see Edward Berkowitz, *Disabled Policy: America's Programs for the Handicapped* (New York: Cambridge University Press, 1987).

7. See Wilma T. Donahue and Clark Tibbits, "The Task before the Veteran and Society," *Annals of the American Academy of Political and Social Science*, vol. 239, *The Disabled Veteran* (May, 1945), ed. Wilma T. Donahue and Clark Tibbits (Philadelphia, American Academy of Political and Social Science), 1–9; Roy R. Grinker and John P. Spiegel, *Men under Stress* (Philadelphia: Blakiston, 1945), 449. These concerns were widespread. See for example Frank Fearing, "Warriors Return: Normal or Neurotic?" *Hollywood Quarterly* 1 (October 1945): 97–109.

8. Charles Reich, "The New Property," *Yale Law Journal* 73 (April 1964): 733–87; see also John Kenneth Galbraith, *The Affluent Society and Other Writings 1952–1967* (New York: Penguin, 2010).

9. "There are two groups of individuals," wrote William Menninger, psychiatrist in the Office of the Surgeon General, "whom psychiatrists have to evalu-

ate that are not sick but are nonetheless noneffective in military service." The men he labeled "can'ts" were "inept and lacking in ability." The "won'ts" were "potentially capable of doing the job required of them" but were unwilling. William Menninger, "The Mentally or Emotionally Handicapped Veteran," in Donahue and Tibbits, *Disabled Veteran*, 20–28.

10. Donahue and Tibbits, "Task before the Veteran and Society."

11. As historian James Sparrow has noted, the commitments coming out of war both reinforced the commitments of New Deal liberalism and extended those commitments in new ways—the GI Bill being the foremost example. See James Sparrow, *Warfare State: World War II Americans and the Age of Big Government* (New York: Oxford, 2011); for "a roof over the head . . . ," see Sam Stavisky, "Where Does the Veteran Stand Today?" *Annals of the American Academy of Political and Social Science*, vol. 259, *Parties and Politics: 1948* (September, 1948), 135; for "sense of inadequacy . . . ," Donahue and Tibbits, "Task before the Veteran and Society"; *Annual Report: Administrator of Veterans Affairs, 1952* (Washington, D.C.: General Printing Office, 1952), 68; for an example of expansion of "service-related" ailments, see Public Law 174 passed by the Eighty-Second Congress, which provided for broader coverage of multiple sclerosis as a disability when diagnosed within two years of separation from active service, *Annual Report: Administrator of Veterans Affairs, 1952*, 67; for Truman's views, see Philip J. Funigiello, *Chronic Politics: Health Care Security from FDR to George W. Bush* (Lawrence: University of Kansas, 2006), 61; for "this means a profound change . . . ," see Box 88, folder: Basic Philosophy of Pensions Supporting Data (1), U.S. President's Commission on Veterans' Pensions (Bradley Commission): Records, 1954–58, Dwight D. Eisenhower Library, Abilene, KS.

12. Ray Cromley, "Doctors Prescribe Less 'Civilization' for Your Chronic Aches and Pains," *Wall Street Journal*, December 8, 1949, 1. Knapp was former president of the American Congress of Rehabilitative Medicine.

13. Ibid.

14. Arthur J. Altmeyer, "The Future of Social Security," *Social Service Review* 27 (September 1953): 267.

15. For the testimony of the director of the Veterans Administration, see Funigiello, *Chronic Politics*, 68. The new disability enactments (Public Law 149; Public Law 174; Public Law 356; Public Law 357; Public Law 427—all passed by the Eighty-Second Congress) are discussed in *Administrator of Veterans Affairs, Annual Report, 1952*, 66.

16. Theda Skocpol, *Protecting Soldiers and Mothers: The Political Origins of Social Policy in the United States* (Cambridge, MA: Harvard University Press,

1982); and Beth Linker, *War's Waste: Rehabilitation in World War I America* (Chicago: University of Chicago, 2011).

17. For "temporarily won the battle . . . ," see "Private Medicine Victory seen in GOP Success," *Los Angeles Times*, December 15, 1952, 9; for "From such dreams . . . ," see "Address at the Alfred E. Smith Memorial Dinner, New York City, October 21, 1954," *Public Papers: Eisenhower*, 936.

18. " Citation Accompanying Medal of Honor Awarded to Private First Class Alford L. McLaughlin—August 18, 1953," *Public Papers of the Presidents: Dwight D. Eisenhower* (Washington, D.C.: United States Government Printing Office, 1953): 174; see also David Gerber, "Heroes and Misfits: The Troubled Social Reintegration of Disabled Veterans in 'The Best Years of Our Lives,'" *American Quarterly* 46 (December 1994): 545–74.

19. Eisenhower, State of the Union address, 1953, 33.

20. For "Holders of the Purple Heart . . . ," see The Military Order of the Purple Heart, Inc. to the Bradley Commission, May 27, 1955, Bradley Commission Papers, box 9, folder: Indexed Replies Copy 1 (2); for "compensation for those . . . ," see Disabled American Veterans letter to Bradley Commission, May 19, 1955, Bradley Commission Papers, box 9, folder: Indexed Replies Copy 1 (2).

21. For "disgusting . . . ," see "VFW Chief Hits Medical Group," *Los Angeles Times*, February 26, 1954, 5; see also "AMA Head Calls VA Free Enterprise Threat," *Los Angeles Times*, October 26, 1953, 34; Lisa McGirr, *Suburban Warriors: The Origins of the New American Right* (Princeton, NJ: Princeton University Press, 2001), 67; for "continued federal encroachment . . . ," see Nate Haseltine, "AMA Claims Legion Aids Socialism," *Washington Post*, August 31, 1954, 2; for "cash-conscious . . . ," see "American Legion Attacks AMA on Free Care Stand," *Los Angeles Times*, September 2, 1954, 18; for "lay off . . . ," see "AMA Is Assailed by VFW Leader," *Washington Post*, March 16, 1954, 13; see also Nate Haseltine, "AMA Claims Legion Aids Socialism," *Washington Post*, August 31, 1954, 2; "Non-Service Veterans Care Under Attack," *Los Angeles Times*, December 29, 1955, 12.

22. "Veto of Bill for the Relief of Fred P. Hines. July 20, 1953," *Public Papers: Eisenhower* (1953), 498.

23. Letter from Eisenhower to General Omar N. Bradley, Chairman, President's Commission on Veterans' Pensions, Concerning a Study of Veterans' Benefits, March 5, 1955, www.presidency.ucsb.edu/ws/?pid=10429.

24. For proposed legislation, see "Social Security Extension Plan Rapped by AMA," *Los Angeles Times*, July 16, 1955, 4; "AMA Blasts Security Bill for Disabled," *Washington Post*, July 23, 1955, 24; "Non-Service Veterans Care under Attack," *Los Angeles Times*, December 29, 1955, 12.

25. Meeting with John Gunther, February 7, 1950, Miller Center, Scripps Archive, University of Virginia, http://millercenter.org/scripps/archive/presidentialrecordings/eisenhower#presidential.

26. McGirr, *Suburban Warriors*.

27. "Thanks to Penicillin . . . He Will Come Home," Henley Laboratories Inc. advertisement, *Life*, August 14, 1944; for studies on drug production in World War II and postwar drug cultures, see Nicholas Rasmussen, *On Speed: The Many Lives of Amphetamines* (New York: NYU Press, 2008); and David Herzberg, *Happy Pills in America: From Miltown to Prozac* (Baltimore: Johns Hopkins University Press, 2010).

28. Oxycodone production around 1948–50 stood at 9 kilograms; by 1960 it was 569 kilograms. Mentioned by Edward Bloomquist, MD, Los Angeles member of the Committee on Dangerous Drugs, California Medical Association in his "The Addiction Potential of Oxycodone (Percodan)," *California Medicine* 99, no. 2 (August 1963): 127–30. See also Nathan Eddy, H. Halbach, and Olav Braenden, "Synthetic Substances with Morphine-Like Effect: Clinical Experience: Potency, Side Effects, Addiction Liability," *Bulletin of the World Health Organization* 17 (1957): 569–863.

29. Peter Bart, "Aspirin Consumption Increases with the Nation's Headaches," *New York Times*, March 26, 1961, F1; John Kenneth Galbraith, *The Affluent Society and Other Writings 1952–1967* (New York: Penguin, 2010); for Frank Erving, see "Attack on Pain," *Time*, March 2, 1959, 32, 34. As Dominique Tobbell has noted, "Retail pharmacists were struggling to meet the demands placed on them by the ever-expanding market of prescription drugs." Dominique A. Tobbell, "'Eroding the Physician's Control of Therapy': The Postwar Politics of the Prescription," in *Prescribed: Writing, Filling, Using, and Abusing the Prescription in America*, ed. Jeremy A. Greene and Elizabeth Siegel Watkins (Baltimore: Johns Hopkins University Press, 2012), 68.

30. Paul DeKruif, "God's Own Medicine," *Reader's Digest*, June 1946, 15; for Senate testimony, see William Moore, "Addict Reveals Use of Dope by Chicago Pupils," *Chicago Daily Tribune*, June 27, 1951, 8; and "Stiffer Sentence for Selling Drugs to Minors Proposed," *Washington Post*, July 26, 1951, 9; for "my first shot of dope . . . ," see David Courtwright, Herman Joseph, and Don Des Jarlais, eds., *Addicts Who Survived: An Oral History of Narcotic Use in America, 1923–1965* (Knoxville: University of Tennessee Press, 1989), 56; for "he had become addicted . . . ," see Harold Hinton, "Three Minors Recount Narcotic Scourge," *New York Times*, June 27, 1951, 19.

31. For "has become the fastest-selling . . . ," see "Wonder Drugs and Mental Disorders," *Consumer Reports*, August 1955, 388; see also

"Don't-Give-a-Damn-Pills," *Time*, February 27, 1956, 98; for deinstitutionalization, see "Importance of Tranquil Drugs Noted: May Outweigh Atomic Power, Psychiatrist Tells Congress," *Baltimore Sun*, February 12, 1958, 3.

32. "'Ideal' in Tranquility," *Newsweek*, October 29, 1956, 63; on Blatnik, see "Washington High Lights—Many Items Face Study," *Christian Science Monitor*, July 15, 1957, 11; and "Promotion of Tranquilizing Drugs to Be Investigated," *Baltimore Sun*, February 9, 1958, 3; "AMA Cover-Up on Ads Charged," *New York Times*, January 29, 1960, 15.

33. Howard Snyder to Alfred Guenther, Supreme Commander, SHAPE, July 9, 1956, from Gettysburg, box 10, folder: Correspondence re DDE EIS thru LEI (3), Howard Snyder Paper, Dwight Eisenhower Library. See also Robert Gilbert, "Eisenhower's 1955 Heart Attack: Medical Treatment, Political Effects, and the 'Behind the Scenes' Leadership Style," *Politics and the Life Sciences* 27, no. 1 (March 2008): 3.

34. For "an unusually large . . . ," John Bonica, *The Management of Pain* (Philadelphia: Lea and Febiger, 1953), 5; for "though it is common . . . ," see Bonica, *Management of Pain*, 135.

35. Ibid., 73. Writing to the medical department of Smith, Kline, and French in 1955, he noted, "In the past I have used the 10mg. 'Dexedrine' Spansule" for postoperative pain, "but I have found that the side effects, particularly depression of appetite and the jittery feeling, with this amount are too great." John Bonica to P. C. Lawson, Medical Department, Smith, Kline and French Laboratories, April 27, 1956, box 67, folder 13, John Bonica Papers, UCLA.

36. For "the leading reason . . . ," see advertisement copy for Lea and Febiger Books, Bonica, *Management of Pain*, in "The Scientist's Bookshelf," *American Scientist* 42 (January 1954): 162. An excellent account of Bonica's role in the field is found in Isabelle Baszanger, *Inventing Pain Medicine* (New Brunswick, NJ: Rutgers University Press, 1998); the Bonica papers document extensively the researcher's relationship with industry. For "I am anxious to use . . . ," see Dr. M. J. Lewenstein, Endo Products, to Bonica, May 1955, Box 67, folder 13, Bonica Papers: "Dear Dr. Bonica . . . I expect to be in Tacoma on Wednesday and should like to discuss with you at that time your paper on Percodan as well as the results which you so far have obtained with Numorphan."

37. For "the neurosurgeon plays . . . ," see "Relief of Pain Due to Cancer of Head and Neck," Thomas E. Douglas Jr., MD, Seattle, WA, *General Practitioner*, November 1952, 65–70; for "there is no fine . . . ," quoted in N. S. Haseltine, "Brain Surgery Is Successful in Easing Pain," *Washington Post*, November 26, 1947, 13; see Walter Freeman, "Psychosurgery for Pain," *Southern Medical Journal*; see also Jack Pressman, *Last Resort: Psychosurgery and the Limits of American Medicine*

(New York: Cambridge University Press, 1998); for "pain ceases to be bothersome ...," see Roy Gibbons, "Search for Pain Killers," *Chicago Daily Tribune*, January 30, 1955, 14; see also "Brain Surgery Successful in Relief of Pain," *Chicago Daily Tribune*, April 19, 1947, 12.

38. Haseltine, "Brain Surgery," 13.

39. For an excellent study of psychosurgery and Freeman's arguments against the notion that lobotomy created "vegetables," see Pressman, *Last Resort*.

40. David Serlin, *Replaceable You: Engineering the Body in Postwar America* (Chicago: University of Chicago, 2004), 4; for "to cut the pain tracts ..." and "from prolonged suffering," see William L. Laurence, "Pain Relief Cited in Brain Surgery," *New York Times*, October 7, 1950, 37; see also "Body Pain Is Ended by Brain Surgery," *New York Times*, June 17, 1948, 27; and Howard W. Blakeslee, "MDs Split on Right to Tinker with Brain," *Washington Post*, March 16, 1947, B7; see also Pressman, *Last Resort*; for "so that the pain ...," see "Personality Shift in Laid to Surgery," *New York Times*, December 14, 1947, 51.

41. For "unbearably severe ..." and "in the aged ...," see William L. Laurence, "Pain Relief Cited in Brain Surgery," *New York Times*, October 7, 1950, 37. They used the technique on a wide range of people—those with a few weeks to live but also those with longer than six months. Reflecting a few years later on what was learned from the less extreme neurosurgical treatment for pain, the cordotomy, a leading neurology researcher, P. W. Nathan, noted that "patients have been seen, who before this operation had to be in hospital and on large doses of morphine, amidone, or pethidine, and were in bed all the time. After the operation their pain could be controlled by mild analgesics ... and they were able to be at home, look after their children, cook, and run their homes." P. W. Nathan, "Results of Antero-lateral Cordotomy for Pain in Cancer," *Journal of Neurology, Neurosurgery, and Psychiatry* 26 (1963): 362; for "cutting the channels ...," see "Two Doctors Report Surgery on Brain Ends Dope Addiction," *Chicago Daily Tribune*, May 3, 1948, 2.

42. For "a sensation rather than ..." and "interesting effects on personality," see William S. Barton, "Brain Surgery Seen as Aid for Christine," *Los Angeles Times*, May 6, 1953, A1; for "certain aspects of personality ...," see Asenath Petrie, "Some Psychological Aspects of Pain and the Relief of Suffering," *Annals of the New York Academy of Sciences* 86 (1960): 13. These aspects of personality transformation must be understood as part of the postwar ideal, touching on all aspects of pathologized identity. As David Serlin observed, here was a society fascinated with the promise of biomedical transformation (through biology, surgery, medicine, and prosthetic engineering) to build a better body and society. Serlin, *Replaceable You*; see also Joanne Meyerowitz, *How Sex Changed: A History of*

Transsexuality in the United States (Cambridge, MA: Harvard University Press, 2004).

43. For "destructive procedures," see Bonica, *Management of Pain*, 164; for "tranquilizers, like alcohol ...," see Ian Stevenson, "Tranquilizers and the Mind," *Harper's Magazine* 215 (1957): 21–27; noted another publication, "Happiness pills and elixirs continue to be sought by those who want the satisfaction of a good life without a life that is good. Instead of grappling with the causes of unhappiness they seek merely to remove the symptoms." "Happiness Pills Are No Answer," *Christian Century*, September 12, 1956, 1044.

44. *Compensation for Service-Connected Disabilities: A General Analysis of Veterans' and Military Disability Benefits, Mortality Rates, Disability Standards in Federal Programs, Workmen's Compensation, and Rehabilitation. A Report on Veterans' Benefits in the United States by The President's Commission on Veterans' Pensions*. Staff Report no. 8, part A, August 3, 1956 (Washington, D.C.: Government Printing Office, 1956), 8.

45. Ibid., 8.

46. Another unnamed physician noted that, "of the chronic diseases, I would certainly exclude arteriosclerosis, arthritis," and other such ailments that were too often presumed to be service connected. *The Veterans' Administration Disability Rating Schedule: Historical Development and Medical Appraisal, A Report on Veterans' Benefits in the United States by the President's Commission on Veterans' Pensions*. Staff Report no. 8, part B, June 18, 1956 (Washington, D.C.: Government Printing Office, 1956): 122–24.

47. Ibid., 227–29.

48. Ibid.; see Bradley Commission Papers, folder 34: Snell, Albert M., p. 16: "These are imponderables which cannot be measured and to include them in the present framework would hopelessly complicate the problem of rating boards."

49. Bradley Commission Papers, folder 34: Snell, Albert M., p. 16.

50. Bradley Commission Papers, box 29, folder 82: Cleveland, Mather.

51. Bradley Commission Papers, box 28, folder 55: Canfield, Norton.

52. Bradley Commission Papers, box 27, folder 31: Burrage, Walter S.

53. "I believe that a man should be a soldier throughout life and not be downed because of some remunerative disability that he can compensate for." Bradley Commission Papers, box 28, folder 47: Bunnell, Sterling.

54. Omar N. Bradley, Clarence G. Adamy, and William J. Donovan, et al., *Veterans' Benefits in the United States: A Report to President by the President's Commission on Veterans' Pensions, The Bradley Commission* (Washington D.C.: Government Printing Office, 1956), 135.

55. For "scars about the face . . . ," see Bradley Commission Papers, box 30, folder: Veterans Administration, 101–3. (physician unnamed); for "the compensation of wound scars . . ." and "loss of physical integrity . . . ," *Veterans' Benefits*, 164.

56. All citations from Bradley Commission Papers. For "some critics . . . ," see box 88, folder; Basic Philosophy of Pensions Work File, p. 11; for "the yardsticks . . . ," box 28, folder 69: Hampton, Oscar P., Jr.; for "in order to conserve . . . ," see box 27, folder 29: Morgan, Hugh J.; for "I doubt if . . . ," see box 28, folder 59: Kuhn, Hedwig S.; Others also defended the system, but one Virginia physician believed that "the Veterans Administration is more liberal in their rating policy than comparable state agencies or liability insurance companies." Medical survey with unnamed VA surgeon, p. 16. Box 30, folder: Veterans Administration, 93–97.

57. All citations from Bradley Commission Papers. For "modern developments . . . ," see box 27, folder 17: Minor, John M.; for Bauer quotes, see box 27, folder 12: Bauer, Walter; see also introductory remarks from Robert Sidney Schwab to commission, with his survey. Box 27, folder 10: Schwab, Robert Sidney.

58. Funigiello, *Chronic Politics*, 93. As Funigiello noted, the aged were a high-risk group from the standpoint of the rising private insurance industry, locked out of the ability to purchase health insurance. "Six million aged lived in families earning less than $3,000 a year . . . and most of those (7 out of 10) had no health insurance" (98). Attempting to smooth political feathers, Eisenhower insisted that the new disability benefit for the elderly should be considered separate from retirement and survivors' benefits, thus "a separate trust fund was established . . . in an effort to minimize the effects of the special problems in this field on the other parts of the program"; for this quote and for "rehabilitate the disabled . . . ," see "Statement by the President upon Signing the Social Security Amendments of 1956. August 1, 1956," *Public Papers: Eisenhower* (1956), 639.

59. *Social Security Amendments of 1954: Report of the Committee on Ways and Means, House of Representatives to Accompany H.R. 9366* (Washington, D.C.: U.S. Government Printing Office, 1954). Criticizing a 1954 court ruling, one legal scholar noted that "insofar as the court relied upon the judgments of the physicians that the claimant was 'disabled' or 'unemployable,' it overlooked the obvious intent of Congress to guard against the subjective judgment of the plaintiff's personal physicians." Landon H. Rowland, "Judicial Review of Disability Determinations," *Georgetown Law Review* 52 (1963–1964): 63; President's Commission on Veterans' Pensions, *Compensation for Service-Connected Disabilities: A General Analysis of Veterans and Military Disability Benefits,*

Mortality Rates, Disability Standards in Federal Programs, Workmen's Compensation, and Rehabilitation, Staff Report, no. 8, part A (Washington, D.C.: Government Printing Office, 1956), 8; for "requests for consideration . . . ," see "Appeals Procedure," *Hearings of House of Representatives Subcommittee on Administration of the Social Security Laws of the Committee on Ways and Means,* Monday, November 9, 1959 (Statement of Joseph E. McElvain, Director of the Office of Hearings and Appeals), 644.

60. Orr, "To Socialize Medicine."

61. Ibid.

62. Stavisky, "Where Does the Veteran Stand Today?," 131, 132.

63. For "it is difficult . . . ," see Louis Orr, "Answer to Letter from Robert A. Bell," *Journal of the American Medical Association* 164 (June 1, 1957): 574; for "the factor that . . ." and "offered their maximum . . . ," see Robert A. Bell, "VA Medical Care Program," *Journal of the American Medical Association* 164 (June 1, 1957): 572–74.

64. For "the performance of the duties . . . ," see Orr, "Answer to Letter from Robert A. Bell," 579; The report saw "new general social security programs as increasingly meeting the economic needs of veterans as well as nonveterans." Michael March (technical adviser to the commission), "President's Commission on Veterans Pensions: Recommendations," *Social Security Bulletin* 13 (August 1956): 13.

65. For "spoiled identity," see Erving Goffman, *Stigma: Notes on the Management of Spoiled Identity* (New York: Simon and Schuster, 1963); for "problems of psychogenic pain," see Henry Albronda, "Psychological Aspects of Pain," *California Medicine* 86 (May 1957): 296.

66. Albronda, "Psychological Aspects of Pain." For broader discussion of postwar psychiatry and psychiatric theory, see Gerald Grob, *From Asylum to Community: Mental Health Policy in Modern America* (Princeton, NJ: Princeton University Press, 1991).

67. Albronda, "Psychological Aspects of Pain."

68. Barbara Wooten, "Sick or Sinful?" *Time,* June 11, 1956, 50.

69. For arthritis evidence, see "The No. 1 Crippler," *New York Times,* September 14, 1959, 28; and "Arthritis Quacks Scored in Report: $250,000,000 Found Spent Yearly on Treatments," *New York Times,* November 10, 1959, 49; see "Don't-Give-A-Damn-Pills," *Time,* February 27, 1956, 98.

70. Melvin M. Belli, "The Adequate Award," *California Law Review* 39 (March 1951): 1. Jim Herron Zamora, "'King of Torts' Belli Dead at 88," *San Francisco Chronicle,* July 10, 1996, www.sfgate.com/cgi-bin/article.cgi?f=/e/a/1996/07/10/NEWS2814.dtl&hw=melvin+belli&sn=004&sc=774; J. L. Barritt,

"Subjective Complaints in Industrial Injuries," *California Medicine* 87 (August 1957): 79.

71. For "no one but the patient . . . ," see Barritt, "Subjective Complaints in Industrial Injuries"; for "to the processes . . . ," see Keith Wailoo, *Dying in the City of the Blues: Sickle Cell Anemia and the Politics of Race and Health* (Chapel Hill: University of North Carolina Press, 2001), 18; For "distinguish between . . . ," see J. L. Barritt, "Subjective Complaints in Industrial Injuries." In Dr. Barritt's view, California legislation made his life easier in one respect: the maximum compensation rate was capped at $40 a week, and so "with an average industrial wage of approximately $90 a week . . . there is usually no . . . incentive for an injured person to intentionally prolong his disability."

72. For "the increasing attention . . . ," see D. H. Werden, "Intervertebral Disc Lesions: Surgical Treatment, End Results, Disability Ratings and Cost in Industrial Accident Injuries," *California Medicine* 86 (February 1957), 84–92; Byron Mork, "Disability under Social Security: Medical Evaluation and Decision as to Rehabilitation," *California Medicine* 87 (October 1957), 256–60.

73. Louis Lasagna, "Introductory Statement on a Symposium on Pain and Its Relief," *Journal of Chronic Diseases* 4, no. 1 (July 1956): 1–3; see also Louis Lasagna, "The Problem of Pain," *Time*, July 30, 1956, 32, 34.

74. Alan Petigny, *The Permissive Society: America, 1941–1965* (New York: Cambridge University Press, 2009).

75. Tracey McCarley, "Psychological Aspects of Pain in Patients with Terminal Cancer," *California Medicine* 99 (July 1963), 17. "This virtue of self-reliance," McCarley continued, "may lead to such tension that pain may be intensified by the consequent increased muscle tension" (17)

76. Albronda, "Psychological Aspects of Pain."

77. Fredric B. Nalven and John F. O'Brien, "Personality Patterns of Rheumatoid Arthritic Patients," *Arthritis and Rheumatism* 7, no. 1 (February, 1964), 18.

78. For "the privileges and exemptions . . . ," see Talcott Parsons, *The Social System* (Routledge, 1951), 437; for "the patient with . . . ," see Frederic W. Rhinelander, "Treatment of Osteoarthritis of the Knees," *Arthritis and Rheumatism* 3 (1960): 561–63; see also Robert A. Herfort, *The Surgical Relief of Pain in Arthritic Disease: The Hip and Knee Joint.* (Springfield, IL: Thomas, 1967); on the sociology of gender and the headache, see Joanna Kempner, "Uncovering the Man in Medicine: Lessons Learned from a Case Study of Cluster Headache," *Gender and Society* 20 (October 2006): 632–56; for Michigan epidemiologist, see Sidney Cobb, "Hostility and Its Control in Rheumatoid Disease," *Arthritis and Rheumatism* 5 (June 1962): 290.

79. See Bradley Commission Papers. As Oscar Hampton wrote, "We have in the Veteran's Hospital now a man aged 69 (he now has a broken hip) who hasn't worked for the past nine years because he had a gastric resection (which to all intents and purposes was successful) because he is able to draw a 100% disability under these provisions." Box 28, folder 69: Hampton, Oscar P., Jr. Glenn Spurling cited the case of a local doctor still earning disability benefits for a low back injury although he had built up "a large and lucrative surgical practice." Box 28, folder 51: Spurling, R. Glenn.

80. Bradley Commission Papers, box 28, folder 41: Altemeier, William A.

Chapter Two: Opening the Gates of Relief

1. Page v. Celebrezze, 311 F.2d 757, (5th Cir. Jan. 9, 1963).

2. The *Kerner v. Flemming* ruling placed the onus on the Social Security Administration (SSA) to show (for even a person with minimal disabilities) that real work opportunities existed. Kerner v. Flemming, No. 52, Dkt. No. 26290, (2d Cir. November 18, 1960). See also Unemployment Insurance Report, no. 571-37, November 29, 1960, folder: Litigation in Kerner Case, 1958–1965, Bureau of Disability Insurance Division of Disability Policy and Procedures, Disability Program policy files, 1938–67, box 8 of 12, RG 0047, records of the Social Security Administration, National Archives and Records Administration; for "and see the oldsters . . . ," see Edwin Brinkley to Senator George Smathers, February 9, 1962. *Retirement Income of the Aging: Hearings before the Subcommittee on Retirement Income of the Special Committee on Aging*, United States Senate, Eighty-Seventh Congress, second session, part 10, Fort Lauderdale, FL, February 15, 1962. (Washington, D.C.: U.S. Government Printing Office, 1962), 907; for "a price we pay . . . ," see *Pain Brochure, 1968*, National Institute of General Medical Sciences, box 58, folder 6, John Bonica Papers, UCLA.

3. For "chiselers," see "Celebrezze Vows More Rehabilitation Emphasis," *Los Angeles Times*, September 24, 1962, 14; see also "Report Shows Total of 102,378 Disabled Persons Rehabilitated," *Atlanta Daily World*, September 13, 1962.

4. For "in 1949 . . . ," see Don Shannon, "Kennedy Rips Nixon 'Promises,' " *Los Angeles Times*, November 4, 1960, 1; for Kennedy and Page, see Landon H. Rowland, "Judicial Review of Disability Determinations," *Georgetown Law Review* 52 (1963–1964): 47. See also Robert Dallek, "The Medical Ordeals of JFK," *Atlantic*, December 2002.

5. Page v. Celebrezze.

6. Collyn A. Peddie, "Lessons from the Master—The Legacy of Judge John R. Brown," *Houston Journal of International Law* 25 (2002–2003): 247.

7. Brown, whose court purview extended to Alabama, Louisiana, Mississippi, and Georgia, became a major force in the era's civil rights rulings as part of the Fifth-Circuit Four. Jack W. Peltason, *Fifty-Eight Lonely Men: Southern Federal Judges and School Desegregation* (Urbana: University of Illinois, 1971); for "those of us . . . ," see "Whites Can't Know Pain of Racial Bias, RFK Says," *Baltimore Afro-American*, November 9, 1963, 13; See also William O. Walker, "The Pain of Race Hate Is Peculiar to the Negro," *Cleveland Call and Post*, May 30, 1964, 6B; for "climb in [her] . . . ," see Harper Lee, *To Kill a Mockingbird* (Philadelphia: J. B. Lippincott, 1960).

8. For New York Circuit ruling, see Kerner v. Flemming; for "if pain is real . . . ," see Page v. Celebrezze.

9. Theberge v. United States, 87, F.2d 697 (2d Cir., 1937).

10. The *Page* ruling was not the first to lean in this liberal direction. Brown found support in Ber v. Celebrezze, 1960 (also an arthritis case), which endorsed the notion that even though the claimant's physical symptoms might have produced pain tolerable to other people, the physical symptoms "nevertheless amply [support] her complaint that in her particular medical case these symptoms were accompanied by pain so very real to her and so intense as to disable her."

11. Brown ruling in Page v. Celebrezze. Here, Brown cited two other cases, Butler v. Flemming, 288 F.2d 591, 595 (5th Cir., 1961); and Hayes v. Celebrezze, 311 F.2d 648 (5th Cir., 1963).

12. For "a significant number . . . ," see Marian Osterweis, Arthur Kleinman, and David Mechanic, eds., *Pain and Disability: Clinical, Behavioral, and Public Policy Perspectives* (Washington, D.C.: National Academy Press, 1987), 55. The quote references G. Zaiser, "Proving Disabling Pain in Social Security Disability Proceedings: The Social Security Administration and the Third Circuit Court of Appeals," *Duquesne Law Review* 22 (Winter 1984): 491–520; for "HEW tries literally . . . ," see The Solicitor General, August 24, 1965, Ralph S. Spritzer, on the case of *Massey v. Celebrezze* (No. 15823, C.A. 6), box 8 of 12, records of the SSA, Bureau of Disability Insurance Division of Disability Policy and Procedures, Disability Program policy files, 1938–1967, NARA; Entry 34, A1 FRC, folder: Litigation. As one Social Security administrator wrote in 1961 (quoting a federal judge), there has been "produced in the mind of the reviewing court an impression that the referees [at HEW] have been inclined to focus too much attention upon any evidence or inference which might justify a denial of claimed benefits and not enough upon other evidence which fairly detracts from its weight." Mr. Abraham, Report of Meeting of Medical Advisory Committee, February 16 and 17, 1961, folder: Disability Insurance Memorandum No. 75, May 31, 1961, box 9 of 12, records of the SSA, NARA; on bureaucracy of relief,

see Ruth O'Brien, *Crippled Justice: The History of Modern Disability Policy in the Workplace* (Chicago: University of Chicago Press, 2001).

13. The Solicitor General, August 24, 1965, folder: Litigation.

14. For new trend, see Albert Averbach, "Projection of Courtroom Trauma," *Tort and Medicine Year Book* 1 (1961): 1–14; for "circling the wounded . . ." and "the doctor and lawyer . . . ," see "Law and Medicine, Text and Source Materials on Medico-Legal Problems by William J. Curran," review by Melvin M. Belli, *Yale Law Journal* 70 (January 1961): 492, 498.

15. Lawrence Galton, "Pain," *Popular Science,* July 1962, 42; Larry W. Myers, "'The Battle of Experts:' A New Approach to an Old Problem in Medical Testimony," *Nebraska Law Review* 44 (1965): 548.

16. For "today's chronic disorders . . . ," "deny that pain . . . ," and "the 'fit' of certain signs . . . ," see Irving Kenneth Zola, "Culture and Symptoms—an Analysis of Patient's Presenting Complaints," *American Sociological Review* 31 (October 1966): 615, 623, 618. See also Jerome L. Singer, "Ethnic Differences in Behavior and Psychopathology: Italian and Irish," *International Journal of Social Psychiatry* 2 (Summer, 1956).

17. Hubert Rosomoff, "Neurosurgical Control of Pain," *Annual Review of Medicine* 20 (1969): 189.

18. Henry K. Beecher, "Increased Stress and Effectiveness of Placebos and 'Active' Drugs," *Science,* July 8, 1960, 91. See also Henry K. Beecher, *Measurement of Subjective Responses* (New York: Oxford University Press, 1959); and Henry K. Beecher, "Anesthesia's Second Power: Probing the Mind," *Science,* February 14, 1947, 164–66; for "the power attributed . . . ," see Henry Beecher, "The Powerful Placebo," *Journal of the American Medical Association* 159 (December 24, 1955): 1606; for "placebos work best . . ." and on the evolution of pain theory and sugar pills as placebos, see "Placebos Can Calm Pains on Occasion, Dentists Are Told," *New York Times,* September 11, 1959, 29.

19. For "a person's reaction . . . ," see "How Much Pain Can You Stand?" *Science Digest,* April 1964, 46–47; for "conditioned anxiety . . . ," see "Feeling No Pain," *Newsweek,* July 8, 1963, 61.

20. For "spectatorial sympathy," see Karen Halttunen, "Humanitarianism and the Pornography of Pain in Anglo-American Culture," *American Historical Review* 100 (April 1995): 303–34; for "do they not feel . . . ," see Patricia McBroom, "Martyrs May Not Feel Pain," *Science News* 89 (June 25, 1966), 505–6; for "how much pain . . . ," see "How Much Pain Can You Stand?," 46.

21. For Calvin's recurring pain, see "Three VA Youngsters Fight Dread Disease Which Killed Brother," *Chicago Daily Defender,* November 14, 1962, 2; for "common Negro disease . . . ," see J. Donald Porter, "5,000 Stricken by Sickle

Cell Anemia Yearly," *Philadelphia Tribune*, January 19, 1960, 1; on pain, race, and racial politics in sickle cell disease, see Keith Wailoo, *Dying in the City of the Blues: Sickle Cell Anemia and the Politics of Race and Health* (Chapel Hill: University of North Carolina Press, 2001); for "nor is 'suffer' . . . ," see John A. Osmundsen, "Gains Are Noted in Sickle Cell Anemia," *New York Times*, March 21, 1965, 51; see also Harry Nelson, "Negroes Unaware of Danger: Doctors Press Warning on Sickle Cell Disease," *Los Angeles Times*, November 1, 1967, A6; Keith Wailoo and Stephen Pemberton, *The Troubled Dream of Genetic Medicine: Ethnicity and Innovation in Tay Sachs, Cystic Fibrosis, and Sickle Cell Disease* (Baltimore: Johns Hopkins University Press, 2007).

22. For writing disapproving of these views on "open society" in 1960 and liberalism, see Wilmoore Kendall, "The 'Open Society' and Its Fallacies," *American Political Science Review* 54 (December 1960): 973; on subjective pain and real pain, see Arthur Kleinman, Veena Das, and Margaret Lock, eds., *Social Suffering* (Berkeley: University of California Press, 1997); on arthritis, see Patricia McBroom, "Martyrs May Not Feel Pain."

23. For "the most famous . . . ," see "Koufax Given Injection to Reduce Pain," *Washington Post*, January 26, 1966, B2; "Koufax Suffers Flare-Up of Arthritis in Left Elbow," *New York Times*, July 30, 1965, 20; for arthritis as marker of disability, see Harold Kaese, "Koufax, Salaun, Joint Sufferers," *Boston Globe*, December 7, 1966, 57; Milton Gross, "Koufax Could Forget the Needle but Not the Constant Pain," *Boston Globe*, November 20, 1966, 51; see also Ruth Gale Elder, "Social Class and Lay Explanations of the Etiology of Arthritis," *Journal of Health and Social Behavior* 14 (March 1973): 28–38; for Eisenhower's wrist, see "Eisenhower's Type of Arthritis Is Mild," *New York Times*, May 20, 1966, 38; for "arthritis cripples . . . ," see "Arthritis among the Poor," *New York Times*, October 14, 1965, 42.

24. For health insurance entitlement, see Faith Perkins, *My Fight with Arthritis* (New York: Random House, 1964); when he signed the bill, Johnson asked Americans to "see past the speeches and the political battles to the doctor over there that's tending the infirm and to the hospital that is serving those in anguish." He credited President Truman, who "planted the seeds of compassion and duty which today have flowered in to care for the sick and serenity for the fearful." "Transcript of Remarks by Truman and Johnson," *New York Times*, July 31, 1965, 9; for "era of the hard sell . . . ," see Senator McNamara, Michigan, in *Frauds and Quackery Affecting Older Americans: Hearings before the Special Committee on Aging*, U.S. Senate Eighty-Eighth Congress, first session, Parts 1–3 (Washington: U.S. Government Printing Office, 1963), 2. See also "Drug Industry Warned about Overcharging Sick and Elderly," *Norfolk New Journal and Guide*

(December 23, 1967), 8; see also Don Colburn, "Pain, Placebos and Profits: Quacks Prey on Elderly 'When They Feel Helpless,' Experts Warn," *Washington Post*, November 27, 1985, H9.

25. For "a billion dollar crippler . . . ," see *Arthritis: Billion Dollar Crippler, Highlights of the Report;* Surgeon General's Workshop on Prevention of Disability from Arthritis (Washington, D.C.: U.S. Government Printing Office, 1966); Howard Rusk, "13 Million Arthritics: Surgeon General Calls for Drive to Combat Effects of Crippling Illness," *New York Times*, August 21, 1966, 95; for "not all who are poor . . . ," see Jacobus tenBroek and Floyd W. Matson, "The Disabled and the Law of Welfare," *California Law Review* 54 (1966): 809. A disability activist, tenBroek became a founder of the National Federation of the Blind. For "repressed hostility . . . ," see Fredric B. Nalven and John F. O'Brien, "Personality Patterns of Rheumatoid Arthritic Patients," *Arthritis and Rheumatism* 7, no. 1 (February, 1964), 18; for "the public . . . ," see "Talks Slated to Expose 'Quackery in Arthritis,'" *New York Times*, September 23, 1962, 79. See also *Committee on Government Operations. Drug Safety. Part 5. Appendixes and Index: Hearings Before the United States House Committee on Government Operations*, Eighty-Ninth Congress, second session, on March 9, 10, May 25, 26, June 7–9, 1966 (Washington: U.S. Government Printing Office, 1966).

26. Stanley W. Jacob, Margaret Bischel, and Robert J. Herschler, "Dimethyl Sulfoxide (DMSO): A New Concept in Pharmacotherapy" *Current Therapeutic Research* 6, no. 2 (February, 1964): 134–35; "Sweet Taste of DMSO," *Newsweek*, December 23, 1963, 68. "Two Concerns Market 'Cure' for Arthritis," *New York Times*, August 18, 1966, 23; see also "Bufferin Accused by F.T.C. over Ads," *New York Times*, January 24, 1967, 10; see also Marjorie Hunter, "Arthritis Pills Barred from U.S.: Homemade Agent Produced in Canada Described as Dangerous by F.D.A.; One Death Is Reported; Federal Agency to Review Public Comments on New Drug-Testing Rules," *New York Times*, October 10, 1962, 49; Norman O. Rothermich, "Coming Catastrophes with Chloroquine?," *Annals of Internal Medicine* 61 (December 64), 1203; "DMSO—Promise and Danger," *New York Times*, April 3, 1965, 28; Joseph Lee Hollander, "The Calculated Risk of Arthritis Treatment," *Annals of Internal Medicine* 62 (May 1965), 1062.

27. Marc Wilson, "A Dubious Arthritis 'Miracle,'" *Baltimore Sun*, January 4, 1976, T1. Datelined Mexicali, Mexico, this report documented the trend of Americans crossing into Mexico for pain relief, "in a dusty alley 200 yards from the United States border."

28. For the emergence of new drugs and findings on psychotoxicity of tranquilizers, see David Herzberg, *Happy Pills in America: From Miltown to Prozac* (Johns Hopkins University Press, 2009), 102, 210; and *Control of Psychotoxic*

Drugs: Hearing Before the Subcommittee on Health of the Committee on Labor and Public Welfare, U.S. Senate, Eighty-Eighth Congress, second session, August 3, 1964 (Washington, D.C.: U.S. Government Printing Office, 1964): 38; for "therapeutic society," see Philip Rieff, *The Triumph of the Therapeutic* (Chicago: University of Chicago Press, 1966); and Katie Wright, *The Rise of the Therapeutic Society: Psychological Knowledge and the Contradictions of Cultural Change* (Washington, D.C.: New Academia, 2010), 15.

29. For "it kills pain . . . ," see John Osmundsen, "Miracle Drug," *New York Times*, February 28, 1965, B6; on the antidotes, as one writer on women's issues for the Negro Press International noted, these "wonder inventions have long since become a familiar pattern in our lives." Pam McAllister, "Women's Talk," *Philadelphia Tribune*, March 27, 1965, 8.

30. For "the nearest thing . . . ," see "DMSO-Promise and Danger," *New York Times*, April 3, 1965, 28; "Crown Zellerbach to Expand DMSO Plant in Louisiana," *Wall Street Journal*, May 21, 1965, 3; on the questioning of the drug, see Robert G. Sherrill, "Razz-Ma-Tazz in the Drug Industry," *Nation*, April 11, 1966, 425–27.

31. On the need for more pain experts, see Sherrill, "Razz-Ma-Tazz in the Drug Industry"; for "not as wonderful . . . ," see Thomas Fenton, "Two Doctors Wary on Wonder Drug," *Baltimore Sun*, September 8, 1965, 46; William M. Carley, "DMSO May Have Caused Death of Woman, Makers of 'Wonder' Drug Warn Doctors," *Wall Street Journal*, September 9, 1965, 6. "DMSO: Demise of a Wonder Drug?," *American Journal of Nursing* 65 (December 1965): 62.

32. On new regulatory actions, as Dan Carpenter has noted, Kelsey "reined in investigators who lacked credibility" and terminated investigational projects on such controversial substances as DMSO and LSD. Daniel Carpenter, *Reputation and Power: Organizational Image and Pharmaceutical Regulation at the FDA* (Princeton, NJ: Princeton University Press, 2010), 287–88; on the launching of DMSO hearings, *Committee on Government Operations. Drug Safety*; for "sensible resumption . . . ," see "Decision on DMSO," *New York Times*, December 29, 1966, 30; Harold M. Schmeck, "DMSO Ban Ended by Drug Agency," *New York Times*, Dec. 23, 1966, 27.

33. J. Harold Brown, "Clinical Experience with DMSO in Acute Musculoskeletal Conditions Comparing a Noncontrolled Series with a Controlled Double Blind Study: Biological Actions of Dimethyl Sulfoxide," *Annals of the New York Academy of Medicine* 141 (March 15, 1967), 496–505.

34. For "persecuted drug . . . ," see "Blackout on DMSO," *Time*, May 5, 1967, 70, 72; on Kelsey and standoff, see Wilson, "Dubious Arthritis 'Miracle.'" Among the drugs offered were cortisone and DMSO; on the new era, see Stanley

W. Jacob, Edward E. Rosenbaum, and Don C. Wood, eds., *Dimethyl Sulfoxide*, vol. 1: *Basic Concepts of DMSO* (New York: Marcel Dekker, 1971); Pat McGrady Sr., *The Persecuted Drug: The Story of DMSO* (New York: Doubleday, 1973).

35. The next decade brought another round of congressional DMSO hearings, promises of the drug's return, and a wide range of officially unapproved uses by consumers who continued to believe in the product. See *DMSO, New Hope for Arthritis? Hearing before the Select Committee on Aging, House of Representatives*, Ninety-Sixth Congress, second session, March 24, 1980. (Washington: U.S. Government Printing Office, 1980); *Committee on Labor and Human Resources. Subcommittee on Health and Scientific Research. Preclinical and Clinical Testing by the Pharmaceutical Industry—DMSO: Hearing Before the Subcommittee on Health and Scientific Research of the Committee on Labor and Human Resources*, United States Senate, Ninety-Sixth Congress, second session, on Examination of the testing of DMSO and FDA's role in the process, July 31, 1980 (Washington: U.S. Government Printing Office, 1980); Barry Tarshis, *DMSO: The True Story of a Remarkable Pain-Killing Drug* (New York: Morrow, 1981); Jane Brody, "Debate Rages on DMSO Despite Its Users' Claims," *New York Times*, May 18, 1983, C1.

36. On Bonica, see Isabelle Baszanger, *Inventing Pain Medicine: From the Laboratory to the Clinic* (New Brunswick, NJ: Rutgers University Press, 1995); on insights into disability, see Jack Olender, "Proof and Evaluation of Pain and Suffering in Personal Injury Litigation," *Duke Law Journal* 1962, no. 3 (Summer 1962): 344–78; In one 1964 case, a staff member at Winthrop Laboratories thanked Bonica for going "to such an extent to prove the innocence of Carbocaine in this case, since we have a pending new drug application" before the FDA. Letter from A. Scribner, senior associate director of medical research, Wintrop Laboratories, to John Bonica, November 24, 1964, Bonica Papers, box 68, folder 37. See also Bonica to A. Scribner, November 20, 1964.

37. C. Richard Chapman, "The Founding Father of the Pain Field," quoted in Ajit Panickar, "Medicine: John Bonica," *Pain News* (Winter 2009), 30, http://www.britishpainsociety.org/bps_nl_winter_2009.pdf.

38. "Relief of Pain," *Time*, May 17, 1963, 93.

39. Ronald Melzack, "Pain: Past, Present, and Future," In *Pain: New Perspectives in Therapy and Research*, ed. M. Weisenberg and B. Tursky (New York: Plenum, 1976), 138.

40. On the gate control concept, see Baszanger, *Inventing Pain Medicine*, 57; David Morris, *The Culture of Pain* (Berkeley: University of California Press, 1991); for "pain is not a fixed . . . ," see Ronald Melzack, "The Perception of Pain," *Scientific American*, February 1961, 49; for "the concept of a . . . ," see

Ronald Melzack and Patrick D. Wall, "Pain Mechanisms: A New Theory," *Science* 50 (1965): 971–79; for pain and perceptions, see Ronald Melzack, "The Puzzle of Pain" (lecture, National Film Board of Canada, 1965). "Psychology Topics for Discussion Groups: Supervised Series by Professor D. O. Hebb," http://www.snagfilms.com/films/title/the_puzzle_of_pain.

41. Melzack and Wall, "Pain Mechanisms." For Wall's comments on MIT and cybernetics, see Martin Rosenberg and Steve McMahon, "Extract from an Annotated Physiology Society Interview with Professor Patrick Wall (1925–2001)," appendix 1 in *Innovation in Pain Management: The Transcript of a Witness Seminar Held by the Wellcome Trust Centre for the History of Medicine at UCL, London, on 12 December 2002*, ed. L. A. Reynolds and E. M. Tansey (London: Wellcome Trust, 2004), 101.

42. For "specificity theory," see Melzack and Wall, "Pain Mechanisms"; for "all fiber endings . . . ," see Melzack and Wall, "Pain Mechanism"; and Ronald Melzack and Patrick Wall, "On the Nature of Cutaneous Sensory Mechanisms," *Brain* 85, no. 2 (June 1962): 337; for failure of current theories, see Melzack and Wall, "Pain Mechanisms."

43. Other scholars echoed these points. See Benjamin Spector, "A Doctor's Dilemma" (commencement address) *Journal of the American Medical Association* 194, no. 2 (October 11, 1965): 154–56. On the increasing value placed on patient attitude in diagnosis, see Harry Nelson, "Patient's Attitude toward Pain Called Aid to Diagnosis," *Los Angeles Times*, March 3, 1966, A1; for "if we can recover . . . ," see R. Melzack and K. L. Casey, "Sensory, Motivation, and Central Control Determinants of Pain: A New Conceptual Model," in *The Skin Senses*, ed. Dan R. Kenshalo (Springfield, IL: Charles C. Thomas, 1968), 423–43; on the blurring the lines among medical therapy, consciousness raising, and revolutionary social protest, see, for example, Erika Dyck, *Psychedelic Psychiatry: LSD from Clinic to Campus* (Baltimore: Johns Hopkins University Press, 2008); William Braden, *The Private Sea: LSD and the Search for God* (Chicago: Quadrangle Books, 1967); and Howard Becker, "History, Culture, and Subjective Experience: An Exploration of the Social Bases of Drug-Induced Experience," *Journal of Health and Social Behavior* 8 (September 1967): 163–76. See also David Kaiser, *How the Hippies Saved Physics: Science, Counterculture, and the Quantum Revival* (New York: Norton, 2011).

44. Robert Shaw, who developed the concept, was not sympathetic to malingerers. He wrote, "Physicians must know that their larger obligation to society for the medical truth, as nearly as it can be defined, must not be subservient to their duty to their individual patient . . . Increased public consciousness of reward through litigation has made the motivation for seeking it and maintaining

maximum disability enormously strong." Robert S. Shaw, "Pathologic Malingering: The Painful Disabled Extremity," *New England Journal of Medicine* 271 (July 2, 1964): 26. See also Delos Smith, "Malingering Said Evil of Times," *Beaver County Times* (PA), July 9, 1964, 5; and Knud Rasmussen, Robert Shaw, and Karl Sparup, "The Terrible Cost of Being Compensated," *Journal of the American Bar Association* 53 (1967): 1136–39.

45. Harry Schwartz, "Pain: Why We Do and Don't Say Ouch!," *New York Times*, June 6, 1971, E12.

46. For "the three problems . . . ," see "Social Security Disability Benefits: Three Current Problems," *Minnesota Law Review* 52 (1967–1968): 169; on the film *Threshold*, see "*Threshold* Film Receives Gold Medal at Festival," *NIH Record* (July 8, 1970). The film, produced by Tracy Ward, Audio Productions, received a gold medal at the Atlanta International Film Festival; by 1971, nearly sixteen million television viewers and seventy-five thousand medical, dental, nursing, and civic groups had seen it. Helen Neal (NIH) to John Bonica, August 6, 1971, box 58, folder 10, Bonica Papers.

47. Mark Zborowski, *People in Pain* (San Francisco: Jossey-Bass, 1969), 31–32.

48. For "preoccupation with the . . . ," see ibid., 110, 114. See also Mark Zborowski, "Cultural Components in Response to Pain," *Journal of Social Issues* 8 (Fall 1952): 16–30; for "transmission of cultural values . . . ," "like the Jewish patient . . . ," and "that he does not want," see Zborowski, *People in Pain*, 3–5, 136, 96.

49. On the interaction of the gay rights and psychiatry in this era, for example, see Ronald Bayer, "Diagnostic Politics: Homosexuality and the American Psychiatric Association," in *Homosexuality and American Psychiatry: The Politics of Diagnosis*, ed. Ronald Bayer (Princeton, NJ: Princeton University Press, 1987); on race and medicine, see Keith Wailoo, "Between Progress and Protest," in *How Cancer Crossed the Color Line*, ed. Keith Wailoo (New York: Oxford University Press, 2011); and on gender and medicine, see, for example, Elizabeth Siegel Watkins, *On the Pill: A Social History of Oral Contraceptives, 1950–1970* (Baltimore: Johns Hopkins University Press, 2001).

50. Zborowski, *People in Pain*, 3–5.

51. On diversifying of pain theory in 1960s, see "Behavioral Sciences Notes: Gate Theory; Animals Raised without Stimulation," *Science News* 92 (December 2, 1967): 542; "Controlling Pain at the Gate," *Science News* 100 (July 3, 1971): 7; for "appealing because . . . ," see John Bonica, "Current Concepts of the Pain Process," *Northwest Medicine* 69 (1970), 661–64. See also Richard A. Sternbach, *Pain: A Psychophysiological Analysis* (New York: Academic Press, 1968); on the

theory's endorsement of diversity, see, for example, Ernest R. Hilgard, "The Alleviation of Pain by Hypnosis," *Pain* 1 (1975), 213–31; Ernest R. Hilgard and Joseph R. Hilgard, *Hypnosis in the Relief of Pain* (Los Altos, CA: William Kaufmann, 1975); R. A. Ersek, "Transcutaneous Electrical Neurostimulation: A New Therapeutic Modality for Controlling Pain," *Clinical Orthopaedics & Related Research* 128 (October 1977): 314–24; Dorothy S. Siegele, "The Gate Control Theory," *American Journal of Nursing* 74 (March 1974): 498–502.

52. Schwartz, "Pain: Why We Do and Don't Say Ouch!"; on popular meaning of gate control theory, see "Pain: Search for Understanding and Relief," *Time*, June 1969, 63–64. As this article noted, it became common wisdom that "mind doctors and body doctors are at last recognizing that in their evolving concern with pain they are really talking about the same thing in different terms" (63). For "bona fide medical . . . ," see Albert Rosenfeld, "The Vital Facts about the Drug and Its Effects," *Life*, March 25, 1966, 30A; for "in evaluating . . . ," see T. P. Hackett, "Pain and Prejudice: Why Do We Doubt That the Patient Is in Pain?," *Anesthesia Progress* (May–June 1971): 55; for "switch off," see "Switching Off the Pain." *Time*, October 1, 1965, 62; and Rosenfeld, "Vital Facts about the Drug," 30A.

53. On P. W. Nathan, see G. D. Schott, "In Memoriam: Peter Nathan," *International Association for the Study of Pain*, http://www.iasp-pain.org/AM/Template.cfm?Section=In_Memoriam1&Template=/CM/HTMLDisplay.cfm&ContentID=1263; for "although the theory . . . ," see P. W. Nathan, "The Gate-Control Theory of Pain: A Critical Review," *Pain* 99, no. 1 (1976): 123–58.

54. On methadone, see Guy P. Seaburg, "The Drug Abuse Problems and Some Proposals," *Journal of Criminal Law, Criminology, and Police Science* 58 (September 1967): 349–75; on critics of methadone, see "Methadone: Cracks in the Panacea," *Science News* 97 (April 11, 1970): 366–67; for "reaction to the excessive . . . ," see Henry L. Lennard, Leon J. Esptein, and Mitchell S. Rosenthal, "The Methadone Illusion," *Science*, May 26, 1972, 881–84; on methadone detractors, see Robert Balzell, "Drug Abuse: Methadone Becomes the Solution and the Problem," *Science* 179, February 23, 1973, 772. Constance Holden, " Methadone: New FDA Guidelines Would Tighten Distribution," *Science*, August 11, 1972, 502.

55. George Herman (correspondent), Vern Diamond (producer), Burton Benjamin (executive producer), "The Mystery of Pain," *CBS News* (special transcript), April 7, 1970, box 58, folder 10, Bonica Papers, UCLA, pp. 1, 6.

56. Harry Schwartz, "Acupuncture: The Needle Pain-Killer Comes to America," *New York Times*, June 4, 1972, E7. See also Margaret E. Armstrong, "Acupuncture," *American Journal of Nursing* 72 (September 1972): 1582–88.

57. On James Reston, see William L. Prensky (letter to the editor), "Reston Helped Open a Door to Acupuncture," *New York Times*, December 9, 1995; on the encounter between American and Chinese medicine, the cover of *JAMA*, December 1971, featured a Chinese acupuncture manikin; for "explain and legitimate . . . ," see Laurence Cherry, "Solving the Mysteries of Pain," *New York Times*, January 30, 1977, SM8.

58. On growth of acupuncture, see Barbara Culliton, "Acupuncture: Fertile Ground for Faddists and Serious NIH Research," *Science*, August 18, 1972, 592–94; Robert Schwartz, "Acupuncture and Expertise: A Challenge to Physician Control," *Hastings Center Report* 11 (April 1981): 5–7; Paul Root Wolpe, "The Maintenance of Professional Authority: Acupuncture and the American Physician," *Social Problems* 32 (June 1985): 409–24; for "after years of injections . . . ," see Eileen Mullan to John Bonica, June 23, 1973, box 66, folder 33, Bonica Papers; for "Dear John . . . ," see Frank Moya, MD, anesthesiology, Miami, to Bonica, November 1972, Bonica Papers, UCLA; on Bonica, see John J. Bonica, "Acupuncture Anesthesia in the People's Republic of China: Implications for American Medicine," *Journal of the American Medical Association* 228 (1974): 1544–51.

59. John Bonica, "Trip to the People's Republic of China," June–July 1973, box 66, folder 52, Bonica Papers.

60. Ibid.

61. For "the gate [control] . . ." and "acupuncture analgesia . . . ," see Harry Nelson, "Researchers Agree on One Point—Acupuncture Works," *Los Angeles Times*, June 15, 1973, A1; for one important analysis of East-West tensions as played out in conceptualizations of the body, see Shigehisa Kuriyama, *The Expressiveness of the Body and the Divergence of Greek and Chinese Medicine* (New York: Zone Books, 2002).

62. For "I am certain . . . ," Secretary of Health, South Dakota, to John Bonica, July 1973, Box 66, Folder 23 ("Acupuncture in other states, 1973–74"), John Bonica Papers; Tom Read, "UW Medic Back from China with Prescription for Future," *Seattle Post-Intelligencer*, July 12, 1973, D1.

63. Ibid.

64. "Needling the China Watchers," *Wall Street Journal*, July 18, 1973, 8. See also Jeremi Suri, "Détente and Its Discontents," in *Rightward Bound: Making America Conservative in the 1970s*, ed. Bruce J. Schulman and Julian E. Zelizer (Cambridge, MA: Harvard University Press, 2008); for "one doctor who . . . ," see "Needling the China Watchers."

65. Box 66, folder 52, Bonica Papers, UCLA. In a letter to the editor of the *Washington Post* (which had misrepresented his views from a *JAMA* article), Bonica wrote, "Since relief of pain and response to treatment are influenced by

many factors, including culture, tradition, education, and background, and because acupuncture is a new therapeutic modality in American medicine, it is essential that it be tested in American patients using well established scientific principles." John Bonica, "Acupuncture's Efficacy," *Washington Post*, July 10, 1974, A31. Asked by *U.S. News and World Report* in 1974, "Dr. Bonica, what is pain? Can science actually define the sensation?" he responded, "If you ask 100 different authorities that question, you would get 100 different answers." See interview transcript, Box 133, folder 5, Bonica Papers, UCLA.

66. For "real" pain, see Baszanger, *Inventing Pain Medicine*, 59; on gate control theory, the *British Medical Journal* concluded that, despite its vagueness as to mechanisms, Melzack and Wall had "enshrined a major medical concept and it has had a powerful impact on research, theory, and treatment." "The Gate Control Theory of Pain," *British Medical Journal* 2 (August 26, 1978): 586–87; See also Sheri Emond, "Therapy Works Where Surgery Fails," *Los Angeles Times*, September 14, 1980, V5.

67. One study that framed developments in pain management in explicitly political terms—albeit framed by the micropolitics of the doctor-patient relationship—was S. Y. Fagerhaugh and Y. Shizuko, *Politics of Pain Management: Staff-Patient Interaction* (Menlo Park, CA: Addison-Wesley, Health Sciences Division, 1977); Philip Sechzer, "Patient-Controlled Analgesia (PCA): A Retrospective," *Anesthesiology* 72 (1990): 735–36. See also M. Keeri-Szanto, "Apparatus for Demand Analgesia," *Canadian Anaesthesiology Society Journal* 18 (1971): 581–82; Philip H. Sechzer, "Objective Measurement of Pain," *Anesthesiology* 29 (1968): 209–10; J. S. Scott, "Obstetric Analgesia," *American Journal of Obstetrics and Gynecology* 106 (1970): 959–78; for Demand Dropmaster, see the discussion in Scott Fishman, *The War on Pain: How Breakthroughs in the New Field of Pain Medicine Are Turning the Tide against Suffering* (New York: Harper Collins, 2000), 47.

68. On learned helplessness, see Martin Seligman, "Learned Helplessness," *Annual Review of Medicine* 23 (1972): 407–12; for "I share your concern . . . ," see letter from Steven Brena to John Bonica, 1982, Box 1, Folder 91 "Brena, Steven," John Bonica Papers.

69. Helen Neal, *The Politics of Pain* (New York: McGraw Hill, 1978). As one report noted, "American doctors are not allowed by law to use heroin which has been banned since 1924. In Britain heroin has been found to be indispensable in 10% of cancer pain largely because less is needed than morphine, it can have fewer side effects and it can be taken orally." Derek Humphry, "Dying Patients—Pain Control: Is Everything Being Done?" *Los Angeles Times*, January 4, 1979, B1. On other alternatives to drugs and surgery ranging from biofeedback to

"grinning and bearing it," see Ronald Kotulak, "How Pain-Killing Drugs Can Cause More Pain," *Chicago Tribune*, September 11, 1977, 1; Marilyn Ferguson, "Use of Mind to Overcome Pain Explored," *Hartford Courant*, November 11, 1973, 4A. "Pain: Medical Science Begins to Take It Seriously," *U.S. News & World Report*, August 1, 1977, 61.

70. For "losers . . . whose learned . . . ," see "Pain: Where Does It Hurt?," *NBC News*, discussed in Clarence Petersen, "Ouch! Hurt Feelings Can Be a Real Pain," *Chicago Tribune*, March 28, 1972, B11. For a later commentary, see H. C. Pheasant, "Backache–Its Nature, Incidence and Cost," *Western Journal of Medicine* 126(1977): 330–32. The phrase "low back loser" built on the work of low-back pain scholars. R. A. Sternbach, R. W. Murphy, W. H. Akeson, and S. R. Wolf, "Chronic Low-Back Pain—the 'Low-Back Loser,'" *Postgraduate Medicine* 53 (May 1973). For "pain is not . . . ," see Miranda v. Richardson 514 F.2d 996 (1st Cir., April 14, 1975) (75 Ford Administration).

Chapter Three: The Conservative Case against Learned Helplessness

1. "'Welfare Queen' Loses Her Cadillac Limousine," *New York Times*, February 29, 1976, 42; Dan Miller, "The Chutzpah Queen: Favorite Reagan Target as Welfare Cheat Remains Unflappable at Trial in Chicago," *Washington Post*, March 13, 1977, 3. For insight on the Reagan years, see Matthew Dallek, *The Right Moment: Ronald Reagan's First Victory and the Decisive Turning Point in American Politics* (Oxford: Oxford University Press, 2004). On welfare politics in this era, see Michael Katz, *In the Shadow of the Poorhouse: A Social History of Welfare in America* (New York: Basic Books, 1986).

2. For "most often collides . . . ," see "Secretary of Collision," editorial, *New York Times*, October 3, 1985, A26; See Robert C. Smith, "The Ascendancy of Ronald Reagan and the Parts Played by Ideology and Race," and "The Reagan Presidency and Race," in *Conservatism and Racism: And Why in America They Are the Same* (Albany: SUNY Press, 2010). See also Dan Carter, *From George Wallace to Newt Gingrich: Race in the Conservative Counterrevolution, 1963–1994* (Baton Rouge: Louisiana State University, 1996).

3. For "weed[ing] out ineligible . . . ," see Memo, July 9, 1981 from John Svahn to Richard Kusserow, entry UD-07W entry 1, Office of the Commissioner, Executive Secretariat, correspondence files, 1981, FRC box 2 of 1, National Archives and Records Administration, Social Security Archives, RG 47; for Peter Ferrara comments, see "Collection: Anderson, Martin Files," CFOA 89, box 5, folder 16 of 20, Office of Policy Development, Ronald Reagan Library. See also Peter Ferrara, *Critical Issues: Social Security Reform* (Washington, D.C.: Heritage Foundation: 1982).

4. See for example, box OA7423: Hemmel, Eric: Files—Policy Development—box 2, folder: social security background (1), April 10, 1981, memo—regarding Peter Ferrara's proposals for social security reform.

5. For HHS roll reduction statistics, see Marian Oseterweis, Arthur Kleinman, and David Mechanic, eds., *Pain and Disability: Clinical, Behavioral, and Public Policy Perspectives* (Washington, D.C.: National Academy Press, 1987), 30; for "they cut my social security . . . ," see Margaret Engel, "U.S. Gets Tough with Disabled, *Washington Post*, September 7, 1982, A1; for volume of pain and disability litigation, see David Lauter, "Disability-Benefit Cases Flood Courts," *National Law Journal* (October 17, 1983): 1.

The legal literature produced in the wake of the Reagan-era disability and pain policy shifts is expansive. See for example, George R. Zaiser, "Proving Disabling Pain in Social Security Disability Proceedings: The Social Security Administration and the Third Circuit Court of Appeals," *Duquesne Law Review* 22 (1983–1984): 491–520; Margaret Rodgers, "Subjective Pain Testimony in Disability Determination Proceedings: Can Pain Alone Be Disabling?" *California Western Law Review* 28 (1991–1992): 173–211; Jon Dubin, "Poverty, Pain, and Precedent: The Fifth Circuit's Social Security Jurisprudence," *St. Mary's Law Journal* 81 (1993–1994): 81–141.

6. Charles R. Morris, "Why Liberal Programs Have Failed," *Los Angeles Times*, September 30, 1984, D1.

7. Laura Kalman, *Right Star Rising: A New Politics, 1974–1980* (New York: Norton, 2011).

8. "Secretary of Collision."

9. For rise in disability payments, see "Don't Disable Social Security," *New York Times*, July 19, 1979, A18; for number of disability awards, see Office of Policy, Social Security Administration, *Trends in the Social Security and Supplemental Security Income Disability Programs*, www.ssa.gov/policy/docs/chart books/disability_trends/secto4.html; for Califano's focus on fraud, see "HEW Revamping Ordered," *Baltimore Sun*, March 9, 1977, A1. Califano predicted that "the savings for U.S. taxpayers related to these reorganization initiatives, especially those involving efforts to eradicate errors, fraud, and abuse, will be at least $1 billion over the next two years and will reach a total of at least $2 billion annually by 1981." For "so wary of offending . . . ," see "Don't Disable Social Security," *New York Times*, July 19, 1979, A18. As many scholars have noted, the new field of law and economics became allied with conservatism in launching such critiques. See, for example, Steven Teles, *The Rise of the Conservative Legal Movement: The Battle for Control of the Law* (Princeton, NJ: Princeton University Press).

10. For Nixon era expansion and consolidation, see James Sparrow, *Warfare State: World War II Americans and the Age of Big Government* (Oxford: Oxford University Press, 2011); for cost and recipient statistics, see Robert Rubinson, "Government Benefits: Social Security Disability, 1987," Annual Survey of American Law (June 1988): 195, 196; for changes in SSDI contributors and recipients, see Rodgers, "Subjective Pain Testimony," 174.

11. "Don't Disable Social Security," *New York Times*, July 19, 1979, A18.

12. For "the largest computer system . . . ," see Grayson Mitchell, "Computer to Aid Welfare Policing," *Los Angeles Times*, May 6, 1979, SC1; in terms of welfare program policing, even before Reagan's electoral victory, Carter himself had "shifted uneasily towards deregulation (of airlines and trucking) as a partial solution to the crisis of stagflation." David Harvey, *A Brief History of Neoliberalism* (New York: Oxford University Press, 2005), 22, 23.

13. Mark I. Whitman, "Carter, a Reluctant Radical," *Baltimore Sun*, September 12, 1980, A17.

14. "Modest Social Security Reform," *Chicago Tribune*, July 25, 1979, A2.

15. "Social Security Disability Amendments of 1980: Statement on Signing H.R. 3236 into Law, June 9, 1980," *Public Papers of the Presidents of the United States: Jimmy Carter, 1980–1981* (Washington, D.C.: Government Printing Office, 1980–1981), 2:1062.

16. For "Governor Reagan's first . . . ," "Medicare and Social Security," October 31, 1980, *Public Papers: Carter*, 3:2578; for "I oppose cutting back . . ." and "I am proud to stand for . . . ," 3:2579. Writing in the wake of the election, Reagan's adviser David Gergen noted of Southern Protestants, "This key vote abandoned Jimmy Carter in large numbers . . . I urge that if President Reagan makes a trip outside Washington in the first months of his Administration that the trip be to the deep South." "First 90 Days Project, 1980" December 29, 1980, memorandum t: Dave Gergen from Rich Williamson regarding thoughts on the first 90 days, in MC197, box 66, folder 6, p. 19, James A. Baker III Papers, RBSC Mudd Library, Princeton University.

17. For "there is the program . . . ," see "The President's New Conference, May 13, 1982," *Public Papers of the Presidents of the United States: Ronald Reagan, 1981–1989* (Washington, D.C.: Government Printing Office, 1981–1989), 1:625; for Reagan's changes to the programs and conservative ascendancy, see Harvey, *Brief History of Neoliberalism*.

18. "Interview with the President, Remarks and a Question-and-Answer Session with a Group of Out-of-Town Editors, October 5, 1981," *Weekly Compilation of Presidential Documents* 17, no. 41 (Monday, October 12, 1981): 1094.

19. Simon Nelson Patten, *The Development of English Thought* (New York: MacMillan, 1899); and E. K. Hunt, "Simon N. Patten's Contributions to Economics," *Journal of Economic Issues* 4 (December 1970): 38–55; on the origins of the disability provision in Social Security, see Social Security Administration, "Vote Tallies," *Social Security*, www.ssa.gov/history/tally56.html; see also James Sparrow, *Warfare State*.

20. Steven Brena, ed., *Chronic Pain: America's Hidden Epidemic* (New York: Antheneum, 1978).

21. For "chronic pain is often . . . ," see S. F. Brena, S. L. Chapman, and R. Decker, "Chronic Pain as Learned Experience: Emory University Pain Control Center," *NIDA Research Monographs* 36 (May 1981): 76–83; for medical proof of pain, see discussions of medical-only determination, Collection: Anderson, Martin files, CFOA 89, box 5, folder: Social Security (6 and 8 of 20), Ronald Reagan Library.

22. On learned helplessness, see Martin Seligman, "Learned Helplessness," *Annual Review of Medicine* 23 (1972): 407–12; Martin Seligman, *Helplessness: On Depression, Development, and Death* (San Francisco: Freeman, 1975); Lyn Y. Abramson, Martin E. P. Seligman, and John D. Teasdale, "Learned Helplessness in Humans: Critique and Reformulation," *Journal of Abnormal Psychology* 87 (1978): 49–74; Stanley L. Chapman and Steven F. Brena, "Learned Helplessness and Responses to Nerve Blocks in Chronic Low Back Pain Patients," *Pain* 14 (1982): 355–64; Adele Thomas, "Learned Helplessness and Expectancy Factors: Implications for Research in Learning Disabilities," *Review of Education Research* 49 (Spring 1979): 208–21; for pain sufferer and disability claims, see Chapman and Brena, "Learned Helplessness and Responses to Nerve Blocks."

23. For "nobody likes welfare . . . ," see Katz, *In the Shadow of the Poorhouse*, 1. See also Michael Katz, *The Undeserving Poor: From the War of Poverty to the War on Welfare* (New York: Pantheon, 1989); for compassion as a misguided liberal construct, see Marvin Olasky, *The Tragedy of American Compassion* (Washington, D.C.: Regnery, 1992); for "malingering may be . . . ," see Rodgers, "Subjective Pain Testimony," 178.

24. For changes to disability rolls, see "U.S. Gets Tough with Disabled," *Washington Post*, September 7, 1982, A1; for "negative fallout . . . ," see May 28, 1981, memo from pollster Richard B. Wirthin to Ed Meese, Jim Baker, and Mike Deaver, folder 13 of 20, Anderson, Ronald Reagan Archives, Loma Linda, CA.

25. For legal appeals, see Robert Pear, "Dispute Continues on Aid to Disabled," *New York Times*, August 12, 1984, 26; for "incorrect denials . . . ," see Fair, 885 F.2d, p. 602, quoted in Rodgers, "Subjective Pain Testimony," 191.

26. See Laura Kalman, *The Strange Career of Legal Liberalism* (New Haven, CT: Yale University Press, 1996), 78; see also Steven M. Teles, *The Rise of the Conservative Legal Movement: The Battle for Control of the Law* (Princeton, NJ: Princeton University Press, 2008); for "people involved with . . . ," see Richard Posner, "The Economic Approach to Law," Texas Law Review 53 (1975): 761–65; for social security cases as tests, see Zaiser, "Proving Disabling Pain."

27. For changing environment for disabled, see Robin Herman, "Easing of U.S. Rules on Aid for Disabled Is Sought," *New York Times*, February 8, 1982, B2; for "an 'in house' ruling," and "there must be . . . ," see Rodgers, "Subjective Pain Testimony," 194; For "many Congressmen say . . . ," see Margaret Engel, "U.S. Gets Tough With Disabled," *Washington Post*, September 7, 1982, A1.

28. For "soften the image," see Robert Pear, "Softening Some Images, If Not Policies," *New York Times*, June 26, 1983, E4; Robert Pear, "Reagan Aide Hails Shift on Disability," *New York Times*, June 8, 1983, A17; for "had no idea . . ." and "number of people exempted . . . ," see Baroody, Michael E., Collection, box 2, folder: Heckler/Women's Op-Ed, HHS news statement, June 1983; Op-Ed—June 7, 1983, "Social Security Disability Review Reform," Ronald Reagan Library.

29. For "a state of legal confusion . . . ," and on disability lawsuits clogging courts see Pear, "Dispute Continues on Aid to Disabled"; on purged claimants, see Margaret Shapiro and Spencer Rich, "Hill Alters Rules for Disability," *Washington Post*, September 20, 1984, A1. As one judge said, "For some unexplained reason, the Secretary insists upon ignoring this court's statements" that she must consider subjective complaints of pain, even if they are not fully corroborated by objective medical evidence. Quoted in Robert Pear, "U.S. Flouts Courts in Determination of Benefit Claims," *New York Times*, May 13, 1984, 1.

30. On purging the rolls, see Robert Pear, "Reagan Reported Prepared to Stop Cuts in Disability," *New York Times*, March 24, 1984, 1. David Lauter, "Social Security's Legal Tactics Hit by 9th Circuit," *National Law Journal* (March 12, 1984): 8; for "the huge SSDI program . . . " and "malingerer hunters," see Charles Lane, "A Disability Primer," *New Republic*, August 12/19, 1985, 18–20; see also Milton Coleman, "Mondale Carries Coals of Compassion to Boston's Castle of Liberalism," *Washington Post*, November 3, 1984, A7; Milton Coleman and David Broder, "'Fairness' Issue Loses Potency," *Washington Post*, October 7, 1984, 1; for "heartless" and quote from Heckler on hardship, see "Social Security Bills Stalled in Congress," *Baltimore Sun*, August 12, 1984, 6A.

31. "1984 Presidential Debate between the President Reagan and Former Vice President Walter F. Mondale," October 7, 1984, *Weekly Compilation of Presidential Documents* 20, no. 41 (Monday, October 15, 1984): 1457–58.

32. "Ronald Reagan TV Ad: 'It's Morning in America Again,'" YouTube video, posted by Andre Morgado, n.d., www.youtube.com/watch?v=EU-IBF 8nwSY.

33. Of course, these issues were not entirely new to the post–World War II era. For scholarship on the nineteenth- and early-twentieth-century politics of pain, labor, and compensation, see Barbara Welke, *Law and the Border of Belonging in the Long Nineteenth Century United States* (Cambridge: Cambridge University Press, 2010); and Barbara Welke, *Recasting American Liberty: Gender, Race, Law, and the Railroad Revolution, 1865–1920* (Cambridge: Cambridge University Press, 2001); for disability assessment system, see David A. Hyman, "Health Care Fraud and Abuse: Market Change, Social Norms, and the Trust 'Reposed in the Workmen,'" *Journal of Legal Studies* 30 (June 2001): 531–67.

34. For "the federal courts . . . ," see Allan Goldhammer and Susan Bloom, "Recent Changes in the Assessment of Pain in Disability Claims Before the Social Security Administration," 3 Soc. Sec. Rep. Serv. 1119 *West's Social Security Reporting Service* January, 1984; for "would rest solely . . . ," see Peter Ferrara, Office of Policy Development Memo, 1981. Ronald Reagan Archives, Loma Linda, CA; Carter thanked J. J. Pickle for his work on H.R. 3236. "Social Security Disability Amendments of 1980: Statement on Signing H.R. 3236 Into Law, June 9, 1980," *Public Papers: Carter*, 2:1062; for "Section 205 . . ." and "the administration proposal . . . ," see Eric Hempel, Memorandum for Martin Anderson and Ed Gray, subject: differences between Congressman Pickle's and the administration's Social Security proposals," May 13, 1981, Social Security Administration file, Ronald Reagan Library. See also "Statement of Honorable J. J. Pickle (D, Texas), chairman of the Subcommittee on Social Security, House Committee on Ways and Means, at meeting of the Social Security Subcommittee, Wednesday, March 25, 1981, draft committee print, Sec. 206, Evaluation of Pain, Ronald Reagan Papers; for "several billions dollars . . . ," see "Statement on Signing a Bill Amending the Social Security Disability Insurance System, January 12, 1983," "H.R. 7093 is Public Law 97-455, approved January 12," *Public Papers: Reagan*, 24:39.

35. On the complicated struggle, see Charles Lane, "A Disability Primer," *New Republic*, August 12, 1985, 19; for "the secretary is not . . . ," see Miranda v. Richardson 514 F.2d 996 (1st Cir., April 14, 1975) (75 Ford Administration); on Reagan's combative approach, a later critique of this policy appears in the *National Law Journal*: "Non-Acquiescence," editorial, *National Law Journal* (June 17, 1985): 14; on nonacquiescence, see David Hedge, *Governance and the Changing American States* (Boulder, CO: Westview Press, 1998).

36. For "they will say . . . ," see "Courts in Conflict," *Los Angeles Times*, December 2, 1980, C10; for "attacked liberal judges . . . ," see William Endicott,

"Meese Hits Liberal Judges, Would End Insanity Pleas," *Los Angeles Times*, April 16, 1981, 1; Jack Nelson, "No. 2 Man: Ed Meese: He, Reagan Think Alike," *Los Angeles Times*, June 14, 1981, 1; for the concern of Reagan supporters, see Rodgers, "Subjective Pain Testimony," 195.

37. Robert Pear, "New York and Other States Defy U.S. Rules for Disability Benefits," *New York Times*, September 12, 1983, A1. As the article also noted, "Over three months, the Governors of New York, North Carolina, Massachusetts, Arkansas, Kansas, West Virginia, and other states have challenged the Reagan Administration's restrictive interpretation of the law."

38. For "pain is an . . . ," see Rodgers, "Subjective Pain Testimony," 198; for "if the regional courts . . . ," 198–99; for Senate bill discussion and dispute within government, see Pear, "Dispute Continues on Aid to Disabled."

39. On patients like Polaski and their influence on health policy, particularly amid Reagan-era activism and calls for both fiscal restraint and patient's rights, see Beatrix Hoffman, Nancy Tomes, Rachel Grob, and Mark Schlesinger, eds., *Patients as Policy Actors* (New Brunswick, NJ: Rutgers University Press, 2011); for "was not supported . . . ," see Polaski v. Heckler 751 F.2d 943 (8th Cir., 1984) Minnesota; for "directly and flagrantly," as well as other details of the Polaski case, see Polaski v. Heckler, 585 F. Supp. 1004, 1013 (D. Minn., 1984); "Judge Orders Benefits Paid," *Washington Post*, April 28, 1984, A12; "HHS Gets Order to Mail Disability Checks," *Washington Post*, July 24, 1984, A13; Edward A. Gargan, "Delay in Restoring Benefits Said to Hurt Disabled," *New York Times*, August 26, 1984, 42; for "state of lawlessness," see "Judge Orders Benefits Paid," *Washington Post*, April 28, 1984, A12; see also "HHS Gets Order to Mail Disability Checks," *Washington Post*, July 24, 1984, A13; Edward A. Gargan, "Delay in Restoring Benefits said to Hurt Disabled," *New York Times*, August 26, 1984, 42; on the temporary halt, see Polaski v. Heckler, No. 84-5085 (8th Cir., Dec. 31, 1984); for the case's movement through the courts, see Civ. No. 4-84-64 (D. Minn., 4th Div., April 17, 1984); Polaski v. Heckler No. 84-5085, 751 F.2d 943, 8 Soc. Sec. Rep. Ser. 178, Unempl. Ins. Rep. CCH 15,666 (8th Cir., Dec. 31, 1984); Polaski v. Heckler, No. 4-84-64, 606 F. Supp. 549 (Dist. Ct., D. Minn., 4th Div., April 12, 1985); Heckler v. Polaski, No. 85-55 (U.S., October Term, 1985).

40. For "that will bring . . . ," see Shapiro and Rich, "Hill Alters Rules for Disability," 1, 3; Congress and the administration both objected to the lack of uniformity across the courts in how disability was evaluated; see Kevin F. Foley, "Establishing Medically Determinable Impairments," *Trial* (April 1, 1999); for "substantially limit . . . ," see Eileen Sweeney, "New Disability Legislation Enacted," *Clearinghouse Review* 18 (1984–1984): 819; on the pain question, the Institute of Medicine Report on pain and disability was published in 1987. Mar-

ian Osterweis, Arthur Kleinman, and David Mechanic, eds., *Pain and Disability: Clinical, Behavioral, and Public Policy Perspectives* (Washington, D.C.: National Academy Press, 1987); on the expert panel, see "Report of the Commission on the Evaluation of Pain," *Social Security Bulletin* 50 (January 1987): 13–44, www .ssa.gov/policy/docs/ssb/v50n1/v50n1p13.pdf. See also Michael Ruppert, "Developments in Social Security Law," *Indiana Law Review* 22 (1988): 401; and Rodgers, "Subjective Pain Testimony," 200.

41. On search for middle ground and polarization, see Rodgers, "Subjective Pain Testimony," 192. In an effort to get beyond the conflicting court rulings on the status of pain, Congress in 1984 enacted a statute that included an express provision for evaluating pain: Social Security Disability Benefits Reform Act of 1984, Pub. L. No. 98-460, § 3(a)(1), 98 Stat. 1794, 1799–1800 (codified at 42 U.S.C. § 423(d)(5)(A) (1988)); discussed in Ellen Smith Pryor, "Compensation and the Ineradicable Problems of Pain," *George Washington Law Review* 59 (January 1991): 239–306, 243.

42. Rodgers, "Subjective Pain Testimony," 195; On administration's upper hand, see Shapiro and Rich, "Hill Alters Rules for Disability," A1.

43. Polaski v. Heckler, No. 84-5085 (8th Cir., Dec. 31, 1984).

44. On the completion of the Polaski story, see "Supreme Court Upholds Disability Ruling," *Atlanta Daily World*, June 18, 1987, 1; on the Polaski standard, see Osterweis, Kleinman, and Mechanic, *Pain and Disability*, 57.

45. Rodgers, "Subjective Pain Testimony," 195. For "apply the requirement . . . ," see Foley, "Establishing Medically Determinable Impairments."

46. Legal scholar Ellen Smith Pryor noted that pain remained an ineradicable problem, "a troublesome and largely unexplored area in the vast world of nontort compensation programs." Pryor, "Compensation and the Ineradicable Problems of Pain," 244. As Pryor noted, "Congress's sunset date of Jan 1, 1987 passed without an alternative" pain standard.

47. Joseph Sobran, "The Averted Gaze: Liberalism and Fetal Pain," *Human Life Review* 10 (Spring 1984): 5–15, cited in Sara Dubow, "Debating Fetal Pain, 1984–2007" in *Ourselves Unborn: A History of the Fetus in Modern America* (New York: Oxford University Press, 2011). See, for example, Joseph Sobran, "The Science, Law, and Politics of Fetal Pain Legislation," *Harvard Law Review* 115 (May 2002): 2010–33. On *The Silent Scream*, see Dena Kelman, "Debate on Abortion Focuses on Graphic Film," *New York Times*, January 25, 1985, B8.

48. For "if every member . . . ," see Kelman, "Debate on Abortion"; see also Ronald Reagan, "Remarks to Participants in the March for Life Rally January 22, 1988," *Weekly Compilation of Presidential Documents* 24, no. 3 (Monday, January 25, 1988): 74.

49. "Remarks at a White House Ceremony for Participants in the National Initiative on Technology and the Disabled, December 3, 1985," *Public Papers: Reagan*, 2:1429.

50. A. H. Lebovits et al., "The Prevalence and Management of Pain in Patients with AIDS: A Review of 134 Cases," *Clinical Journal of Pain* 5 (1989): 245–48; for "became associated with . . . ," see 1990 interview sponsored by Center for Applied Christian Ethics, Wheaton College (undated), "Dr. C. Everett Koop on HIV/AIDS," YouTube video, posted by cacewheatoncollegeil on November 19, 2008, www.youtube.com/watch?v=ivdBODl7YTg.

51. For "yuppie flu," see Muhammad Yunus, "Fibromyalgia Syndrome: A Need for Uniform Classification," *Journal of Rheumatology* 10 (December 1983): 841–44; see also D. L. Goldenberg, "Fibromyalgia Syndrome: An Emerging but Controversial Condition," *Journal of the American Medical Association* 257 (May 22, 1987): 2782–87; Muhammad Yunus, "Fibromyalgia Syndrome: New Research on an Old Malady," *British Medical Journal* 289 (February 25, 1989): 474; Lawrence K. Altman, "Chronic Fatigue Syndrome Finally Gets Some Respect," *New York Times*, December 4, 1990, C1; Robert Aronowitz, "From Myalgic Encephalitis to Yuppie Flu: A History of Chronic Fatigue Syndromes," in *Making Sense of Illness* (New York: Cambridge University Press, 1998); Susan Greenhalgh, *Under the Medical Gaze: Facts and Fictions of Chronic Pain* (Berkeley: University of California Press, 2001); for "whether patients have . . . ," see Philip M. Boffey, "Fatigue 'Virus' Has Experts More Baffled and Skeptical Than Ever" *New York Times*, July 28, 1987, C1; see also Jane Brody, "Chronic Fatigue Syndrome," *New York Times*, July 28, 1988, B6; for CFS exemplification and other discussion, see Marilyn Dunlop, "MDs Pinpoint 'Yuppie Plague' Virus," *Toronto Star*, February 14, 1987, H2; "Study Says 'Yuppie Disease' May Just Be Depression," *St. Petersburg Times*, May 11, 1988, 7A. For the SSA's interpretation of CFS, see Providing Medical Evidence to the Social Security Administration for Individual with Chronic Fatigue Syndrome: A Guide for Health Professionals (Social Sec. Admin. Pub. No. 64-063, Feb. 1996), discussed in Foley, "Establishing Medically Determinable Impairments"; Dara E. Purvis, "A Female Disease: The Unintentional Gendering of Fibromyalgia Social Security Claims," *Texas Journal of Women and Law* 21 (Fall 2011): 85–118; for "potential for manipulation . . . ," see Foley, "Establishing Medically Determinable Impairments," quoting from the 1991 case Cline v. Sullivan, 939 F.2d 560, 568 (8th Cir., 1991).

52. For "millions," see Rovner, *Washington Post*, May 28, 1986, H9. Colman McCarthy, "Abortion: The Pain Debate," *Washington Post*, February 26, 1984, 42.

53. For "stage two . . . ," see "Republican Governors Association—Remarks at a Dinner for Members. October 7, 1986," *Weekly Compilation of Presidential*

Documents 22, no. 41 (Monday, October 13, 1986): 1353; for "many years ago . . . ," see "Remarks at a Rally for Senator James T. Broyhill, October 8, 1986," *Weekly Compilation of Presidential Documents* 22, no. 41 (Monday, October 13, 1986) 1353.

54. Bowen insisted that he "did nothing illegal," pointing out that DMSO was approved for investigational uses in drug therapy. Spencer Rich and Cristine Russell, "Reagan to Nominate Bowen for HHS," *Washington Post*, November 8, 1985, A3. On the politics of DMSO in the early 1980s, see Phillip W. Davis, "An Incipient 'Wonder Drug' Movement: DMSO and the Food and Drug Administration," *Social Problems* 32 (December 1984): 197–212; and Linda Garmon, "Judging DMSO: There's the Rub," *Science News* 122 (December 18–25, 1982): 398–99, 408. As one news account reported, "Bowen said he also gave his wife capsules containing the active ingredient in marijuana to ease her pain." For this and "why can't [a] dying person . . . ," see Jon Van, "Used Banned Drugs on Cancer: Doctor," *Chicago Tribune*, February 14, 1981, 1; on accusations from the Religious Right, fourteen antiabortion groups hurled these charges after Bowen was nominated. Rich and Russell, "Reagan to Nominate Bowen for HHS," A3; for involvement of U.S. Supreme Court, see "Supreme Court Upholds Disability Ruling," 1.

Chapter Four: Divided States of Analgesia

1. For Miller's decision and communication with Kevorkian, see "People of the State of Michigan, Plaintiff, v. Jack Kevorkian, Defendant," *Issues in Law and Medicine* 9 (1993): 189–208; Michigan v. Kevorkian, No.: CR-92-115190-FC (Mich. Cir. Ct., July 21, 1992); for "suicide-machine," see Susan K. Jezewski, "Can a Suicide Machine Trigger the Murder Statute?" *Wayne Law Review* 37 (1990):1931–50.

2. Jezewski, "Can a Suicide Machine."

3. Geoffrey N. Fieger, "Commentaries: The Persecution and Prosecution of Doctor Death and His Mercy Machine," *Ohio Northern University Law Review* 20 (1993–1994): 659–71.

4. For "even if they [these measures] . . . ," see Paul Hoffman, "Pope Grants Use of Pain Reliever," *New York Times*, February 25, 1957, 1; for polarization in 1990s cultural politics, see George Lakoff, *Moral Politics: How Liberals and Conservatives Think* (Chicago: University of Chicago Press, 1996).

5. On the rise of evangelical religious groups and their turn to the Republican Party, see Paul Boyer, "The Evangelical Resurgence in 1970s American Protestantism," in *Rightward Bound: Making America Conservative in the 1970s*, ed. Bruce Schulman and Julian Zelizer (Cambridge, MA: Harvard University Press, 2008).

6. John Dillin, "Lawyers' Alert! Outsiders Line Up to Challenge Congressional Incumbents," *Christian Science Monitor*, January 14, 1994, 1.

7. For "I'm tired of apologizing . . . ," see Ruth SoRelle, "Computerized Pump Spells R-E-L-I-E-F for Intense Pain: Program Allows Patients to Get the Medication as They Need It," *Houston Chronicle*, June 30, 1986, 1; C. Stratton Hill Jr., "Pain Management in a Drug-Oriented Society," supplement, *Cancer* 63 (June 1, 1989): 2383–86; for Congress rejection, see *A Bill to Amend the Controlled Substances Act to Authorize the Use of Heroin for Terminally Ill Cancer Patients: Hearing before the Subcommittee on Health and the Environment of the Committee on Interstate and Foreign Commerce*, Ninety-Sixth Congress, second session on H.R. 7334, September 4, 1980 (Washington: U.S. Government Printing Office, 1980); for Hill's advocacy, see D. M. Thorpe, "Texas Intractable Pain Treatment Act of 1989," *Dimensions in Oncology Nursing* 4, no. 1 (Spring 1990): 33–34. "Cancer Society Chief Admits Its Neglect of Poor," *Houston Chronicle* (April 3, 1989), B8.

8. "Cancer Society Chief Admits Its Neglect of Poor," *Houston Chronicle*, April 3, 1989, B8.

9. Ibid.

10. "Special Session to Cover Three More Topics Added by Clements," *Houston Chronicle*, June 28, 1989, A22; as the article noted, the state's lieutenant governor, Bill Hobby, also strongly supported the proposed Intractable Pain Treatment Act aimed at overriding the "Texas Medical Practices Act, which raises questions about physicians prescribing drugs for patients with incurable pain."

11. For "no physician may be subject . . . ," see Texas Civil Statutes/Title 70: Health Public/Art. 4495c Intractable Pain Treatment Act (November 1, 1989); for "the war on drugs . . . ," see C. S. Hill, "The Intractable Pain Treatment Act of Texas," *Texas Medicine* 88, no. 2 (May 1992): 70–72; Dianna Hunt, "Living with Pain: Doctors' Insensitivity, Legal Fear Cause Needless Suffering," *Houston Chronicle*, December 15, 1991, 1; Hugh McIntosh, "Regulatory Barriers Take Some Blame for Pain Undertreatment," *Journal of the National Cancer Institute* 83 (1991): 1202–4; Dianna Hunt, "Wider Use of Painkillers Urged: Patients' Hospital Stays Could Be Shortened, Experts Say," *Houston Chronicle*, March 6, 1992, 10; Laura E. Keeton, "Officials Give Conflicting Opinions about Painkiller," *Houston Chronicle*, August 25, 1992, A12; C. Richard Stasney and C. Stratton Hill, "Pain Control and the Texas State Board of Medical Examiners," *Texas State Board of Medical Examiners Newsletter* 15, no. 1 (Spring/Summer 1993): 1.

12. David L. Ralston, "Pain Management: Texas Legislative and Regulatory Update," *Journal of Law, Medicine, and Ethics* 24 (1996): 328–37.

13. For middle road, see Anne C. Roark, "Coalition Forms to Ease Pain of Cancer," *Los Angeles Times*, February 16, 1992, 3; Hill, "Pain Management in a Drug-Oriented Society," 2383–86. Hill defined a drug-oriented society as "a society that considers drugs paramount in treating illness and solving a wide variety of physical and emotional problems." Others in the field decried an overregulation of drugs. See "Relieving Patient Pain in a Regulated Environment: A Medical Dilemma for the 1990s," *Journal of Pain and Symptom Management* 5 (February 1990); Robert T. Angarola and David E. Joranson, "State Controlled Substances Laws and Pain Control," *APS Bulletin* 2 (1992), 10–11, 15; Robert T. Angarola and David E. Joranson, "Wins and Losses in Pain Control," *APS Bulletin* 3 (1993), 8–9.

14. On the pain summit and for "we should create . . . ," see "Summit on Effective Pain Management: Removing Impediments to Appropriate Prescribing," *Los Angeles Times*, March 18, 1994; Shari Roan, "A World of Hurt," *Los Angeles Times*, March 29, 1994, E2; Harvey Rose, "Anatomy of a Pain Summit," *Sacramento Medicine* (November 1994); see also "Cancer Painkillers," *Orlando Sentinel*, August 1, 1993, G7; for "nurses' refusal to administer . . . ," see Ben A. Rich, "Physicians' Legal Duty to Relieve Suffering," *Western Medical Journal* 175 (September 2001): 151–52; on moral and political questions, see, for example, Michael R. Flick, "The Due Process of Dying," *California Law Review* 79 (July 1991): 1121–67; and "Physician-Assisted Suicide and the Right to Die with Assistance," *Harvard Law Review* 105 (June 1992): 2021–40.

15. Dr. William Hurwitz, "The Police State of Medicine," remarks before the Drug Policy Foundation, October 18, 1997, New Orleans, LA, www.druglibrary.org/schaffer/asap/policestate.htm.

16. Commenting on changes in late 1980s and early 1990s, Ann Alpers noted that "the past decade has marked a sharp increase in the number of physicians prosecuted for criminal negligence based on arguably negligent patient care." Ann Alpers, "Criminal Act or Palliative Care? Prosecutions Involving the Care of the Dying," *Journal of Law, Medicine, and Ethics* 26 (1998): 308–11. See also P. R. Van Grunsven, "Criminal Prosecutions of Health Care Providers for Clinical Mistakes and Fatal Errors: Is 'Bad Medicine' a Crime?" *Journal of Health and Hospital Law* 29 (1996): 107; for "high," see Drug Reform Coalition Network, "Defend Chronic Pain Treatment," *Activist Guide*, June 5, 1996; for "I was charged . . ." and "hearing might well be . . . ," see Hurwitz, "Police State of Medicine"; for "arrested in his office . . . ," see Rose, "Anatomy of a Pain Summit."

17. For limited understanding discussion, see D. E. Joranson, C. S. Cleeland, D. E. Weissman, and A. M. Gilson, "Opioids for Chronic Cancer and Noncancer Pain: A Survey of State Medical Board Members," *Federation Bulletin* 79 (1992):

15–49; the "while most respondents . . . ," study is described in the following way in David E. Joranson, Aaron M. Gilson, June L. Dahl, and J. David Haddox, "Pain Management, Controlled Substances, and State Medical Board Policy: A Decade of Change," *Journal of Pain and Symptom Management* 23, no. 2 (February 2002): 138–47; for "treated like addicts . . . ," see Hurwitz, "Police State of Medicine."

18. Hill, "Pain Management in a Drug-Oriented Society," 2383–86; for Oregon's Death with Dignity legislation, see Joshua M. Wiener, "Oregon's Plan for Health Care Rationing: Bold Initiative or Terrible Mistake?" *Brookings Review* 10 (Winter 1992): 26–31.

19. For extensive analysis of the PAS controversy, see Neil M. Gorsuch, *The Future of Assisted Suicide and Euthanasia* (Princeton, NJ: Princeton University Press, 2006).

20. Lisa Belkin, "Doctor Tells of First Death Using His Suicide Device," *New York Times*, June 6, 1990, A1.

21. For "we take it as obvious . . . ," see Marvin Zalman, John Strate, Denis Hunter, and James Sellars, "Michigan's Assisted Suicide Three Ring Circus—an Intersection of Law and Politics," *Ohio Northern University Law Review* 23 (1997): 919; for "moral entrepreneur," see Juanne N. Clarke, "The Physician as Moral Entrepreneur," *Journal of Religion and Health* 21 (Winter 1982): 290–306; and also Howard Becker, *Outsiders: Studies in the Sociology of Deviance* (New York: Free Press, 1963): 147–53.

22. For the principle of double effect, see Raanan Gillon, "The Principle of Double Effect and Medical Ethics," *British Medical Journal* 292 (January 19, 1986): 193–94; for "lives of horrible desperation," see "People of the State of Michigan, Plaintiff, v. Jack Kevorkian, Defendant," *Issues in Law and Medicine* 9 (1993): 189–208.

23. For "introduced a package . . . ," see Marvin Zalman et al., "Michigan's Assisted Suicide Three Ring Circus," *Ohio Northern University Law Review* 23 (1997): 913. Tim Richard, "Pain Management Bills to Cut Assisted Suicide," *Birmingham-Bloomfield Eccentric*, June 13, 1996, A12; for "nothing in this section . . . ," see April 8, 1994, Florida Statutes, chap. 458, Medical Practice, § 458.326, Intractable Pain, Authorized Treatment; for "safe harbor," see Allen R. Grossman and D. C. Mackey, "Narcotic Prescription for Pain Management in Florida: The Physician and the Law," *Journal of the Florida Medical Association* 83, no. 10 (December 1996): 673–74. See also M. Skinner, "Aspects of the Problem in Treating Chronic Pain: Florida Pain Management Guidelines," *Journal of the Florida Medical Association* 84 (February 1997): 85–86; for the emerging question, see "Narratives of Pain and Comfort: Dr. M's Story," *Journal of Law, Medicine, & Ethics* 24 (1996).

24. For "explaining that he would . . . ," see Drug Reform Coalition Network, "Defend Chronic Pain II," *Activist Guide*, December 9, 1996; for "effort to characterize . . . ," see New York State Task Force on Life and Law, "When Death Is Sought: Assisted Suicide and Euthanasia in the Medical Context (Supplement to the Report)," http://wings.buffalo.edu/bioethics/suppl .html#.

25. For "I don't think . . . ," see Allan Parachini, "Bringing Euthanasia Issue to the Ballot Box," *Los Angeles Times*, April 10, 1987, G1; for "was a precedent . . . ," see Dirk Johnson, "Foes of Abortion View 'Right to Die' as Second Battle over Life and Death," *New York Times*, July 31, 1990, A8.

26. "State of Michigan in the Circuit Court for County of Oakland. People of the State of Michigan, plaintiff, v. Jack Kevorkian, defendant. Case No. CR-92-115190-FC," *Issues in Law and Medicine* 9 (1993): 189–208. See discussion of PAS cases in Janet M. Branigan, "Michigan's Struggle with Assisted Suicide and Related Issues as Illuminated by Current Case Law: An Overview of People v. Kevorkian," *University of Detroit Mercy Law Review* 72 (1994–1995): 959–87; Benton Kirk Morris, "Physician Assisted Suicide: The Abortion of the Nineties," *Law and Psychology Review* 20 (1996): 215–29; Terry Brantley, "People v. Kevorkian: Michigan's Supreme Court Leads the Way in Declaring No Fundamental Right to Assist Another in Suicide," *Mercer Law Review* 47 (1995–1996): 1191–99; Katherine C. Glynn, "Turning to State Legislatures to Legalize Physician-Assisted Suicide for Seriously Ill, Non-terminal Patients after *Vacco v. Quill* and *Washington v. Glucksberg*," *Journal of Law and Policy* (1997): 329–62. See also "In the United States District Court for the District of Oregon," *Issues in Law and Medicine* 12 (1996): 79–92.

27. James M. Hoefler, "Diffusion and Diversity: Federalism and the Right to Die in the Fifty States," *Publius* 24 (Summer 1994): 153–70.

28. For initiative rejection, see Alexander Morgan Capron, "At Law: Even in Defeat, Proposition 161 Sounds a Warning," *Hastings Center Report* 23 (January–February 1993): 32–33.

29. For the new and ongoing battles, see Brad Knickerbocker, "Oregon's Suicide Measure Draws Hippocratic Fire," *Christian Science Monitor*, November 14, 1994, 1; for "to ensure that seriously ill . . . ," see California Department of Public Health, Proposition 215, www.cdph.ca.gov/programs/mmp/pages/compassionateuseact.aspx; for DEA warnings, see Dave Hogan, "AMA Endorses Legislation to Block Assisted-Suicide Law" *Oregonian*, June 25, 1999, B01.

30. For district court findings, see the case, Compassion in Dying v. Washington, No. 94-35534, 79 F.3d 790 (9th Cir., 1996), http://caselaw.findlaw.com /us-9th-circuit/1139892.html.

31. For "the enemies . . . ," see Drug Reform Coalition Network, "War on Pain Control" *Activist Guide*, October 26, 1996; on persecution in the face of the "just say no" rhetoric surrounding drugs and permissiveness, one doctor's article answered back: S. Z. Pantilat, "Just Say Yes: The Use of Opioids for Managing Pain at the End of Life," *Western Journal of Medicine* 171(1999): 257–59. On a 2000 National Public Radio program, "The People's Pharmacy," hosts noted, "The "just say no" campaign has had a consequence . . . In our efforts to discourage people from taking illicit drugs, we've also made people in pain fear legitimate pain control and adequate pain medication." For "the chilling effect . . . ," see Drug Reform Coalition Network, "War on Pain Control."

32. For "feel their pain . . . ," see Schottenstein, Zox, and Dunn, "Ohio Enacts New Intractable Pain Legislation," *Ohio Health Law Update* 3 (September 1997); for "comply with acceptable pain . . . ," see David E. Joranson, Aaron M. Gilson, June L. Dahl, and J. David Haddox, "Pain Management, Controlled Substances, and State Medical Board Policy: A Decade of Change," *Journal of Pain and Symptom Management* 23, no. 2 (February 2002), 142–43; for "opening the door . . . ," see David Joranson and Aaron Gilson, "State Intractable Pain Policy: Current Status," *American Pain Society Bulletin* 7 (1997).

33. See Vacco v. Quill, 117 S. Ct. 2293 (1997); for analysis of the Supreme Court's ruling, see George J. Annas, "The Bell Tolls for a Constitutional Right to Physician-Assisted Suicide," *New England Journal of Medicine* 337 (October 9, 1997): 1098–1103.

34. For "compassion is a proper . . . ," see Compassion in Dying v. Washington. See also discussion in Morris, "Physician Assisted Suicide"; for Ohio's Supreme Court, see National Catholic Bioethics Center chart of state-by-state policies, www.ncbcenter.org/document.doc?id=177; for the Florida State Supreme Court ruling, see Ben F. Overton and Katherine E. Giddings, "The Right of Privacy in Florida in the Age of Technology and the Twenty-First Century: A Need for Protection from Private and Commercial Intrusion," *Florida State University Law Review* 25 (1997): 30. The Florida case is Krischer v. McIver, 22 *Florida Law Weekly* S443 (Fla. 1997); for Supreme Court, see Don Marquis and Alexander Capron, "The Ultimate Pain Relief," *Hastings Center Report* 25 (November–December 1995): 2–3.

35. "Courts in Conflict," *Los Angeles Times*, December 2, 1980, C10.

36. Daniel Rodgers, *Age of Fracture* (Cambridge, MA: Harvard University Press, 2011), 11.

37. On the AMA amicus brief and the court, the principle is often associated with Aquinas and with Roman Catholic moral theology. See discussion in

relation to American law and compassionate death in Richard S. Kay, "Causing Death for Compassionate Reasons in American Law," *American Journal of Comparative Law* 54 (Fall 2006): 693–716. See also Kenneth L. Vaux, "The Theologic Ethics of Euthanasia," *Hastings Center Report* 19 (January–February 1989): 19–22; for "the recognition . . . ," see Yale Kamisar, "Assisted Suicide and Euthanasia: An Exchange," *New York Review of Books*, November 6, 1997, www.ny books.com/articles/archives/1997/nov/06/assisted-suicide-and-euthanasia-an-exchange/.

38. "Dennis. C. Vacco, Attorney General of New York, et al., Petitioners, v. Timothy E. Quill et al., No. 95-1858. Washington, D.C., Wednesday, January 8, 1997. Oral Argument before Supreme Court of the United States," *Issues in Law and Medicine* 12 (1996–1997): 417–39; "State of Washington, Christine O. Gregoire, Attorney General of Washington, Petitioners, v. Harold Glucksberg, M.D., Abigail Halperin, M.D., Thomas A. Preston, M.D., and Peter Shalit, M.D., Ph.D., Respondents," *Issues in Law and Medicine* 12 (1996–1997): 295–321; One reaction to opinions in the *Glucksberg* case, for example, came from the New York State Task Force, which took issue with the judges who had alleged that pain relief when pushed too far was akin with euthanasia.

39. For "the . . . challenging task . . . ," see O'Connor, concurring opinion, Cruzan v. Director, Missouri Department of Health, 497 U.S. 261, No. 88-1503 (U.S., June 25, 1990), www.law.cornell.edu/supct/html/historics/USSC_CR_0497 _0261_ZC.html. See also Kathryn Tucker, "In the Laboratory of the States: The Progress of *Glucksberg*'s Invitation to States to Address End-of-Life Choice," *Michigan Law Review* 106 (June 2008): 1593–1612; and Michael P. Allen, "Justice O'Connor and the 'Right to Die': Constitutional Promises Unfulfilled," *William and Mary Bill of Rights Journal* 14, no. 3 (2006): 821, http://scholarship.law .wm.edu/wmborj/vol14/iss3/3; for "right," see Joanne Lynn and George Annas, "Legislation and End-of-Life Care," letter to the editor, *Journal of the American Medical Association* 283 (June 14, 2000): 2933. They cite R. A. Burt, "The Supreme Court Speaks: Not Assisted Suicide but a Constitutional Right to Palliative Care," *New England Journal of Medicine* 337 (1997): 1234–36; for "there is no dispute . . . ," see National Council on Disability, "Assisted Suicide: A Disability Perspective," *Issues in Law and Medicine* 14 (1998): 273–300. A National Council on Disability position paper on the fallibility of prognosis, among other topics, is useful here: Robert L. Burgdorf, "Assisted Suicide: A Disability Perspective," *Issues in Law and Medicine* 14 (1998): 273–300. On the Supreme Court ruling in *Glucksberg*, see Burt, "Supreme Court Speaks"; for "Justices Breyer and O'Connor . . . ," see Yale Kamisar, reply to Ronald Dworkin, "Assisted Suicide and Euthanasia: An Exchange," *New York Review of Books*, November 6, 1997,

www.nybooks.com/articles/archives/1997/nov/06/assisted-suicide-and-euthana
sia-an-exchange/.

40. In two 1997 cases, Washington v. Glucksberg, 117 S. Ct. 2258, and
Vacco v. Quill, 117 S. Ct. 2293, the Supreme Court invited further debate by the
states. See A. Alpers and B. Lo, "The Supreme Court Addresses Physician-Assisted
Suicide: Can Its Rulings Improve Palliative Care?" *Archives of Family Medicine* 8
(May–June 1999): 200–205. The authors noted, "The Court's reasoning may
help physicians resolve substantial ethical dilemmas regarding the provision of
narcotics given in high dosages, the care of incompetent patients, and the suffering caused by symptoms other than pain." On states following their own paths,
see D. E. Joranson and A. M. Gilson, "State Intractable Pain Policy: Current Status," *American Pain Society Bulletin* 7, no. 2:7–9.

41. On the Suicide Funding Restriction Act, see "Oregon's Assisted Suicide
Law Stands, but Debate Continues," *AIDS Policy and Law* 12, no. 221 (November 28, 1997): 18; for "I feel your pain . . . ," see President William Jeffer-
son Clinton, "Statement upon Signing the Assisted Suicide Funding Restoration
Act of 1997 (April 30, 1997)," *Public Papers of the Presidents of the United
States, William J. Clinton* (Washington, D.C.: Government Printing Office,
1997), 515.

42. For "The Lethal Drug Abuse Prevention Act . . . ," see National Right to
Life News, "Action Request—U.S. Senators to Cast Four Crucial Votes Important
to the Pro-Life Movement after the August Recess," August 12, 1998, back cover,
www.nrlc.org/news/1998/NRL8.98/back.html; for "If we've learned anything . . . ,"
see 144 Cong. Rec. E2148 (October 13, 1998), www.gpo.gov/fdsys/pkg/CREC
-1998-10-13/html/CREC-1998-10-13-pt1-PgE2147-2.htm.

43. For "legitimate medial purpose," see Robert Pear, "House Backs Ban on
Using Medicine to Aid in Suicide," *New York Times*, October 28, 1999: for "it
has certainly . . . ," see *Controlled Substances Act Amendments: Hearing on H.R.
2260 before the Subcommittee on the Constitution of the Committee on the Judiciary*, House of Representatives, 106th Congress, first session (Statement of
Richard Doerflinger, associate director for Policy Development, secretariat for
Pro-Life Activities, National Conference of Catholic Bishops), June 24, 1999.
http://commdocs.house.gov/committees/judiciary/hju62489.000/hju62489
_of.htm.

44. On the Pain Relief Promotion Act, see Vida Foubister, "Some Fear Authority Shift in Pain Treatment Bill," *American Medical News* (November 15,
1999); regarding the Hyde-Nickles bill, the North Carolina Medical Society
voiced concerns that the pending federal bill would cause the DEA to "intrude
more on doctor's offices." For "I am strongly pro-life . . . ," see Rep. Ron Paul

(R-Texas), "Providing for Consideration of H.R. 2260, Pain Relief Promotion Act of 1999," 145 Cong. Rec. (October 27, 1999): 27068.

45. For AMA opinion and "bad bill on dying . . . ," see David Orentlicher and Art Caplan, "The Pain Relief Promotion Acts of 1999: A Serious Threat to Palliative Care," *Journal of the American Medical Association* 283 (January 12, 2000), 255–58; J. P. Freer, "Congress and the Pain Relief Promotion Act," *Western Journal of Medicine* 172 (2000): 5–6; "A Bad Bill on Dying," *Washington Post*, February 16, 2000, A22; "An Improved Pain Relief Bill," editorial, *American Medical News*, May 22/29, 2000; for increasingly split physician opinions, see "Legislation and End-of-Life Care," letters to the editor, *Journal of the American Medical Association* 283 (June 14, 2000): 2934–35.

46. John A. Kitzhaber, "Congress's Medical Meddlers," *Washington Post*, November 2, 1999, A21; "Senators Playing Doctor," editorial, *Washington Post*, September 19, 2000, A22; John Hughes, "Assisted Suicide Battle Could Complicate Session Finale," *Associated Press State & Local Wire*, October 16, 2000; Jim Myers, "Senate GOP Sinks Work of OK Leaders," *Tulsa World*, December 10, 2000.

47. For litigation, see Ashbel S. Green, "Ashcroft Buttresses Suicide Law Challenge," *Oregonian*, September 24, 2002, A01; for "a classic states' rights . . . ," see Patrick J. Kapios, "Oregon v. Ashcroft 192 F. Supp. 2D 1077 (D. Or. 2002)," *Journal of Gender, Social Policy, and the Law* 11 (2002–2003): 223–36.

48. Michael J. Kennedy, "Libertarian Plods On—Alone and Unheard," *Los Angeles Times*, May 10, 1988, 12.

49. See Sandra H. Johnson, "Introduction: Legal and Regulatory Issues in Pain Management," *Journal of Law, Medicine, and Ethics* 26 (1998): 265–66; J. David Haddox and Gerald M. Aronoff, "Commentary: The Potential for Unintended Consequences from Public Policy Shifts in the Treatment of Pain," *Journal of Law, Medicine, and Ethics* 26 (1998): 350–52; Tim Jost, "Public Financing of Pain Management: Leaky Umbrellas and Ragged Safety Nets," *Journal of Law, Medicine, and Ethics* 26 (1998): 290–307; Ann M. Martino, "In Search of a New Ethic for Treating Patients with Chronic Pain: What Can Medical Boards Do?" *Journal of Law, Medicine, and Ethics* 26 (1998): 332–49.

50. See for example, Diane E. Hoffmann and Anita J. Tarzian, "Achieving the Right Balance in Oversight of Physician Opioid Prescribing for Pain: The Role of State Medical Boards," *Journal of Law, Medicine, and Ethics* 31 (2003): 21–40; Pain and Policy Studies Group, University of Wisconsin Comprehensive Cancer Center, "Achieving Balance in Federal and State Pain Policy: A Guide to Evaluation," July 2000, www.medsch.wisc.edu/painpolicy/eguide2003/index/eguide2003 .pdf. See also Barry Meier, "The Delicate Balance of Pain and Addiction," *New*

York Times, November 25, 2003, F1. In New York State, for example, the moderate Republican governor George Pataki signed new legislation in August 1998 changing the legal definition of "addict" and "habitual user" to exclude cancer patients and others who used controlled substance for legitimate medical use. Previously, practitioners who "prescribed controlled substances for long-term medical need, such as cancer pain, were required to report their patients to the Department [of Health] as 'addicts' or 'habitual users.'" New York State Controlled Substances Law, 1998.

Chapter Five: OxyContin Unleashed

1. *The Rush Limbaugh Show*, Premiere Radio Networks. October 5, 1995. Quoted in Lynne R. Webster and Beth Dove, *Avoiding Opioid Abuse While Managing Pain* (North Branch, MN: Sunrise River Press, 1007), 7. See also Clarence Page, "Call for Treatment Instead of Jail," *Chicago Tribune*, November 19, 2003, 29.

2. "Internet Pharmacies: Hydrocodone, an Addictive Narcotic Pain Medication Is Available without a Prescription through the Internet," *Testimony before the Permanent Subcommittee on Investigations, Committee on Governmental Affairs, U.S. Senate* (Statement of Robert J. Cramer, managing director, Office of Special Investigations, United States General Accounting Office), June 17, 2004. Amy Cadwell, "In the War on Prescription Drug Abuse, E-Pharmacies are Making Doctor Shopping Irrelevant," *Houston Journal of Health Law and Policy* (2007): 85–126.

3. Robert Brenner, *The Boom and the Bubble: The U.S. in the World Economy* (New York: Verso, 2002).

4. G. Cohen, "The 'Poor Man's Heroin': An Ohio Surgeon Helps Feed a Growing Addiction to OxyContin," *U.S. News and World Report* 130 (2001): 27.

5. For discussion of drug regulation, see Daniel Carpenter, *Reputation and Power: Organizational Image and Pharmaceutical Regulation at the FDA* (Princeton: Princeton University Press, 2010); for "the 1962 reforms . . . ," see Allan Parachini, "The Medical Community Ponders 'a Touchy Subject,'" *Los Angeles Times*, July 9, 1981, G1. As the author noted, "However, aids have tried to distance themselves from that statement—which Reagan made during the transition after the 1980 presidential election."

6. For "we stand on the threshold . . . ," see Reagan, State of the Union address, 1985, *Public Papers of the Presidents: Ronald Reagan* (Washington, D.C.: United States Government Printing Office, 1985), 131; for deregulation and bringing drugs to market, see Stan Chock and Albert R. Karr, "Reagan Starts Moving on Deregulation," *Wall Street Journal*, February 19, 1981, 56; for Sch-

weiker's actions, see Cristine Russell, "Loss of FDA's Independence Feared as Sch-weiker Tightens Reins," *Washington Post*, September 1, 1982, A8.

7. Feder Barnaby, "The Boom in Arthritis Drugs," *New York Times*, April 23, 1982, D1.

8. For sedentary lifestyle, see Philip M. Boffey, "Pain Victims' Care Faulted by Panel," *New York Times*, May 22, 1986, B14; for "headaches are a malady . . . ," see Jon Van, "Pain Research Gives Bad Ratings to TV," *Chicago Tribune*, October 22, 1985, 5.

9. For Lilly's Oraflex, see Feder, "Boom in Arthritis Drugs"; for "some wild rides . . . ," see Stan Kulp, "Stiff Competition: Number of Antiarthritic Drugs Grows Rapidly," *Barron's National Business and Financial Weekly*, June 18, 1982, 26; for Oraflex popularity, see "Arthritis Drug Oraflex Withdrawn from Market," *Chicago Tribune*, August 5, 1982, 1; for Oraflex sales figures, see "Lilly Halts World Sales of Arthritis Drug, Plans $11.4 Million Charge Against Net," *Wall Street Journal*, August 5, 1982, 4; for patient enthusiasm, see "Once a Day Arthritis Treatment Gets the Nod," *Atlanta Daily World*, May 9, 1982, 5.

10. For problems with Oraflex, see "Arthritis Drug Oraflex Withdrawn from Market," 1; "At Least Eight Deaths Tied to Arthritis Drug," *Baltimore Sun*, July 31, 1982, A5; for impact on the company, see "Lilly Halts World Sales of Arthritis Drug," 4; "Lilly Says Grand Jury Now Is Investigating Firm's Oraflex Drug," *Wall Street Journal*, April 24, 1984, 49.

11. For Lilly's argument, see "Lilly Halts World Sales of Arthritis Drug," 4; for "out of fear . . . ," see "U.S. Toughens Plan for Quicker Review of Drug Products," *Wall Street Journal*, October 19, 1982, 12.

12. "U.S. Refused to Prosecute Lilly Officials," *Baltimore Sun*, August 29, 1985, 19A; for Conyers, see Philip Shenon, "U.S. Is Said to Have Dropped Three Officials from Lilly Case," *New York Times*, August 29, 1985, A20.

13. For Democrats' charge, see "Justice Department Defends Handling of Lilly Case," *Los Angeles Times*, September 12 1985, D4; for "the agency's need . . . ," see Morton Mintz, "Drug Approval Hit," *Washington Post*, July 21, 1987, H6. Zomax had been withdrawn from the market in the spring of 1983, and congressional hearings had found that while the FDA had received reports of more than two thousand allergic reactions, key officials at the agency failed to act because they remained unaware of those reports. As a 1985 *New York Times* editorial concluded, "The prescriptions for avoiding more Oraflex scandals are obvious enough . . . The FDA must be tougher in insisting on getting the data it needs to protect the public. As for the Justice Department, its failure to prosecute the case its staff lawyers had built is a disservice to the drug industry, the FDA's

reporting system and the public." "Arthritis at the Justice Department," *New York Times*, September 14, 1985, 22.

14. For Toradol concerns, see C. J. Pearce, F. M. Gonzalez, and J. D. Wallin, "Renal Failure and Hyperkalemia Associated with Ketorolac Tromethamine," *Archives of Internal Medicine* 153, no. 8 (April 26, 1993): 1000–1002; R. P. Murray and R. C. Watson, "Acute Renal Failure and Gastrointestinal Bleed Associated with Postoperative Toradol and Vancomycin," *Orthopedics* 16, no. 12 (December 1993): 1361–63; for "anti-arthritis wonder drug," see Morton Mintz, "Arthritis Drug Naprosyn May Be Taken off Market," *Washington Post*, September 13, 1976, A8; for increasing concerns over Toradol, see T. L. Yarboro Sr., "Intramuscular Toradol, Gastrointestinal Bleeding, and Peptic Ulcer Perforation: A Case Report," *Journal of the National Medical Association* 87, no. 3 (March 1995): 225–27. In 1996, *JAMA* published a study that revealed significantly increased risk of bleeding after use of Toradol at high doses or after prolonged use. Brian Strom et al., "Parenteral Ketorolac and Risk of Gastrointestinal and Operative Site Bleeding: A Postmarketing Surveillance Study," *Journal of the American Medical Association* 275 (1996): 376–82; see also Luis Alberto Garcia Rodriguez, "Risk of Hospitalization for Upper Gastrointestinal Tract Bleeding Associated with Keterolac, Other Nonsteroidal Anti-Inflammatory Drugs, Calcium Antagonists, and Other Antihypertensive Drugs," *Archives of Internal Medicine* 158 (1998): 33–39.

15. For industry profit speculation, see N. R. Kleinfeld, "Arthritis: Building an Industry on Pain," *New York Times*, August 18, 1985, F1; for "competitors financial aches," see Michael Millenson, "New Pain Relievers May Give Competitors Financial Aches," *Chicago Tribune*, May 27, 1984, H1; for "an arrogant and unconscionable effort," see Patti Domm, "Tylenol to Get Rival," *Baltimore Sun*, May 28, 1984, D8.

16. Dale Gieringer, "The FDA Continues to Commit Regulatory Malpractice," *Wall Street Journal*, March 27, 1985, 34.

17. For "a Federal grand jury . . . ," see Richard Wood, chair, Eli Lilly and Company, "Of Eli Lilly and the Short Life of Oraflex on the U.S. Market," *New York Times*, October 12, 1985, 26; for Lola Jones and "we're a little disappointed . . . ," see "Oraflex Death Brings Award of $6 Million," *Los Angeles Times*, November 22, 1983, B5.

18. For "frivolous lawsuits," see Caryle Murphy, "Eli Lilly Co. Cleared in Va. Death," *Washington Post*, September 10, 1985, D6; for industry victory, *National Childhood Vaccine Injury Act of 1986, House Committee on Energy and Commerce*, report 99-908 part 1 (Washington D.C.: Government Printing Office, 1986).

19. For "threatened to transform . . . ," see George Annas, "Faith (Healing), Hope and Charity at the FDA: The Politics of AIDS Drug Trials," *Villanova Law Review* 34 (1989): 771–97; for "lurching from one crisis . . ." and "three FDA employees . . . ," see Bruce Ingersoll and Gregory Stricharchuk, "Generic-Drug Scandal at FDA Is Linked to Deregulation Drive," *Wall Street Journal*, September 13, 1989, A1; see also Richard Berke, "Deregulation Has Gone Too Far, Many Tell the New Administration," *New York Times*, December 11, 1988, 1.

20. Pilar Kraman, *Drug Abuse in America—Prescription Drug Diversion* (Washington, D.C.: Council of State Governments, 2004); for "one New Mexico . . . ," see Pete Stark, "Not All Drug Lords Are Outlaws," Op-Ed, *New York Times*, August 12, 1990, E21.

21. For "prescription drug abuse . . . ," "how the legal distribution . . . ," and "a patient will present . . . ," see David Pesci, "Connecticut Q and A: William Ward, Ferreting Out Illegal Use of Legal Drugs," *New York Times*, July 3, 1994, CN3; for "doctors who help . . . ," see Tim Golden, "Doctors Are Focus of Plan to Fight New Drug Laws," *New York Times*, December 23, 1996, A10.

22. For changing advertising, see Lawrence K. Altman, "Prescription Drugs Are Advertised to Patients, Breaking with Tradition," *New York Times*, February 23, 1982, C1; for AMA concerns, see Michael Millenson, "New Pain Drug Ordered Too Readily, Group Says," *Chicago Tribune*, March 7, 1983, 3.

23. Elisabeth Rosenthal, "Maybe You're Sick. Maybe We Can Help," *New York Times*, April 10, 1994, E2; for "a major concern . . . ," see Louis A. Morris and Lloyd G. Millstein, "Drug Advertising to Consumers: Effects of Formats for Magazine and Television Advertisements," *Food Drug Cosmetics Law Journal* 39 (1984): 497–503; see also Louis A. Morris et al., "Miscomprehension Rates for Prescription Drug Advertisements," *Current Issues and Research in Advertising* 9 (1986): 1, 93–117; for other manufacturer concerns, see Mary Jane Sheffet and Steven W. Kopp, "Advertising Prescription Drugs to the Public: Headache or Relief?" *Journal of Public Policy and Marketing* 9 (1990): 42–61; for "increasing price competition . . . ," see Richard B. Schmitt, "Prescription Drug Ads Stir New Wave of Court Battles," *Wall Street Journal*, October 4, 1994, B10. As this article noted, "In mid-August [1994], for example, a federal judge in Hartford, Conn., ordered Pfizer, Inc., to overhaul a campaign that criticized a new hypertension drug developed by the Miles unit of Bayer AG. The Miles drug, known as Adalat, threatened to undercut an established Pfizer treatment called Procardia."

24. See, for example, "Percodan Drug Bill Signed by Governor," *Los Angeles Times*, May 19, 1965, 23; and Nan Robertson, "U.S. Tightens Rule on Sale of a Drug," *New York Times*, December 29, 1963, 20.

25. For sales and "if Grandma is placed . . . ," see Barry Meier and Melody Petersen, "Sales of Painkiller Grew Rapidly, but Success Brought a High Cost," *New York Times*, May 5, 2001, A1. See also Christine L. Pasero, Margo McCaffery, and Lynda F. McKitrick, "Pain Control: Planning for Breakthrough Cancer Pain," *American Journal of Nursing* 96 (June 1996): 24; for "if the drug . . . ," see David Musto, "Boon for Pain Sufferers, and Thrill Seekers," review of *Pain Killer: A 'Wonder' Drug's Trail of Addiction and Death*, by Barry Meier, *New York Times*, December 17, 2003, E9.

26. For controlled release pill and "the interference of pain . . . ," see S. H. Roth, R. M. Fleischmann, F. X. Burch, F. Dietz, B. Bockow, R. J. Rapoport, J. Rutstein, P. G. Lacouture, "Around-the-Clock, Controlled-Release Oxycodone Therapy for Osteoarthritis-Related Pain: Placebo-Controlled Trial and Long-Term Evaluation," *Archives of Internal Medicine* 160 (2000): 853–60.

27. For "a rash of armed . . . ," see National Public Radio, "OxyContin Robberies," *All Things Considered*, August 23, 2001, www.npr.org/templates /story/story.php?storyId=1127845; for "ground zero . . . ," see Walt Schaefer, "OxyContin Use Said Likely to Spread," *Cincinnati Enquirer*, February 10, 2001, http://enquirer.com/editions/2001/02/10/loc_oxycontin_called.html; see also Debbie Cenziper, "OxyContin Can Ease Pain, but for Abusers, It's Deadly," *Charlotte Observer*, July 7, 2002; for the rise of methamphetamine, see Timothy Egan, "Meth Building Its Hell's Kitchen in Rural America," *New York Times*, February 6, 2002, A14; and Jo Thomas, "Illegal Drug's Manufacture Puts Rural Areas at Risk," *New York Times*, November 11, 2000, A9.

28. For "brought relief to . . . ," see Frank R. Wolf, chair, Virginia, introducing the December 11, 2001 hearing. *Subcommittee of the Committee on Appropriations, House of Representatives*, 107th Congress, first session, part 10, Oxy-Contin (Washington, D.C.: U.S. Government Printing Office, 2002), 3; for "as an academician . . . ," see J. David Haddox, letter to the editor, *New York Times*, March 9, 2001, A18; for arguments about exaggerated clinical fears, see *Interim Report: OxyContin C-II (Oxycodone HCl, Controlled-Release) Tablet and the Public Health (Purdue Pharma, December 7, 2001); Attachment 2 in Subcommittee of the Committee on Appropriations, House of Representatives*, 107th Congress, first session, part 10, OxyContin (Washington, D.C.: U.S. Government Printing Office, 2002).

29. For litigation and OxyContin revenues, see Tim O'Brien, "OxyContin Suits Coming Up Empty: Purdue Pharma's Litigation Strategy Costly, but Effective," *Connecticut Law Tribune*, October 27, 2003, 3; for deaths in Florida, see Vanita Gowda, "Not What the Doctor Ordered," *Governing* 16 (January 2003):

34; and Kraman, *Drug Abuse in America*; for regulators' focus, see T. Roche, "The potent perils of a miracle drug," *Time* 157 (2001): 47.

30. For physician targeting, see Jill Barton, "Rush: I'm an Addict," *Philadelphia Daily News*, October 11, 2003, 2; Robyn E. Blumner, "Limbaugh Scandal Puts OxyContin on Trial," *St. Petersburg Times*, October 19, 2003, 7D; and Ralph Vartabedian, "Doctors Become Targets in Drug War," *Chicago Tribune*, October 23, 2003, 22; for "the first time . . ." and "media-induced hysteria," see Ronald T. Libby, "Treating Doctors as Drug Dealers: The DEA's War on Prescription Painkillers," *Cato Institute Policy Analysis Series*, no. 545, June 6, 2005. www.cato.org/publications/policy-analysis/treating-doctors-drug-dealers-deas -war-prescription-painkillers and Melinda Ammann, "The Agony and the Ecstacy," *Reason* 34, April 2003, 28–34.

31. For "upscale junkies," see Matthew Sweeney and Philip Messing, "Upscale Junkies—White-Collar Abuse of Oxycontin Skyrockets," *New York Post*, February 14, 2004, 19; for "college-aged kids," see Natalie Hopkinson, "Addicted to 'Oxy': One Man's Struggle," *Washington Post*, October 26, 2003, D1; for "migrating out of . . . ," see "Painkiller Sales Doubled in 8 Years," *Bennington Banner* (Vermont), August 21, 2007; for "over the past several years . . . ,"see Limbaugh quoted by Barton, "Rush: I'm an Addict," 2; for "refreshing honesty," see Howard Kurtz, "Limbaugh, Unbowed," *Washington Post*, November 18, 2003, C1; for "beyond the damage . . . ," see Blumner, "Limbaugh Scandal Puts OxyContin on Trial," 7D.

32. United States House of Representatives Committee on Governmental Reform—Minority Staff Special Investigations Division, *FDA Enforcement Actions against False and Misleading Prescription Drug Advertisements Declined in 2003* (Washington D.C.: Government Printing Office, January 2004), 3.

33. Ibid., 4.

34. For "radio antennas . . . ," "bar code . . . ," and "we get calls . . . ," see Gardiner Harris, "Tiny Antennas to Keep Tabs on U.S. Drugs," *New York Times*, November 15, 2004, A1; for "Purdue pledged . . . ," see Robert Trigaux, "Strong Dose of Hype for OxyContin Inexcusable," review of *Pain Killer*, by Barry Meier, *St. Petersburg Times*, November 10, 2003, 1E.

35. Amy Pavuk, "DEA: Walgreens Pushed Sales of Oxycodone," *Orlando Sentinel*, June 29, 2013, A1.

36. For the industry defense, see Joseph Prater, "West Virginia's Painful Settlement: How the OxyContin Phenomenon and Unconventional Theory of Tort Liability May Make Pharmaceutical Companies Liable for Black Markets," *Northwestern University Law Review* (Spring 2006): 1418; for "it appeared that the plaintiffs . . . ," see Richard C. Ausness, "Product Liability's Parallel Universe:

Fault-Based Liability Theories and Modern Products Liability Law," *Brooks Law Review* 635 (2008–2009): 652.

37. For resistance to high prices, see Milton Freudenheim and Melody Petersen, "The Drug Price Express Runs into a Wall," *New York Times*, December 23, 2001, BU1; for the settlement, see Prater, "West Virginia's Painful Settlement," 1425.

38. Vioxx was one of the products heavily promoted by DTCA. See Julie M. Donohue, Maria Cevasco, and Meredith B. Rosenthal, "A Decade of Direct-to-Consumer Advertising of Prescription Drugs," *New England Journal of Medicine* 357 (August 16, 2007): 674. When the drug was withdrawn from the market in 2004, these authors noted, calls increased to place limits on the practice of DTCA, "particularly for new drugs, a view that was reiterated" in other reports; for SEC concerns, see Andrew Pollack, "Justice Dept. and S.E.C. Investigating Merck Drug," *New York Times*, November 9, 2004, C1.

39. On Kaiser and Bextra, see Gardiner Harris, "Big Health Plan Suspends Use of Painkiller," *New York Times*, January 29, 2005, C1. On Enron and corporate malfeasance, see Kurt Eichenwald, "A Mini-Enron in Every Corner," *New York Times*, May 29, 2005, B1. See also Barnaby Feder, "Merck's Actions on Vioxx Face New Scrutiny," *New York Times*, February 15, 2005, C1.

40. For adverse events, see David Spurgeon, "Serious Adverse Events Double in Seven Years in U.S.," *British Medical Journal* 335 (September 22, 2007): 585; for "the United States accounted for . . . ," see International Narcotics Control Board, *Report of the International Narcotics Control Board for 2008* (New York: United Nations, 2009), 20.

41. For Merck settlement, see Alex Berenson, "Merck Is Said to Agree to Pay $4.85 Billion for Vioxx Claims," *New York Times*, November 9, 2007, A1; for Pfizer settlement, see Stephanie Saul, "Pfizer in $894 Million Drug Settlement," *New York Times*, October 18, 2008, B2; for Vioxx revenue and claims, see Karl Stark, "Merck Offers Billions for Vioxx Claims," *McClatchy Tribune Business News*, November 10, 2007; Barry Meier, "Judge to Rule on Plea Deals of Executives in OxyContin Case," *New York Times*, July 20, 2007, C2.

42. 1.Press Release from Jill Kozeny for Chairman Chuck Grassley to Reporters and Editors, September 22, 2006.

43. On the legal wrangling over Bush era torture policy, see Jane Mayer, *The Dark Side: The Inside Story of How the War on Terror Turned into a War on American Ideals* (New York: Anchor, 2009); "Vice President of Torture," editorial, *Washington Post*, October 26, 2005, A18; Josh White and Charles Babbington, "House Supports Ban on Torture," *Washington Post*, December 15, 2005, A1; Jeffrey Rosen, "Conscience of a Conservative," *New York Times*, September

9, 2007, E40; Maureen Dowd, "Cheney, King of Pain," *New York Times*, May 17, 2009, WK13; "The Torture Report," *New York Times*, December 18, 2009, A42; Paul Krugman, "King of Pain," *New York Times*, September 16, 2006, A27.

44. Gina Pace, "Family Endures Pain of Soldier's Sacrifice," *Citrus Times* (Florida), July 26, 2006.

45. Gregg Zoroya, "Troops' Pain Meds Raise Concerns," *USA Today*, October 21, 2008, 1A; see also Elizabeth Weise, "Soldiers in Iraq Carry Extra Load: Back Pain," *USA Today*, November 21, 2005, 6D; Gregg Zoroya, "Abuse of Pain Pills Concerns Pentagon; Senate Eyes Leap to 3.8 M Prescriptions," *USA Today*, March 17, 2010, 1A.

46. For "has lost its way . . . ," see Senator Charles Grassley to Andrew C. von Eschenback, acting commissioner, FDA, September 20, 2006 (press release), www.finance.senate.gov/newsroom/chairman/release/?id=86589465-6ce7-426c -9972-2e2c22b31200; for "companies routinely promise . . . ," see Robert Pear, "Senate Approves Tighter Policing of Drug Makers," *New York Times*, May 10, 2007, A1.

47. For "it is an irony . . . ," see Sandy Rovner, "Panel Finds Hospitals Stingy with Pain Drugs," *Washington Post*, May 28, 1986, H9. See, for example, A. G. Rogers, "The Underutilization of Oxycodone," *Journal of Pain & Symptom Management* 6 (1991): 452; for discussion of the pain divide, see Sean R. Morrison, Sylvan Wallenstein, Dana K. Natale, Richard S. Senzel, and Lo-Li Huang, "'We Don't Carry That': Failure of Pharmacies in Predominantly Nonwhite Neighborhoods to Stock Opioid Analgesics," *New England Journal of Medicine* 342, no. 14 (April 6, 2000): 1023–26. As the authors noted, an array of "studies of diverse populations of patients have found that unrelieved pain is highly prevalent, especially among minority groups." See also R. Bernabei et al., "Management of Pain in Elderly Patients with Cancer," *Journal of the American Medical Association* 279 (1998): 1877–82; C. S. Cleeland, R. Gonin, and A. K. Hatfield, "Pain and Its Treatment in Outpatients with Metastatic Cancer," *New England Journal of Medicine* 330 (1994): 592–96. On minority differences, see C. S. Cleeland et al., "Pain and Treatment of Pain in Minority Patients with Cancer: The Eastern Cooperative Oncology Group Minority Outpatient Pain Study," *Annals of Internal Medicine* 127 (1997): 813–16; K. Todd, N. Samaroo, and J. R. Hoffman, "Ethnicity as a Risk Factor for Inadequate Emergency Department Analgesia," *Journal of the American Medical Association* 269 (1993): 1537–39; and D. D. McDonald, "Gender and Ethnic Stereotyping and Narcotic Analgesic Administration," *Research in Nursing and Health* 17 (1994): 45–49; for "physicians sometimes think . . . ," see W. P. Buchanan, Peter C. Ungaro, and Jane E. Ranney, "Objective Laboratory Parameters in the Diagnosis of Sickle-Cell Pain Crisis,"

North Carolina Medical Journal 49 (November 1988): 583–84. See also Keith Wailoo, *Dying in the City of the Blues: Sickle Cell Anemia and the Politics of Race and Health* (Chapel Hill: University of North Carolina Press, 2001); and Keith Wailoo and Stephen Pemberton, *The Troubled Dream of Genetic Medicine* (Baltimore: Johns Hopkins University Press, 2008).

48. For minorities' pain, see, for example, Benny J. Primm et al., "Managing Pain: The Challenge in Underserved Populations," *Journal of the National Medical Association* 96 (September 2004): 1152–61; for more on race and the politics of pain, see Wailoo, *Dying in the City of the Blues*; for Knox Todd, see Knox Todd, Tony Lee, and Jerome Hoffman, "The Effect of Ethnicity on Physician Estimates of Pain Severity in Patients with Isolated Extremity Trauma," *Journal of the American Medical Association* 271, no. 12 (March 23, 1994); for Atlanta disparities, see Todd et al., "The Effect of Ethnicity"; and Cleeland et al., "Pain and Its Treatment in Outpatients."

49. The trend persisted; a 2003 study found the same "racial and ethnic disparities in emergency department analgesic prescription." J. H. Tamayo-Sarver et al., "Racial and Ethnic Disparities in Emergency Department Analgesic Prescription," *American Journal of Public Health* 93 (2003): 2067–73; for "inadequate prescribing . . . ," see Charles Cleeland, Rene Gonin, Luis Baez, Patrick Loehrer, and Kishan Pandya, "Pain and Treatment of Pain in Minority Patients with Cancer: The Eastern Cooperative Oncology Group Minority Outpatient Pain Study," *Annals of Internal Medicine* 127, no. 9 (November 1, 1997): 813–16.

50. For "major public health problem," see *Summary of the Capitol Hill Breakfast Briefing on Pain Management*, sponsored by the Honorable Tom Harkin, May 7, 1997, www.docstoc.com/docs/48489459/Pain-Management; for gender difference, see Diane E. Hoffmann and Anita J. Tarzian, "The Girl Who Cried Pain: A Bias against Women in the Treatment of Pain," *Journal of Law, Medicine, and Ethics* 29 (2001): 13–27; Nancy Wartik, "Hurting More, Helped Less?" *New York Times*, June 23, 2002, M1; Christine Miaskowski, "Women and Pain," *Critical Care Nursing Clinics of North America* 9 (1997): 453–58; for "more inclined than men . . . ," see Peg Rosen, "The Pain Truth," *Good Housekeeping*, May 2003, 83–84, 86, 88.

51. For an example of this attitude from the 1920s, see E. Libman, "Observations on Sensitiveness to Pain," *Transactions of the Association of American Physicians* 41 (1926): 305. Libman pronounced that "prizefighters, Negroes, and American Indians, as groups, failed to react to noxious stimuli of intensity great enough to induce reaction of discomfort in the average white city dweller."

52. Morrison et al., "'We Don't Carry That.'"

53. For "one of the saddest ...," see Drug Reform Coalition Network, "War on Pain Control," *Activist Guide* (October 26, 1996); for costs, see *Summary of the Capitol Hill Breakfast Briefing on Pain Management,* sponsored by the Honorable Tom Harkin (May 7, 1997); for "pain is our nation's ...," see Ronald Carson, "Drugs and Pain," *Washington Post,* August 21, 1998, A23; see also "Nickles Introduces Pain Relief Promotion Act" (press release), June 17, 1999 www.gpo.gov/fdsys/pkg/BILLS-106s1272is/pdf/BILLS-106s1272is.pdf; see also Ron Wyden, Gordon Smith, and Darlene Hooley's legislation reintroducing the Conquering Pain Act, June 13, 2001, www.govtrack.us/congress/bills/108 /s1278/text; A. Meisel, L. Snyder, and T. Quill, "Seven Legal Barriers to End-of-Life Care: Myths, Realities, and Grains of Truth," *Journal of the American Medical Association* 284 (2000): 2483–88. See Stephen J. Ziegler and Nicholas P. Lovrich Jr., "Pain Relief, Prescription Drugs, and Prosecution: A Four-State Survey of Chief Prosecutors," *Journal of Law, Medicine, and Ethics* 31 (2003): 75–100.

54. For "in such cases ...," see Christine L. Pasero and Peggy Compton, "Pain Control: When Does Drug-Seeking Behavior Signal Addiction?" *American Journal of Nursing* 97 (May 1997): 17–18; D. E. Weissman and J. D. Haddox, "Opioid Pseudoaddiction," *Pain* 36 (1989): 363–66; see also A. Hegarty and R. K. Portenoy, "Pharmacotherapy of Neuropathic Pain," *Seminars in Neurology* 14, no. 3 (1994): 213–24; for new theory of pain behavior, see Knox H. Todd, "Chronic Pain and Aberrant Drug-Related Behavior in the Emergency Department," *Journal of Law, Medicine, and Ethics* (Winter 2005): 761–69.

55. For "pill mills," see Bob LeMendola and Larry Lebowitz, "Doctor Pushed Pills, Agents Say at Least 8 Patients Died," *Ft. Lauderdale Sun Sentinel,* April 2, 1999, 1A; Jennifer C. Kerr, "Bush Anti-Drug Plan Targets Painkillers," *Cincinnati Post,* March 1, 2004, A1; on new hospital regulations, Barbara Acello, "Meeting JCAHO standards for pain control," *Nursing* 30 (March 2000): 52; "JCAHO Begins Surveying for New Pain Standards," *Hospital Peer Review* 25 (May 2000): 67–68; "JCAHO Publishes Pain Assessment and Management: An Organizational Approach," *Journal of Clinical Engineering* 25 (July–August 2000): 199; D. M. Phillips, "JCAHO Pain Management Standards Are Unveiled. Joint Commission on Accreditation of Healthcare Organizations," *Journal of the American Medical Association* 284 (July 26, 2000): 428–29; Susan Okie, "New Medical Standard Brings Pain into Focus," *Washington Post,* January 8, 2001, A3.

56. On environment for Limbaugh's use, see Teresa Lane, "Alleged 'Pill Mill' Leads to Charges," *Palm Beach Post,* July 4, 2003, 1B; "Too Many Pills, Too Many Deaths," *Palm Beach Post,* August 8, 2003, 16A; on Limbaugh's defense,

see "Judge Unseals Medical Records of Limbaugh," *New York Times*, December 24, 2003.

57. Harris Gardiner, "FDA to Place New Limits on Prescription of Narcotics," *New York Times*, February 10, 2009, A13.

58. For "more people than heroin . . . ," see Charles Ornstein and Tracy Weber, "Senate Panel Investigates Drug Companies' Ties to Pain Groups," *Washington Post*, May 8, 2012; for "guides for patients . . . ," see letter to medical groups including Johnson and Johnson, Endo Pharmaceutical, American Pain Society, and others, from Sens. Baucus and Grassley Regarding Potential Ties of Opioid Manufacturers, May 8, 2012, www.finance.senate.gov/newsroom/chairman/release /?id=021c94cd-b93e-4e4e-bcf4-7f4b9fae0047. As the committee saw the matter, the country was experiencing "an epidemic of accidental deaths and addiction resulting from the sale and use of powerful narcotic painkillers such as Oxycontin (oxycodone), Vicodin (hydrocodone), and Opana (oxymorphone). According to CDC data, 'more than 40% (14,800)' of the '36,500 drug poisoning deaths in 2008' were related to opioid-based prescription painkillers." Peter Whoriskey, "The Prescription Painkiller Binge," *Washington Post*, December 31, 2012, A1.

59. For "powerful voice . . . ," see Clarence Page, "Call for Treatment Instead of Jail," *Chicago Tribune*, November 19, 2003, 29; for "the Democrats still cannot . . . ," see "Judge Unseals Medical Files of Limbaugh," *New York Times*, December 24, 2003, A18.

60. Ben Fishel, "Confronted by Caller, Limbaugh Denied Any Similarity between His OxyContin Issue and Kennedy's 'Cover Up,' " *MediaMatters*, May 8, 2006, http://mediamatters.org/research/200605080015.

Conclusion: Theaters of Compassion

1. Javier Moscoso, *Pain: A Cultural History* (New York: Palgrave MacMillan, 2012), 43.

2. Talal Asad, *Formations of the Secular: Christianity, Islam, Modernity* (Stanford, CA: Stanford University Press, 2003), 4.

3. Daniel T. Rodgers, *Contested Truths: Keywords in American Politics since Independence* (New York: Basic Books, 1987), 10.

4. Sara Dubow, *Ourselves Unborn: A History of the Fetus in Modern America* (New York: Oxford University Press, 2011).

5. See Unborn Child Pain Awareness Act, S. 356 and H.R. 3442.

6. New Jersey Compassionate Use Medical Marijuana Act, January 11, 2010. See also "Marijuana and Medicine: Assessing the Science Base—a Summary of the 1999 Institute of Medicine Report," *Archives of General Psychiatry* (June 2000).

7. This section of the conclusion expands on a previously published essay. Keith Wailoo, "Can Reform Spell Relief?" *American Prospect*, July 2010.

8. The Patient Protection and Affordable Care Act (2010), 466, www.gpo .gov/fdsys/pkg/BILLS-111hr3590enr/pdf/BILLS-111hr3590enr.pdf.

9. Robert Pear, "Expecting Presidential Veto, Senate Passes Child Health Measure," *New York Times*, November 2, 2007, A23.

10. For two models of how morality and religion intersect with the political Left and Right in America, see James A. Marone, *Hellfire Nation: The Politics of Sin in American History* (New Haven, CT: Yale University Press, 2003); and George Lakoff, *Moral Politics: How Liberals and Conservatives Think* (Chicago: University of Chicago Press, 2002).

11. "Congressman Mike Rogers' Opening Statement on Health Care Reform," YouTube video, posted by RepMikeRogers on July 16, 2009, www.you tube.com/watch?feature=player_embedded&v=G44NCvNDLfc.

12. Committee on Advancing Pain Research, Care and Education, Institute of Medicine, *Relieving Pain in America: A Blueprint for Transforming Prevention, Care, Education, and Research* (Washington, D.C: National Academies Press, 2011), x. See also R. Gallagher, "What Should All Physicians Know about Pain Medicine? Workgroup Report, the First National Pain Medicine Summit—Final Summary Report," *Pain Medicine* 11:1450–52.

13. *Relieving Pain in America*, xii.

14. Eric Lichtblau, "Economic Slide Took a Detour at Capitol Hill," *New York Times*, December 27, 2011, 1.

15. "Pain and Disability: Clinical, Behavioral, and Public Policy Perspectives; Report on the Commission of the Evaluation of Pain," *Social Security Bulletin* 50, no. 1 (January 1987): 22.

16. Asad, *Formations of the Secular*, 83.

Index

disabilities *(cont.)*
25–27; veterans' groups and, 25–26,
47. *See also* Social Security disability
insurance
disability studies, 66, 219–20n4
Disabled American Veterans (DAV),
25, 47
DMSO (dimethyl sulfoxide), 71, 72–75,
74, 129
doctors. *See* physicians
doctor shopping, 5, 170, 181, 198
Dodd, Christopher, 209
Dole, Bob, 119
Donahue, Wilma, 17
double effect, principle of, 147–48, 156,
157, 167, 207
drug companies. *See* pharmaceutical
industry
Drug Enforcement Administration
(DEA): Bush administration and, 188;
Hurwitz and, 141–42; Hyde-Nickles
bill and, 160–61; medical marijuana
and, 181; PAS and, 151–52; war on
drugs and, 135
drug offenders, selective prosecution of,
176–77
Drug Reform Coalition Network, 152,
197
drugs. *See* medication; prescription drugs
Dubrow, Sara, 124, 206

Eisenhower, Dwight: heart attack of,
32, 69; SSDI and, 3–4, 57; veterans'
benefits and, 16, 17, 23–25, 26–27,
44–45; views on liberalism and
conservatism, 28
elderly: arthritis and, 70–76; disability
benefit for, 27, 45, 48, 229n58
Eli Lilly and Oraflex, 174–76, 179
end-of-life care: compassion and, 129,
131, 132–35, 140, 143, 186, 206; pain
relief and, 134–35, 144–48, 150,
156–58, 182; Religious Right and,
162–63; social disparities and, 171
Ervin, Frank, 30
ethnicity: African Americans and sickle
cell disease, 68–69; pain complaints
and, 65, 66, 68, 81–84, 86, 196; pain
relief and, 194–95

euthanasia: alternatives to, 37, 140;
Bowen and, 129–30; fears of, 147.
See also Kevorkian, Jack; physician-
assisted suicide

Fagerhaugh, Shizuko, 10
FDA. *See* Food and Drug Administration
Federalism, 150, 206
Federal Trade Commission, 72
Federation of State Medical Boards,
200–201
Ferrara, Peter, 99–100
"fetal pain," 6, 9, 123–25, 128, 134,
140, 150, 160, 165, 167, 196, 205–6,
208, 209
Florida: Graves case in, 186–87;
Intractable Pain Treatment Act, 148;
Limbaugh case in, 5, 170, 183, 187,
199; OxyContin in, 184, 186; PAS in,
154; Purdue Pharma in, 189
Food and Drug Administration (FDA):
deregulation and, 173–78, 188, 193;
direct-to-consumer advertising and,
182, 188; market surveillance and,
178, 192; pain drugs and, 5, 72,
73–75, 169, 170, 174–78, 180, 183
Fortune Cookie, The (film), 202, 212
Fountain, L. H., 73
fraud: conservatism and, 1–3, 7, 9, 100;
liberalism and, 102–8; overview of,
212–13; of pain complaints, 1–2, 9,
93–97; in pain relief, 70–71; Reagan
war on, 108–15; Son of Sam as
example of, 107–8, 204; welfare, 98,
101, 104. *See also* malingering
Freeman, Walter, 36–37, 39
Frist, Bill, 163
Fungiello, Philip, 45

Galbraith, John Kenneth, 30
gate control theory, 77–79, 80, 85–86,
87, 91, 95, 207
gender, 60–61, 65, 126, 195–96. *See also*
masculinity, social codes of
Glucksberg, Harold, 165
Glucksberg, William, 152, 154
Glucksberg case, 154–55, 156–57
Goffman, Erving, 49
Goldhammer, Alan, 115

liberalism *(cont.)*
medical views on, 28, 43–44, 55, 79,
80–81, 86, 87–95; Mill and, 11; pain
and, 18, 48, 63–64, 79, 81, 94–95,
100, 102–8, 122–23, 126–29, 147,
166, 185, 200; tensions within, 101,
171, 220n6. *See also* Carter, Jimmy;
Clinton, Bill
libertarian perspectives, 76, 85, 128,
133, 135–36, 138–39, 155–56, 161,
169, 186–87, 199, 206
Limbaugh, Rush: admission of drug
dependence by, 187; as doctor
shopping, 5, 170; liberalism of
Clinton and, 1; OxyContin and, 5–6,
168, 170–71
lobotomies, 35–39, 79
Long, Russell, 119
Longmore, Paul, 149
Lutz, Harold, 110

malingering, 41–42, 53, 79–80, 93–97,
100
Mao Tse-Tung, 87, 94
marijuana, medical, 151, 181, 206
marketing of painkillers: aspirin, 30;
direct-to-consumer advertising, 169,
181–82; DMSO, 74; negligent, 189–90;
in 1950s, 29–32; OxyContin, 186–99.
See also consumerism in drug market
masculinity, social codes of, 17–18, 21,
41, 50, 81–84
Matson, Floyd, 71
McCarthy, Joseph, 47
McGill Pain Questionnaire, 95
McGirr, Lisa, 28
McLaughlin, Alford, 24, 34
Mechanisms of Pain Management
(Bonica), 33–35
Medicaid, 70, 158, 180, 190
Medicare, 2, 3, 58, 70–71, 93, 97, 105,
106, 108, 158
medication, opiate, 153. *See also*
marketing of painkillers; pharmaceuti-
cal industry; prescription drugs;
regulation of drugs; *specific
medications*
Meese, Edwin, 111, 118
Melzack, Ronald, 77–79, 80, 88, 95

Merck and Vioxx, 190–92
methadone, 86, 88, 94, 95, 127, 183
methamphetamine, 180, 184
Miakowski, Christine, 196
Michigan, 147–48, 154
Military Order of the Purple Heart, 25
Mill, John Stuart, 11
Miller, Sherry, 131, 132, 133, 146
Miltown, 31, 58, 172
Minor, John, 44
Miranda, Manuel, 97
Miranda case, 117
Mondale, Walter, 113–14
morals, 65–66
Morgan, Hugh, 43
morphine, 15, 29, 30, 38, 67, 86, 88, 95,
132, 144, 183, 186
Moscoso, Javier, 202
Motrin, 174, 175, 178
Mullan, Eileen, 88

Nader, Ralph, 175
Naprosyn, 177–78
Nathan, P. W., 85–86
National Association of Disability
Examiners, 115
National Childhood Vaccine Injury Act,
179
National Initiative on Technology and
the Disabled, 125
National Institute of General Medical
Sciences, *Threshold*, 81, 82
National Institute of Nursing Research,
197
National Institutes of Health: Ad Hoc
Committee on Acupuncture, 91, 92;
Institute of Medicine study and, 211
National Recipient System, 104
National Rehabilitation Association, 115
Neal, Helen, 96
New Jersey Compassionate Use Medical
Marijuana Act, 206
New York, 81, 84, 95, 107, 142, 148,
154, 157, 197, 262n50
Nickles, Don, 159, 160
Nixon, Richard M., 59–60, 87–88, 95,
103, 104, 159
North Carolina, 141, 161
Nussbaum, Martha, 10

PAS. *See* physician-assisted suicide

Paul, Ron, 138, 161

penicillin, 29, 44

People in Pain (Zborowski), 81–84, 196

Percodan, 29, 30, 169, 182–83

Pernick, Martin, 196

personality: arthritic, 55–56; learned helplessness and, 96, 109–10; lobotomy and, 37, 38–39; medication and, 31–32; pain tolerance and, 67; and response to pain, 86

perverse incentives, 9, 53, 103–4

Pfizer and Bextra, 191, 192

phantom limb pain, 16, 33, 49, 78

pharmaceutical industry: experts for, 34–35; government regulation and oversight of, 71, 72–73, 173, 190, 238n35; marketing by, 30, 32, 169, 170, 173, 179–86, 199; market share of antiarthritic drugs, *175*; non-profit organizations and, 200–201; pain-killers as financial lifeblood of, *172*; postwar, 29; self-interest of, 197–98; U.S. Department of Justice and, 176–77, 190–91. *See also* prescription drugs; Purdue Pharma

pharmacies: in nonwhite neighborhoods, 194, 197; online, 6, 169, 187; Walgreen's, 189

physician-assisted suicide (PAS): in California, 140; Congress and, 158–59; debate over, 150; Glucksberg challenge to ban on, 152, 154–55, 156–57; irony of, 153; Left and, 149; libertarian and states' rights claims for, 155–56; pain care reform and, 140–41; pain defense and, 132, 144–50; Supreme Court and, 156–57. *See also* Kevorkian, Jack

physicians: acupuncture therapy and, 88–89, 91–92; authority of, 65, 95, 154; conservative practice of, 138, 142; doctor shopping, 5, 170, 181, 198; education in pain care, 8, 138, 142, 185, 190, 210, 211–13; frustrations of, 52–53; as gatekeepers, 41, 50, 53, 76; legal oversight of, 95, 135, 139, 141–43, 160; liberal views and practice of, 60, 66, 80, 87, 89, 135,

136–37; pain persona and, 46, 49–50, 53–54; in politics, 136–38, 151, 153–54; survey comments from, 40–42, 43–44. *See also* American Medical Association

Pickle, J. J., 117, 118, 120

Pius XII (pope), 134

placebos, 67

Polanco, Richard, 139, 140

Polaski, Lorraine, 101, 119–20

Polaski v. Heckler, 119–20, 122, 208

politics of pain: in China, 89–91, 94; disability and, 53–54; at end of life, 134–35; government role and, 58–59; in 1970s, 96–97; overview of, 6–12; OxyContin and, 199–201; party ideology and, 61, 203–4; political parties and, 155–56, 166–67; Reagan era and, 123, 126–30; theaters of compassion and, 202–8; veterans and, 18–19, 21–22, 25, 27–28, 44; and worthiness for relief, 48–49. *See also* conservatism; courts; liberalism

Portnoy, Russell, 200

Posner, Richard, 111

prescription drugs: adverse events from, 191; diversion of, 6, 170, 180–81, 184; overmedication with, 194–99. *See also* medication; regulation of drugs; *specific drugs*

pseudoaddiction, 198, 207

Public Citizen Health Research Group, 175

Public Law 748 (1948), 22

Purdue Pharma, 182, 183, 184–85, 188–90, 191–92, 200

Purvis, Dara, 126

Quill, Timothy, 154

race. *See* ethnicity

radicalization of pain relief, 76–87

Reagan, Nancy, *107*

Reagan, Ronald, *107*; administration of, 97–102, 108–15, 118, 123; Carter and, 105–6; courts and, 117–19, 129; election of, 106; "fetal pain" and, 123–25; HHS and, 98–99; legacy of, 123–28; "nonacquiescence" policy of,